Teaching IOM
Implications of the Institute of Medicine Reports for Nursing Education
Third Edition

Anita Finkelman, MSN, RN, and
Carole Kenner, PhD, RNC-NIC, NNP, FAAN

nurses books.org THE PUBLISHING PROGRAM OF ANA

AMERICAN NURSES ASSOCIATION

SILVER SPRING, MARYLAND
2012

i

Library of Congress Cataloging-in-Publication Data

Finkelman, Anita Ward.
    Teaching IOM : implications of the Institute of Medicine reports for nursing education / Anita Finkelman and Carole Kenner. — 3rd ed.
    p. ; cm.
    Includes bibliographical references and index.
    ISBN 978-1-55810-454-9 (softcover : alk. paper)— ISBN 978-1-55810-459-4 (eBook, PDF format) — ISBN 978-1-55810-460-0 (eBook, PDF format) — ISBN 978-1-55810-461-7 (eBook, Mobipocket format)
    1. Institute of Medicine (U.S.) 2. Nursing—Study and teaching—United States. I. Kenner, Carole. II. American Nurses Association. III. Title. IV. Title: Implications of the Institute of Medicine reports for nursing education. V. Title: Teaching Institute of Medicine.
    [DNLM: 1. Institute of Medicine (U.S.). 2. Education, Nursing—methods—United States. 3. Health Care Reform—United States. 4. Professional Competence—United States. 5. Quality Assurance, Health Care—United States. 6. Safety Management—United States. WY 18 F499t 2012]
    RT71.F46 2012

2012007894

The opinions in this book reflect those of the authors and do not necessarily reflect positions or policies of the American Nurses Association (ANA).

American Nurses Association
8515 Georgia Avenue, Suite 400
Silver Spring, MD 20910-3492
1-800-274-4ANA
http://www.NursingWorld.org

Published by Nursesbooks.org
The Publishing Program of ANA
http://www.Nursesbooks.org/

ISBN-13: 978-1-55810-454-9   1-55810-458-5   SAN: 851-3481   07/2012

First printing: July 2012

Contents

Part 4. Nursing Education and the IOM Reports: Critical Issues and the Implications for the Curriculum

Part 5. Incorporating the Core Competencies into Nursing Education

Part 6. References, Glossary, Acronyms and Abbreviations, and Appendices

Acknowledgments

First we would like to thank our families: Fred, Shoshannah, and Deborah Finkelman and Lester Kenner. Thanks to Elizabeth Karle for assistance with administrative matters. Finally, a special thanks to Rosanne O'Connor Roe and Eric Wurzbacher for all their help in preparing this manuscript and Francine Bennett for her help in marketing, and to all of Nursesbooks.org. Our patients and our students over many years have provided us with guidance and encouraged us to develop new ideas that will improve patient care and our teaching.

About the American Nurses Association

The American Nurses Association (ANA) is the only full-service professional organization representing the interests of the nation's 3.1 million registered nurses through its constituent/state nurses associations and its organizational affiliates. The ANA advances the nursing profession by fostering high standards of nursing practice, promoting the rights of nurses in the workplace, projecting a positive and realistic view of nursing, and by lobbying the Congress and regulatory agencies on healthcare issues affecting nurses and the public.

About Nursesbooks.org, The Publishing Program of ANA

Nursesbooks.org publishes books on ANA core issues and programs, including ethics, leadership, quality, specialty practice, advanced practice, and the profession's enduring legacy. Best known for the foundational documents of the profession on nursing ethics, scope and standards of practice, and social policy. Nursesbooks.org is the publisher for the professional, career-oriented nurse, reaching and serving nurse educators, administrators, managers, and researchers as well as staff nurses in the course of their professional development.

About the Authors

Anita Ward Finkelman MSN, RN, a nurse educator and consultant, is visiting faculty at Northeastern University, Bouvé College of Health Sciences and School of Nursing. She was an Assistant Professor of Nursing at the University of Oklahoma College of Nursing and served as Director of Undergraduate Curriculum and Associate Professor/Clinical Nursing at the University of Cincinnati College of Nursing. Her BSN is from Texas Christian University, master's degree in psychiatric–mental health nursing clinical nurse specialist from Yale University, and post-master's graduate work in healthcare policy and administration from George Washington University. Additional work in the area of health policy was completed as a fellow of the Health Policy Institute, George Mason University. Ms. Finkelman's more than 35 years of nursing experience includes clinical, educational, and administrative positions, and considerable experience developing online courses and curriculum. She has authored many books and journal articles, served on editorial boards, and lectured on administration, health policy, education, and psychiatric–mental health nursing, both nationally and internationally, particularly in Israel for Hebrew University Hadassah School of Nursing, Haifa University, where she served on the interprofessional advisory committee for the first Evidence-Based Practice Center in Israel, and Ben Gurion University in Beer-Sheba, Israel, where she has developed a collaborative healthcare profession study-abroad program with Northeastern University and serves as guest lecturer. She also is a consultant to publishers and healthcare organizations in areas of distance education and development of Internet products. Recent textbook publications include *Professional Nursing Concepts: Competencies for Quality Leadership*, coauthored with Carole Kenner (2013, Jones and Bartlett, 2nd ed.), *Leadership and Management for Nurses: Core Competencies for Quality Care* (2012, Pearson Education, 2nd ed.), *Case Management for Nurses* (2011, Pearson Education), and a number of other books, chapters, and journal articles on leadership and management, health policy, education, international health care, community health, and psychiatric–mental health nursing. She is a member of the *Home Healthcare Nurse* editorial board.

Carole Kenner, PhD, RN-NIC, NNP. FAAN, is currently the President of the Council of International Neonatal Nurses and Dean/Professor at Northeastern University School of Nursing, Associate Dean Bouvé College of Health Sciences, Northeastern University. She has almost 30 years of neonatal/pediatric/women's health experience. Dr. Kenner has published about 20 textbooks and more than 100 journal articles. Her textbook *Comprehensive Neonatal Care* is in its fourth edition and has won the American Journal of Nursing and American Publishing awards throughout its years in print. Her *Neonatal Care Handbook* was just translated into Chinese. The second edition of her co-edited textbook with Dr. Jacqueline McGrath, *Developmental Care of Newborns & Infants: A Guide for Health Professionals,* won the 2011 American Journal of Nursing award. She has taught for more than 25 years, developed master's-level programs in the United States and abroad, and has lectured in more than 20 countries. In 2011 she received the Audrey Hepburn award for contributions to the health and welfare of children, presented by Sigma Theta Tau International. She serves on the National Nursing Advisory Committee of the March of Dimes and the Boston Board of the March of Dimes. She is the founder of the Council of International Neonatal Nurses, which represents more than 60 countries and is the first international organization to represent neonatal nursing. Dr. Kenner received her BSN from the University of Cincinnati, and an MSN from Indiana University with a specialty degree in Perinatal Clinical Nurse Specialist (CNS)/Neonatal Nurse Practitioner (NNP). In 1988 she received her doctorate in nursing from Indiana University with a minor in curriculum design and higher education.

Authors' Preface

This third edition of *Teaching IOM: Implications for Institute of Medicine Reports for Nursing Education* continues the dialogue begun with the first two editions of 2007 and 2009. We have had many opportunities through presentations at conferences and workshops across the United States and abroad to talk with many nurse educators, staff development professionals, and clinicians from healthcare organizations about the implications of the Institute of Medicine reports. This has led us to expand the book.

We appreciate all of the support we have received, both praising the project and adding to our thinking on this critical process. Throughout this book and also in the IOM reports there has been an important factor: *We could not do this alone.* We need more dialogue and more collaboration—partnerships among nurses, particularly between nurse educators and nurses in practice and partnerships with our colleagues in other healthcare professions. Our students and patients require this. We are a practice profession, and this is where our emphasis should be.

What is different about the third edition? Most obviously, it has become two books. The longer one, titled *Teaching IOM,* is again primarily for college, university, and staff educators. The other we have called *Learning IOM*: it is a shorter version of *Teaching IOM,* and is for use by students, whether undergraduate or graduate. We have done this largely in response to the many educators who have requested such a version.

Retaining the same format and structure of the first two, this edition is updated and expanded. We have identified and incorporated numerous newer IOM reports that are relevant to nursing. We have expanded the content on clinical implications and general nursing education issues as well as healthcare reform and the connection of the reports to nursing standards. The content on the five healthcare core competencies has been expanded, with more content and examples on teaching–learning strategies. While these strategies are more explicitly emphasized and interwoven into *Teaching IOM,* they have also informed both titles. These strategies are aligned with the Carnegie Foundation's

2010 report *Educating Nurses: A Call for Radical Transformation,* which promotes student engagement and movement away from lecture-driven education.

Teaching IOM, as the previous two editions, is supplemented by digital material. For this edition, it is delivered online with the purchase of the larger book. This in effective comprises an all-digital manual of supplemental teaching–learning materials that are focused on key content related primarily to quality improvement initiatives.

We continue to be committed to the importance of the IOM reports and projects for nursing, and recognize the great need for nursing to make changes in nursing education to better serve our students and consequently their employers—but more importantly, to provide quality care for all patients who require it and support health in our communities. In addition, the content has relevance for staff educators who must assure that staff are competent in the five healthcare profession core competencies.

We look forward to further dialogue with you, as this is the way we all grow and improve.

Anita and Carole

Foreword to the Second Edition

By Patricia Benner, PhD, RN, FAAN

Anita Ward Finkelman and Carole Kenner have created a synthesis of the Institute of Medicine (IOM) reports on patient safety and best practices, and have developed sound educational approaches for teaching the IOM Core Competencies for Nursing. They draw on other key works in the field of healthcare policy and delivery systems to translate the policy mandates for a safer healthcare system to an insightful educational guide to curriculum and pedagogical development in nursing. This book provides an integrative and useful approach to translating the IOM and Institutes of Health Patient Safety Initiatives into a one-volume work that nurse educators, students, staff nurses, and nurse executives will find essential to teaching and implementing the urgently needed improvements in healthcare quality and safety. This work is central to the current societal discussions, debates, and legislation on developing a more inclusive, less expensive, and higher quality health care in the United States.

Each IOM report from the of the National Academies of Science has provided needed perspectives, theory, and research evidence on improving the quality and safety of health care in the United States. In all the reports, nurses have been acknowledged as at the "sharp end" of patient care, in that they are the ones who are closest and most continuous in their care of patients. Nurses are often cited as the patient's last line of defense in preventing erroneous treatments and medications. Traditionally, patient safety has been central to the nursing role, but now the issues are more complex. The points of possible error have grown, and both prevention and intervention require system-level strategies that nurses must help develop, implement, and oversee.

Undergraduate and graduate nursing students need to be better equipped with the knowledge and skills to develop healthcare policies aimed at improving patient safety and quality of care. They also need knowledge and skills in how to design healthcare delivery systems that will prevent patient care errors and patient harm and promote continuous quality improvement in local systems. Patient care mistakes do not start out to be mistakes, but they do become mistakes at fault lines and at areas of limited attentiveness and monitoring. Weick and Sutcliffe (2001) note that while it is impossible to prevent all errors, highly reliable complex organizations that engage in high-risk work can improve their quality so long as they deliberately acknowledge that failure is an ever-present possibility, try to imagine all the pitfalls and errors that might happen, and make changes accordingly. Such organizations also pay attention to "near misses" so that they can prevent similar incidents from recurring in the future.

This book also effectively draws on the work by Linda Cronenwett and her colleagues (2007) who, with a sponsoring grant by the Robert Wood Johnson Foundation entitled "Quality and Safety Education for Nurses (QSEN)" (www.QSEN.org) translated the IOM competencies for continually improving patient safety and quality into strategies with implementation goals for nursing education. Further strategies for teaching the knowledge, skills, and attitudes needed for improving patient safety and quality from IOM and the QSEN are developed in this book. Nurse educators will find the teaching–learning instructional materials that accompany this book to contain useful classroom teaching strategies. In sum, this is an invaluable, even indispensable resource for those who teach nursing students at any level, and for staff nurses and administrators on how to create higher quality and safer healthcare delivery systems.

References

Cronenwett, L., Sherwood, G., Barnsteiner, J., Disch, J., Johnson, J., Mitchell, P., et al. (2007). Quality and safety education for nurses. *Nursing Outlook, 55*(3), 122–131.
Weick, K. E., & Sutcliffe, K. M. (2001). *Managing the unexpected: Assuring high performance in an age of complexity*. San Francisco, CA: Jossey-Bass.

Dr. Patricia Benner, PhD, RN, FAAN, Professor Emerita, University of California, San Francisco; visiting professor at University of Pennsylvania in Philadelphia, is an internationally known nursing expert. Her seminal 1984 work *From Novice to Expert* has been fundamental to the development of educational and continued competencies in nursing evaluation. Benner serves as the lead scholar on two upcoming reports. One, from the Carnegie Foundation for the Advancement of Teaching, will describe clinical knowledge development of nurses and finally provide evidence to support teaching–learning excellence. The other, a National Council of State Boards of Nursing project, *The Taxonomy of Root Cause Analysis for Practice Responsibility* (TERCAP), examines the taxonomy of nursing error and presents a data collection instrument. Dr. Benner's career has changed the face of nursing education, especially through her work on the basis of the professional development of a nurse.

Relevance of the IOM Reports to Nursing Education

The Institute of Medicine (IOM) of the National Academies serves as the source for science-based advice on matters of biomedical science, medicine, and health. A nonprofit organization created in 1970, the IOM is not part of the federal government, so it can ensure scientifically informed analysis and independent guidance. It cannot make laws or regulations; it can only advise and thus influence policy decisions. The IOM's mission is to improve health by providing "unbiased, evidence-based, and authoritative information and advice concerning health and science policy to policy-makers, professionals, leaders in every sector of society, and the public at large" (IOM, 2008a). The IOM uses experts to examine problems and then publishes reports on the results and its recommendations.

Why should nurse educators pay attention to the IOM? In its 1983 report *Nursing and Nursing Education: Public Policy and Private Actions,* the IOM recommended that nursing research be included in mainstream health research. This recommendation led to the creation of the National Center for Nursing Research in 1993, which became the National Institute of Nursing Research (NINR). The IOM has had a major impact on nursing. Its reports and recommendations do make a difference in healthcare policy and practice, funding, and education. The IOM reports are at the center of the current restructuring of healthcare systems and the movement toward interprofessional team collaboration, and they influence funding from research, education, and health policy agencies and professional organizations. They should therefore be at the core of all nursing education programs.

The IOM *Quality Chasm* series is highly relevant to nursing, as are the IOM's subsequent reports. Each report can be applied to practice and thus has implications for nursing education, both at the academic level and in staff development and continuing education. It is important to note that the IOM report on healthcare education focuses on healthcare professions education, not specific healthcare professionals. The goal is a consistent framework across healthcare professions education that emphasizes interprofessional collaborative care rather than working in isolation.

The IOM reports must also be viewed within the nursing context. How the reports are viewed by nurses and whether they are implemented by the nursing profession is influenced by the current status of nursing practice and education, which may impede integration of critical, current views of health care and the need for change and improvement. Why is this so? There has long been a wall between nursing education and nursing practice, and over time this wall has grown higher and wider. As a profession, we wanted to be academically oriented, and there is nothing wrong with this, but have we gone too far? Nurse educators have separated themselves from practice. We visit the practice arena to teach and then return to our schools. Typically, students do not have role models who practice, but rather teachers who strictly teach nursing. The landmark report on nursing education (Benner, Sutphen, Leonard, & Day, 2010) indicates that students do not think that they are taught by clinically competent faculty. Practice is not always the focus of nursing education—but we are a practice profession.

Educators and practitioners sometimes try to communicate. But educators often feel that they know what should be taught, even though they have long been out of practice or only practice intermittently. This is a dangerous stand to take, and may have led us to poorly serve our students and the employers who hire our graduates. This also is not effectively serving our consumers—patients and their families. The IOM reports require that we (not just nurses, but all healthcare professionals) take a serious look at changes, but perhaps we are too satisfied with the status quo. The demolition of that wall is long overdue. This will be difficult and painful. Practice will have to become a part of education. The IOM reports and their recommendations indicate that healthcare professionals need to do more together—education and practice—to improve care. The IOM reports on quality provide the platform for improvement in health care. This book is predicated on change and acceptance of the need to move forward and work more collaboratively with our colleagues from all healthcare professions.

Nursing Organizations and Quality Issues in Health Care

The American Nurses Association's (ANA) *Nursing's Social Policy Statement* identifies the following as one of the major social concerns in health care and nursing. "Quality health care is a human right for all. To improve the quality of care, healthcare professionals must address these complex issues: increasing costs of care, health disparities; and the lack of safe, accessible, and available healthcare services and resources" (ANA, 2010b, p. 4). The ANA has long strongly supported the IOM quality initiative and recognizes that nursing must assume a major role in the quality improvement process. In 1998, the ANA House of Delegates approved an action report, *Shared Accountability in Today's Work Environment.* Prepared before the landmark 1999 IOM report on patient safety, the ANA action report (ANA, 1998; pp. 27–28) emphasized four strategies:

▌ Educate policy-makers and the public on the effects of downsizing, restructuring, and reorganizing that can lead to breakdowns in safety and quality.

- Work with other healthcare organizations to identify and correct system errors that lead to patient injuries.
- Support the role of the professional nurse in correcting system errors through quality improvement initiatives, and protect the nurse by enacting whistleblower legislation.
- Educate regulators and accrediting bodies on the dangers of the criminalization of healthcare errors.

These strategies, which are similar to the IOM report recommendations (1999), demonstrate that the nursing profession is committed to quality care.

The ANA action report considered practice and healthcare delivery. But another critical factor that can have a long-term effect on quality care is what nursing students are learning about patient quality. This is the major focus of our book. Maddox, Wakefield, and Bull (2001) discuss the need for changing educational experiences. They pose several questions for the nursing profession about care that is in sync with the IOM reports:

- Do nurses and other members of the healthcare delivery team have the same expectations for individual performance in the interdisciplinary healthcare team?
- Do nurse educators have the working knowledge and experience of technical and human factors (including organizational) required in setting new expectations and in facilitating learning experiences for interprofessional teams? Nurse educators need to understand cultural differences in patient populations and the workforce: cultural factors such as the structure of the organization; the significance of the institution's mission and core values on the enterprise; financing of health care; and billing, coding, and reimbursement issues are a few areas of knowledge. Other technical issues include patient information systems, monitoring equipment, new hospital equipment and safety issues in its use, and the relation of the Health Insurance Portability and Accountability Act (HIPAA) to patient information and access to medical records.
- Do we teach and model effective relationship management and communication skills when facing power gradients? (*Power gradients* are differences in status and influence between health professionals—mainly between nurses and physicians. In many instances power or perceived power of an individual is related to status, educational level, and financial impact on the organization, as well as the legitimate or perceived authority of the individual.)

We have not yet resolved these issues. These questions suggest the need for more research to increase nursing's understanding of quality of care and its relationship to nursing care and the role of nurses.

Both the American Nurses Association and the American Academy of Nursing (AAN) have both been involved in work on quality. They have provided nursing representation to the National Quality Forum (NQF). The ANA has taken the lead in designing the quality indicators used in nursing's report card for benchmarking healthcare delivery systems' quality of care through the National Database of Nursing Quality Indicators® (NDNQI), which is discussed in Part 5 in *Teaching IOM*, Part 4 in *Learning IOM*. In late 2008, the AAN sent out a press release about its commitment to transforming the healthcare system and supporting the National Priorities Partnership, which is a diverse coalition of 29 organizations led by NQF (AAN, 2008). The national priorities identified by the partnership, and clearly influenced by the IOM work, are:

 ▎ *Patient and family engagement* to provide patient-centered, effective care;
 ▎ *A healthy population* to bring greater focus on wellness and prevention;
 ▎ *Safety* breakthroughs to eliminate errors wherever and whenever possible;
 ▎ *Care coordination* to provide patient-centered, high-value care;
 ▎ *Palliative care* to guarantee appropriate and compassionate care for patients with advanced illness; and
 ▎ *Reducing overuse* to achieve effective, affordable care.

The Agency for Healthcare Research and Quality (AHRQ) has been involved in healthcare quality for some time within the Department of Health and Human Services (HHS). It has issued several requests for proposals aimed at clinical reduction of errors, or policies that promote patient safety and quality of care. The AHRQ plays a critical role in promoting the IOM *Quality Chasm* series. It administers the National Healthcare Quality Report and the National Healthcare Disparities report, which are discussed later in this book.

In 2008, the American Association of Colleges of Nursing (AACN) included the IOM healthcare profession core competencies in its newest version of *The Essentials of Baccalaureate Education for Professional Nursing Practice*. This was significant, as the addition of this information should affect nursing curricula. Despite this endorsement of the IOM reports by the ANA, AAN, National Institute of Nursing Research (NINR), AHRQ, and AACN, there are health professionals who continue to question the need for IOM information to be included in curricula—change has been slow. But the IOM reports (*Quality Chasm* series and other related reports) are changing every aspect of healthcare delivery and patient care. The business of our educational institutions is to produce graduates capable of rendering safe, quality care. Educational institutions are driven to diversify financial resources through service learning, educational programs, and research grants because of the shortage of funding streams. Given the mounting evidence that IOM findings are driving funding (research and program grants), we should be more aware of these reports and guide our students to understand their importance. Staff also need to be updated on this information and apply it.

The authors of this text realize that to achieve this goal, information must be presented in a concise, usable fashion for educators to present and students to learn. To meet this goal, *Teaching IOM* emphasizes strategies for integrating the IOM material into the curriculum, updating and expanding this information that is so critical to professional nursing. That integration at the point of education remains the core purpose of this text.

Overview of the Third Edition

This third edition has become two books. *Teaching IOM* is primarily for faculty in educational and staff educators in practice settings. It is supplemented by a digital manual of teaching–learning materials. *Learning IOM* is a shorter version of *Teaching IOM* and is primarily for students, either undergraduate or graduate. The two books are outlined briefly below: the teaching–learning manual is outlined in greater detail.

Outline of *Teaching IOM* and *Learning IOM*

As noted above, the student version is a distillation of the larger book for educators, instructors, and practitioners. The two books are organized identically in their first three parts; each has the same set of appended reference material at the end of the book. The fifth part of *Teaching IOM* corresponds to the fourth part of *Learning IOM*:

- Part 1 sets the context for the book with an overview of the critical IOM reports, as well as some of their clinical implications.
- Part 2 discusses healthcare reform and its connection to the quality improvement initiative.
- Part 3 provides information about the implications of the IOM quality reports and nursing standards.
- Part 4 describes an overview of nursing's general educational strategic responses and critical issues and integration of the IOM core competencies into the curriculum. (This content is in *Teaching IOM* only.)
- Part 5 (Part 4 in *Learning IOM*) is the longest and most detailed part of each book, and is arranged by the five core competencies named in the 2003 report *Health Professions Education*. *Teaching IOM* also presents throughout this part a variety of specific strategies for integrating safety and quality into nursing education. Many are referenced directly to the teaching–learning modules, which are in the selection of digital instructional materials.
- References, appendices, glossary, list of abbreviations and acronyms, and index.

Outline of the Teaching–Learning Instructional Resources

This material provides faculty and staff educators with an all-digital selection of teaching–learning modules and other resources focused on teaching and learning about quality improvement. It is a supplement to the larger *Teaching IOM*.

Teaching–Learning Strategies: Overview
- Learning Objectives
- Presentations
- Teaching Tips and Techniques
- Cases for Further Exploration
- Teaching–Learning Activities: Exemplars

Teaching–Learning Modules

1. Adverse Events
2. Benchmarking
3. Centers for Medicare and Medicaid Services: Never Events
4. Change and Quality Improvement
5. Checklists
6. Chronic Care Management Model
7. Clinical Decision Support Systems
8. Clinical Guidelines and Clinical Pathways
9. Comparative Effectiveness Research (CER)
10. Core Competencies Relevance to Care Delivery
11. Culture of Safety or Just Culture
12. Disclosure of Errors
13. Disease Management
14. ERMs/EHRs and Quality Improvement
15. Errors in Health Care
16. Failure Modes with Effects Analysis (FMEA)
17. Failure to Rescue
18. Falls and Quality Care
19. Handoffs
20. Healthcare Informatics and Safety
21. *Healthy People* 2020
22. High Reliability Organizations
23. Increasing Quality by Improving Workplace Practice
24. Integrating the Patient and Family in Quality Improvement
25. IOM Reports: Development and Impact
26. The Joint Commission
27. Medication Reconciliation
28. National Healthcare Disparities Monitoring
29. National Healthcare Quality Monitoring
30. Patient-Centered Care
31. Plan-Do-Study-Act (PDSA)
32. Quality Care and Model for Improvement
33. Quality Improvement Monitoring and Reporting Methods
34. Rapid Response Team

35. Risk Management and Utilization Review

36. Role of the Nurse in Quality Improvement: Leadership to Improve Care

37. Root Cause Analysis

38. Safety and Human Factors

39. Situation, Background, Assessment, Recommendation (SBAR)

40. Sentinel Events

41. Surveillance

42. Teams and Quality Improvement

43. TeamSTEPPS

44. Transforming Care at the Bedside (TCAB)

45. Workarounds

Additional Instructional Materials

Teaching–Learning Experiences
Health Literacy
 ▌ Use of Interpreters
 ▌ Health Education and Health Literacy
 ▌ The Healthcare Delivery System and Health Literacy
 ▌ Health Literacy and Nursing Assessment and Interventions
Team-Based Learning
Work and Workspace Design to Prevent and Mitigate Errors
 ▌ Design of Work Hours
 ▌ Design of Work Processes and Workspace
 ▌ Medications
 ▌ Transfers
Quality: Six Aims of Quality Care
National Healthcare Quality Report Matrix
Competency: Recruitment and Training
Clinical Content and Experiences
Priority Areas of Care: Education Strategies
High-Risk Areas
Occupational Health
Teaching the IOM: Exam Questions and Answers
Sample Discussion and Essay Questions
Additional Readings
Additional References: Evidence-Based Practice and Research
 Annotated Links
 Sample Evidence-Based Practice Assignment

Presentations *(Individual PowerPoint files)*
    Evidence-Based Practice
    Healthcare Diversity
    Healthcare Quality
    Healthcare Safety
    Public Health: Safety and Quality
    Transforming Care at the Bedside (TCAB)

Part 1

The IOM Reports: Summaries, Recommendations, and Implications

Introduction

In 1997, President Clinton established a short-term commission called the Advisory Commission on Consumer Protection and Quality in the Healthcare Industry. The purpose of this commission was to advise President Clinton about healthcare delivery system changes related to quality, consumer protection, and the availability of needed services (Wakefield, 1997). The commission investigated many aspects of quality care and the changes needed to improve care, and published a report of its findings in 1999 (*Quality First: Better Healthcare for All Americans*); however, the commission had no idea that it was opening Pandora's Box and that its work would lead to a comprehensive examination of U.S. health care. This initiative produced numerous healthcare quality recommendations, including the need for change in healthcare professions education. Appendix A lists the commission's recommendations. The Institute of Medicine (IOM) was asked to further examine healthcare quality, respond to issues identified in the Presidential Commission's report, and identify strategies to improve healthcare quality over the next 10 years. As a result of this, the IOM has produced numerous reports collectively referred to as the *Quality Chasm* series. Many of these earlier reports are described in the following sections, as are more current reports that focus on quality care, best practices for better health, leadership, diversity and disparity, research- and evidence-based practice, public health, nursing, healthcare education, and many other issues that are highly relevant to nursing education and practice.

Quality Care

Since 1999, the IOM has published many major reports that focus primarily on quality care. Each of these reports is summarized in this part. The Institute of Medicine is a nonprofit organization, based in Washington, D.C., that was established in 1970. It acts as an advisor to the nation to improve health by providing evidence-based advice to policy makers, professionals, educators, and the public. The IOM cannot make law or regulations; rather, it makes recommendations. When it examines a problem area, it invites a panel of experts to work on the problem and then publishes the experts' final report. The title "Institute of Medicine" does not imply that this group focuses only on medicine. Its focus is on health care, and because of this, it may be time to consider a name change to the Institute for Health Care or something similar. Regardless of the title, though, the work of the IOM is highly significant for nursing education and practice, as is demonstrated in the following information about some of its landmark reports on the quality of care and subsequent discussion on the implications of those reports.

To Err Is Human (1999)

To Err Is Human describes the national patient safety problem and has significantly influenced the public's view of health care. Ensuring patient safety requires a comprehensive approach, and we cannot rely on a single solution. This report emphasizes that the workplace must not focus on punishing individuals for errors. Instead, root-cause analysis, a standardized method of analyzing errors, must be conducted to determine individual practice and system problems that result in errors. The expectation is that healthcare organizations will then use these data to eliminate or at least reduce the system problems that compromise patient safety. Safe care does not imply that the care is thereby of higher quality; however, safe care does increase the likelihood of quality care. It would be easy to say that a strong regulatory and enforcement approach is the strategy for solving this problem, but use of appropriate technology is another means to reduce errors. A national mandatory reporting system for errors will also provide useful information to improve safety. Finally, in any of the recommended strategies, leadership is critical.

Next to recognition of the high level of errors, the most important conclusion from the report is the need to change to a nonpunitive, blame-free environment. If a survey asked healthcare providers what is the most common type of error, the prevailing response would probably be that individual providers make errors. Providers would also point out that they are at risk if they report errors. This is a simplistic view of errors and avoids addressing the more significant effect of systems and processes on errors. "Building safety into processes of care is a more effective way to reduce errors than blaming individuals" (IOM, 1999, p. 4). It is much easier to blame an individual, and this punitive approach has been a tradition in healthcare organizations. It has left us with an environment of fear in which individual staff members are reluctant to report errors or near misses. It ignores the critical fact that errors also provide important information about how the system is working, and keeps practitioners from using this information to improve care. Latent or unnoticed errors are the most problematic errors, and they can later lead to more complex errors. It is, however, much easier to address active errors, which are more visible, and miss the latent errors or errors that are not under the control of the direct care staff, such as equipment problems, environmental issues, and management decisions.

To Err Is Human concludes by identifying five critical principles in the design of safe healthcare systems: (1) provide leadership, (2) respect human limits in process design, (3) promote effective team functioning, (4) anticipate the unexpected, and (5) create a learning environment. All of the report's recommendations are described in Appendix B. One of the recommendations was to continue to examine healthcare quality, as the reported error rate was most likely a low estimate due to the variation in how hospitals defined and/or tracked errors. This recommendation led to the next IOM reports.

Crossing the Quality Chasm (2001)

Following the publication of *To Err Is Human,* the next three IOM reports considered a new health system for the 21st century. The first of the three, *Crossing the Quality Chasm* (IOM, 2001a), describes the nation's healthcare system as requiring fundamental change. At the same time, it recognizes that the system *has* experienced rapid changes, such as new medical science, new technology, and near-immediate availability of information. Nevertheless, the healthcare system is fragmented and poorly organized and does not use its resources efficiently. This report identifies quality as a system property with six important improvement aims: Health care should be (1) safe, (2) effective, (3) patient-centered, (4) timely, (5) efficient, and (6) equitable. All healthcare constituents or stakeholders, including policy makers, purchasers, regulators, health professionals, healthcare trustees and management, and consumers, must commit to a national agenda emphasizing these six aims for improvement. The goal is to raise the quality of care to unprecedented levels. The recommendations from this report are included in Appendix C. In addition, the report states 10 rules to guide major stakeholders to reach positive outcomes through collaboration. These rules are drawn from the work of Donald Berwick, M.D. (2008), who also notes the fundamental differences between the new rules and the current system. These differences are discussed in Part 5.

Envisioning the National Healthcare Quality Report (2001)

After completing a more in-depth description of the healthcare problem, the IOM recommended that care be monitored routinely. After extensive exploration of the quality of health care in the United States, the IOM was then challenged regarding what to do with this information and how to monitor quality. This report takes the process a step further by proposing a system for annually collecting data to monitor the quality of the nation's healthcare system. There was need for a framework to use for monitoring healthcare quality. *Envisioning the National Healthcare Quality Report* (IOM, 2001b) describes a model framework for data collection, and that framework is now used to monitor quality of care annually, though it has been modified since the original version was developed. This analysis is now compiled annually by the Agency for Healthcare Research and Quality (AHRQ).

"The National Healthcare Quality Report should serve as a yardstick or the barometer by which to gauge progress in improving the performance of the healthcare delivery system in consistently providing high-quality care" (IOM, 2001b, p. 2). The focus of the report is not public health, but instead how the healthcare system performs in providing personal health care (health care for the individual). In addition, the report discusses health care from a broader perspective than the performance of individual providers such as hospitals. The report should not duplicate systems that many individual healthcare organizations currently use to measure their own performance. The quality report should assist policy makers and should also be accessible and relevant to consumers, purchasers, providers, educators, and researchers. The design of the annual quality report builds on the definition of *quality* used in the various IOM reports. *Quality* is "the degree to which health services for individuals and populations increase the likelihood of desired health outcomes and are consistent with current professional knowledge" (IOM, 1990, p. 21).

The quality report follows the most common approach to quality care assessment, derived from Donabedian's (1996) three elements of quality: (1) structure, (2) process, and (3) outcomes. It is clear that health care quality does not mean that all desired outcomes will necessarily be reached; also, a patient who receives care below the quality standard may still reach the desired outcomes. In addition, the approach selected for the report recognizes the influence of the patient: The patient's desired outcome and preferences influence treatment and healthcare consumerism. The quality report matrix is discussed in Part 5.

The first annual report was published online in 2003 by the Agency for Healthcare Research and Quality. It is a rich source of data, with current updates that can be used to create course content, learning activities, and student examination of data. The current annual national healthcare quality report can be accessed at the AHRQ site: www.ahrq.gov/qual/qrdr10.htm

Priority Areas for National Action: Transforming Healthcare Quality (2003)

Priority Areas (IOM, 2003f) add another building block to the national initiative to improve the quality and safety of health care. This report begins by recognizing that not every aspect of care can be assessed annually—and that attempting to do so would not offer any advantage. The increase of chronic conditions in the United States has had a major impact on the system and is an important consideration in identifying the priority areas. More people are living longer and with chronic illnesses, mostly because of advances in medical science and technology. Many of these patients also have comorbid conditions that increase the complexity of their problems and require more collaborative health care. Three criteria are used to select the priority areas: (1) impact or extent of burden, (2) improvability or extent of the gap between current practice and evidence-based practice, and (3) inclusiveness or relevance of an area to a broad range of individuals.

Earlier reports identify serious quality and safety concerns in healthcare delivery; however, every part of care cannot be evaluated. The report initially specified 19 priority areas. Over time, the priority areas change as new needs arise and outcomes in priority areas improve; however, the annual report framework should not change greatly unless it proves to be inadequate. The priorities are discussed in more detail in Part 5.

Patient Safety: Achieving a New Standard of Care (2003)

Patient Safety (IOM, 2003e) discusses in more detail one recommended strategy for improving patient safety, defined as "freedom from accidental injury." Patient safety improvement requires major changes in safety and quality of care. Multiple stakeholders must commit to these changes, which includes a revamping of patient information systems. This report continues the examination of safety issues and relates to the recommendations found in *To Err Is Human* (IOM, 1999). In the process of giving health care, providers need to: (1) access complete patient information; (2) understand the implications of environmental factors such as waiting time to receive care, bed availability, and so on; (3) use information about infectious diseases to decrease patient risk; and (4) appreciate the implications of chronic illness and how these may affect care needs. Each of these elements depends on accurate, timely, and accessible information in the form of a comprehensive electronic health record/electronic medical record (EHR/EMR). The EHR supports the implementation of best practices and evidence-based care and facilitates standardization of care where appropriate. Additional discussion about informatics is found in Part 5.

Preventing Medication Errors (2006)

The first report in the *Quality Chasm* series, *To Err Is Human* (IOM, 1999), sounded the alarm for healthcare providers and for consumers that there are too many errors in the healthcare system. *Preventing Medication Errors* takes the next step by proposing a methodology to prevent medication errors (IOM, 2006d). The report focuses on several aspects of medication errors. First is the drug development system, along with regulation and distribution issues. Second, the report reviews the literature on the incidence and costs of medication errors and prevention strategies. Using all this information as background, the report then proposes a comprehensive approach for reducing medication errors. This plan requires changes in the healthcare practice of physicians, nurses, pharmacists, and other healthcare providers, as well as the Food and Drug Administration (FDA), hospitals and other healthcare organizations, and health-related government agencies. With an estimated minimum of 1.5 million preventable adverse drug events (ADEs) a year in hospitals and long-term care facilities, there is much to do to improve care. These errors are expensive, with an estimated average cost per ADE of $8,750 per hospital stay. Not all ADEs are preventable, but many are. Part 5 includes additional information on ADEs. The plan for change begins with a greater emphasis on the patient–provider relationship—pushing patients to take a more active role in medical care with more education about their medications, and providing opportunities for them to ask questions and to question medication decisions. As will be noted later, this will lead to a greater emphasis on patient-centered care (PCC). Greater standardization of patient medication information is also needed.

The second component is the use of information technologies for prescribing and dispensing medications to reduce medication errors. The third area of concern is the need to improve labeling and packaging of medications. Finally, the plan covers policy issues such as funding for research about medication error prevention and greater efforts by regulatory agencies to guide and enforce standards to reduce medication errors.

Advancing Quality Improvement Research: Challenges and Opportunities (2007) and The State of QI and Implementation Research (2007)

Crossing the Quality Chasm (IOM, 2001a) discussed the need for improvement in healthcare quality. It was followed by *Envisioning the National Healthcare Quality Report* (IOM, 2001b), which describes the framework and process for a national healthcare quality report. We now have an active annual report that is accessible via the Internet. However, just recognizing that there is a problem in healthcare quality and collecting annual data on the status of that quality is not sufficient to improve care. *Advancing Quality Improvement Research* (IOM, 2007a) and *The State of QI and Implementation Research* (IOM, 2007h) explore examples of quality improvement (QI) focusing on the non-healthcare service sector (for example, Six Sigma and Lean Sigma); the integrated healthcare delivery system (for example, Kaiser Permanente); the hospital perspective; and the nursing perspective.

Much remains to be understood about quality improvement and methods to analyze improvement. Some of these methods are case reports, systematic reviews, controlled trials, and hybrid quantitative and qualitative reports. This area of research differs from other types in what is considered the "gold standard." Some experts claim that randomized controlled trials (RCTs) do not effectively assess complex social contexts; other experts do not agree. Part 5 explores this further. Numerous barriers may obstruct quality improvement and quality improvement research (Institute of Medicine, 2007h):

- QI has many purposes. The purpose of research is very different from experiential learning, which is also an important part of QI.
- The specific context is important when attempting to generalize across settings.
- It is unclear where QI research belongs in academic settings. It should be interprofessional, but this is difficult to implement.
- Most staff involved in QI projects do not have traditional research backgrounds.
- Ethical oversight is critical for research, but it is not clear how this applies to QI. Is QI human subject research, and does it thus require institutional review boards (IRBs)?
- There are methodological differences between the biological sciences and the social sciences. QI is not based on tightly controlled conditions of clinical interventions, so it is more difficult to generalize from QI studies.
- Much of the published QI research has been poorly conducted.
- There is a lack of common vocabulary for QI and implementation research terms.

Diversity and Disparity

The following IOM reports focus on the critical concern of equality in health care.

Unequal Treatment: Confronting Racial and Ethnic Disparities in Health Care (2003)

Unequal Treatment (IOM, 2003g) indicates that bias, prejudice, and stereotyping can lead to disparities in health care. We need greater education, standardized data collection to further understand the problem, and policies and procedures to eliminate inequities. This was the report that led to the recommendation of monitoring disparities. Healthcare organizations (HCOs) have increased staff training on this topic, and it is included in many curricula, but is this making a difference in practice? Disparities in health care are not caused only by a lack of education about culture, so one should not expect that education alone will make the difference. It is a multifaceted problem and requires multiple strategies—many of which will affect the delivery process.

Unequal Treatment focuses on disparities in health care and their impact on the nation's public health, identifying major concerns about racial, ethnic, geographic, and socioeconomic inequities. Healthcare disparities occur consistently across a variety of illnesses and delivery services. The findings of the Sullivan Commission (2004), though not one of the IOM reports, are relevant. That commission examined disparities in health care and concluded that a key contributor to this growing problem is disparity in the nation's health professional workforce. This imbalance impedes minorities' access to health care and undermines understanding of their needs. The Sullivan commission suggested that the solution is to increase the number of minority health professionals. This translates into increased admission into professional schools, something the United States has historically failed to accomplish. Today, with increased competition for positions in nursing, this problem can only grow. Many minority students do not have a strong basic education prior to entering college. If they are admitted, they often do not graduate. At-risk students should receive assistance to give them a greater chance of completing the program.

The problem of disparity in the nursing profession is slowly resolving. Data from the American Association of Colleges of Nursing (AACN) indicate that representation of students from minority backgrounds increased in all types of nursing programs in 2009, growing to 26.3% in entry-level baccalaureate programs, 25.6% in master's programs, and 23.0% in research-focused doctoral programs (2010, p. 4). The percentage of men in nursing programs increased some, with the following representation: 10.8% of students in baccalaureate programs, 9.1% in master's nursing programs, and 7.3% in doctoral research-focused programs and 8.1% in practice-focused programs. This does not mean that we do not have a diversity problem, as we still need to increase diversity more—but we are headed in the right direction.

Nursing education has tended to stress content related to specific cultural groups as the primary method for improving knowledge of disparities, but this may actually lead to more stereotyping and oversimplification of culture (Betancourt, Green, Carrillo, & Park, 2005). Johnson (2005) states that you need both the generic and the specific approaches. Health Resources and Services Administration's (HRSA)curriculum project on culture, *Transforming the Face of Health Professions through Cultural and Linguistic Competence Education*, is an excellent resource for faculty, accessible at www.hrsa.gov/culturalcompetence/cultcompedu.pdf (HRSA, 2008). This course and materials focus on patient-centered care and skills needed to understand the patient's values, beliefs, and behaviors relevant to the healthcare delivery process for the patient, regardless of the setting, and to ensure effective, efficient, and timely care for all patients. Additional content on diversity is found in other parts of this book.

Guidance for the National Healthcare Disparities Report (2002)

Guidance for the National Healthcare Disparities Report outlines the annual National Healthcare Disparity Report, which is published by the AHRQ and is available on the Internet at www.ahrq.gov/qual/qrdr10.htm. It tracks four measurements: socioeconomic status, access to the healthcare system, healthcare services and quality, and geographic disparities in health care. The *Guidance* report is a companion to the National Healthcare Quality Report. It provides a comprehensive national overview of disparities in health care as they affect racial, ethnic, and socioeconomic groups and priority populations. Similar to the National Healthcare Quality Report, the annual disparities report flows from the earlier IOM reports on diversity and disparity in health care. This report also correlates with the quality framework. The framework used to assess measures of healthcare disparities is described in Part 5.

Health Literacy: A Prescription to End Confusion (2004)

Nearly half of all American adults—90 million people—have difficulty understanding and using health information, and there is a higher rate of hospitalization and use of emergency services among patients with limited health literacy, as reported in *Health Literacy* (IOM, 2004a). Limited health literacy may lead to billions of dollars in avoidable healthcare costs. Health literacy is much more than a measure of reading skills. It also includes writing, listening, speaking, arithmetic, and conceptual knowledge. *Health literacy* is defined as "the degree to which individuals have the capacity to obtain, process, and understand basic information and services needed to make appropriate decisions regarding their health" (IOM, 2004a, p. 2). Even well-educated people with strong reading and writing skills may have trouble understanding a medical form or healthcare provider instructions regarding a drug or procedure. This is a critical topic for nursing students, both undergraduate and graduate, and for staff education. Additional content is discussed in Part 5.

Promoting Health Literacy to Encourage Prevention and Wellness: Workshop Summary (2011)

Health literacy has an impact on the use of preventive services. This report emphasizes the need for public health professionals to do less telling people what they should do and more emphasizing the value of prevention to individuals and the community. Health literacy plays a critical role in a person's ability to understand important prevention information. Health and well-being are addressed by primary prevention and secondary prevention, but they are also influenced by non-health issues such as residence location, work, family, economics, and so on. "People need simple instructions about what they need to do to stay healthy and avoid disease. They need ways to measure or score themselves on how well they are doing" (Institute of Medicine, 2011g, p. 8). Those who have an illness need information for self-management.

There is another viewpoint of health literacy that is very important today given the U.S. problem with healthcare disparities. "Health literacy is about health equity. Those who lack health literacy do not have the same opportunity to achieve health as those who are health literate, and therefore, improving health literacy can have a significant impact on health disparities" (2011g, p. 27). This report provides examples of strategies that have been used to promote health literacy and improve health promotion.

America's Healthcare Safety Net: Intact but Endangered (2007)

The "safety net" is the "default system of care for more than 44 million low-income Americans with no or limited health insurance as well as many Medicaid beneficiaries and people who need services" (IOM, 2007b, p. 49). Since this statement was made, the

U.S. healthcare system has expanded, and there is more advanced treatment for patients than ever before. Safety-net organizations provide care to the uninsured, Medicaid patients, and vulnerable populations. Some provide the care because it is mandated by law or stated as part of an organization's mission. In many cases the providers serve a mix of patients: some belong to these vulnerable populations and others do not. The IOM investigation into the healthcare system found it fragmented, consisting of a patchwork of service settings such as clinics, physician offices, and multiple healthcare organizations. It is also not financially secure. Several safety-net hospitals have closed over the last few years, while others are struggling to maintain services. Who, then, provides care in the safety-net system, and for how long? The most common providers are public hospitals, local health departments, community health centers, academic healthcare centers (not all but most), and specialty services such as AIDS clinics and school health clinics.

The safety-net system varies from state to state, and it has managed to survive, although services and quality have been questioned. However, a number of factors may stress these organizations' already weak financial support and have a major impact on the healthcare safety net (IOM, 2007h):

- As the number of uninsured people increases, there is more need for safety-net services. Healthcare reform over time will reduce the number of uninsured, but not completely.
- The direct and indirect subsidies that have helped to finance uncompensated care are eroding (for example, a decrease in federal Medicaid funds to states). Some providers are no longer able to provide "charity care" because it is harder to transfer these costs to paying patients. With the increase in unemployment, there are more people without coverage, only increasing the stress on the safety-net system.
- Hospitals that care for a large number of Medicaid patients are unable to improve care as rapidly as hospitals that have better funding (Reinberg, 2008). With greater emphasis on performance, these safety-net hospitals experience a secondary impact when their lower performance means they get less funding. Less funding means less improvement—and the cycle continues.

The IOM report discusses policy issues, the healthcare safety-net system, forces affecting the system, and the future viability of the system. Additional discussion about the safety-net system is found in Part 5.

Leadership

Leadership By Example: Coordinating Government Roles in Improving Healthcare Quality (2003)

This report explores the characteristics of an infrastructure that will foster quality care (IOM, 2003d). Six government programs—Medicare, Medicaid, State Children's Health Insurance Program (SCHIP), Department of Defense (DOD) TRICARE and TRICARE for Life programs, Veterans Health Administration (VHA), and Indian Health

Services (IHS) program—are examined for quality enhancement processes. These six programs serve about a third of all Americans. The difficulty with implementation of the recommendations in the IOM reports has been the lack of reliable, valid indicators of quality. This analysis stresses the need for the U.S. government to lead in establishing quality performance measures and improving safety and quality of care. The federal government serves in four healthcare delivery roles, which makes it uniquely suited to move the quality initiative forward.

▮ It serves as *regulator* when it sets minimum acceptable performance standards.
▮ It is the largest *purchaser* of care through six major government health programs, and thus can have a major impact on other purchasers of care.
▮ As a *provider* of care for veterans, military personnel and their dependents, and Native Americans, the federal government can implement model quality improvement programs and gather data about their outcomes—programs that could then be used by other providers.
▮ Finally, it is a *research sponsor,* particularly in applied health services research.

The report's recommendations are included in Appendix D.

Public Health

The IOM recognizes the importance of the U.S. public health system. An examination of the system is found in the following IOM reports.

The Future of the Public's Health in the Twenty-first Century (2003) *and* Who Will Keep the Public Healthy? (2003)

The Future of the Public's Health in the Twenty-first Century (IOM, 2003a) and *Who Will Keep the Public Healthy?* (IOM, 2003h) deal with public health. Reports discussed earlier, *Unequal Treatment: Confronting Racial and Ethnic Disparities in Healthcare* (IOM, 2003g) and *Guidance for the National Healthcare Disparities Report* (IOM, 2002), also relate to public health. These four reports discuss the problems in the public health system and offer recommendations for improvement. Part of the current atmosphere of change is the need to instill a vision of public health, which has been identified as *healthy people in healthy communities* (HHS, 2012). This vision of the future of public health recognizes that "health is a primary good because many aspects of human potential such as employment, social relationships, and political participation are contingent on it" (IOM, 2003a, p. 2). Public health affects citizens, their lifestyle, income, work status, mortality and morbidity, education, and family life. But public health has frequently been overlooked in the broad view of the nation's health. The key points of the action plan in *The Future of the Public's Health,* found in Appendix E, include a population health approach, public health systems, infrastructure, partnerships, accountability, evidence, and communication.

Who Will Keep the Public Healthy? (IOM, 2003h) addresses public health needs in a world of globalization, rapid travel, scientific and technological advances, and demographic changes. Effective response to public health problems requires well-prepared professionals. "A public health professional is a person educated in public health or a related discipline who is employed to improve health through a population focus" (*Orlando Business Journal*, 2008, p. 4).

The Association of Schools of Public Health predicts that by 2020 the United States will need 250,000 additional public health workers; as a consequence, there is more interest in public health among all healthcare professionals (*Orlando Business Journal*, 2008). According to the IOM, the traditional core components of public health are still important: epidemiology, biostatistics, environmental health, health services administration, and social and behavioral science. Other areas are also important for current and future public health professions and should be included in nursing curricula. The report's recommendations are found in Appendix F.

Leading Health Indicators for *Healthy People 2020*: Letter Report (2011)

The Department of Health and Human Services (HHS) requested that the IOM develop and recommend 12 leading health indicators and 24 objectives to assist HHS in its determination of leading indicators and objectives for *Healthy People 2020* (2011g). This report is a good example of how the IOM quality reports are connected to other initiatives such as *Healthy People*. The mission of *Healthy People 2020* (HHS, 2012) is to:

▋ Identify nationwide health improvement priorities;
▋ Increase public awareness and understanding of determinants of health, disease, disability, and opportunities for progress;
▋ Provide measurable objectives and goals applicable at national, state, and local levels;
▋ Engage multiple sectors to take actions to strengthen policies and improve practices that are driven by the best available evidence and knowledge; and
▋ Identify critical research evaluation and data collection needs.

The IOM identified the leading indicators and objectives from the new Healthy People 2020's 42 topic areas and nearly 600 objectives. The overarching goals for the 2020 version are:

▋ Attain high-quality, longer lives free of preventable disease.
▋ Achieve health equity; eliminate disparities.
▋ Create social and physical environments that promote good health.
▋ Promote quality of life, healthy development, and healthy behaviors across life stages.

From these many topics and objectives, the IOM identified the leading indicators and their related objectives, as described in Exhibit 1-1. The IOM used a conceptual

E X H I B I T 1 - 1 The IOM and *Healthy People 2020*: Topics, Indicators, and Objectives

Topics	Indicators	Objectives
Access to Care	Proportion of the population with access to healthcare services	1. Increase the proportion of persons with health insurance (AHS 1). 2. Increase the proportion of persons with a usual primary care provider (AHS 3). 3. (Developmental) Increase the proportion of persons who receive appropriate evidence-based clinical preventive services (AHS 7).
Healthy Behaviors	Proportion of the population engaged in healthy behaviors	4. Increase the proportion of adults who meet current federal physical activity guidelines for aerobic physical activity and for muscle-strengthening activity (PA 2). 5. Reduce the proportion of children and adolescents who are considered obese (NWS 10). 6. Reduce consumption of calories from solid fats and added sugars in the population aged 2 years and older (NWS 17). 7. Increase the proportion of adults who get sufficient sleep (SH 4).
Chronic Disease	Prevalence and mortality of chronic disease	8. Reduce coronary heart disease deaths (HDS 2). 9. Reduce the proportion of persons in the population with hypertension (HDS 5). 10. Reduce the overall cancer death rate (C 1).
Environmental Determinants	Proportion of the population experiencing a healthy physical environment	11. Reduce the number of days the Air Quality Index (AQI) exceeds 100 (EH 1).
Social Determinants	Proportion of the population experiencing a healthy social environment	12. (Developmental) Improve the health literacy of the population (HC/HIT 1). 13. (Developmental) Increase the proportion of children who are ready for school in all five domains of healthy development: physical development, social-emotional development, approaches to learning, language, and cognitive development (ENC 1). 14. Increase educational achievement of adolescents and young adults (AH 5).
Injury	Proportion of the population that experiences injury	15. Reduce fatal and nonfatal injuries (IVP 1).
Mental Health	Proportion of the population experiencing positive mental health	16. Reduce the proportion of persons who experience major depressive episodes (MDE) (MHMD 4).
Maternal and Infant Health	Proportion of healthy births	17. Reduce low birth weight (LBW) and very low birth weight (VLBW) (MICH 8).
Responsible Sexual Behavior	Proportion of the population engaged in responsible sexual behavior	18. Reduce pregnancy rates among adolescent females (FP 8). 19. Increase the proportion of sexually active persons who use condoms (HIV 17).
Substance Abuse	Proportion of the population engaged in substance abuse	20. Reduce past-month use of illicit substances (SA 13). 21. Reduce the proportion of persons engaging in binge drinking of alcoholic beverages (SA 14).
Tobacco	Proportion of the population using tobacco	22. Reduce tobacco use by adults (TU 1). 23. Reduce the initiation of tobacco use among children, adolescents, and young adults (TU 3).
Quality of Care	Proportion of the population receiving quality healthcare services	24. Reduce central-line-associated bloodstream infections (CLABSI) (HA 1).

Source: Institute of Medicine, *Leading Health Indicators for Healthy People 2020, Letter Report* (2011g). Reprinted with permission.

framework in identifying these elements: the life course perspective or life stage and the health determinants and health outcomes. The IOM report discusses each of the indicators in detail.

Research and Evidence-Based Practice

The IOM recognizes the importance of research and evidence-based practice (EBP) in several of its reports, and it identified EBP as one of the five healthcare professions core competencies. All of these reports are excellent resources for faculty and students.

Knowing What Works in Health Care: A Roadmap for the Nation (2008)

The IOM has strongly emphasized the need for evidence-based practice and the need to identify diagnostic, treatment, and prevention services—how they work and under what conditions. Another important issue is how different healthcare providers handle specific problems. Cost is yet another factor in clinical decisions, and should be considered, particularly as it relates to best practice. Quality is integral to all of these concerns. This IOM report noted that "the nation must significantly expand its capacity to use scientific evidence to assess 'what works' in health care. This report recommends an organizational framework for a national clinical effectiveness assessment program" (IOM, 2008b, p. 1). The report describes effective evidence as knowledge that is explicit, systematic, and replicable and notes that it must be related to the "real world" perspective. The major health policy challenges related to this recommendation for a national clinical effectiveness assessment program are (IOM, 2008b, pp. 3, 5):

- *Constraining healthcare costs.* A significant proportion of healthcare costs are directed to care that has not been shown to be effective and may actually be harmful.
- *Reducing geographic variation in the use of healthcare services.* Variations in treatment patterns often reflect deviations from accepted care standards or uncertainty and disagreement regarding what those standards should be. Uncertainties about what works and for whom means that patients cannot always be assured that they will receive the best, most effective care.
- *Improving quality.* To promote quality health care, scientific knowledge should be employed, but the evidence base needed to support effective care is in many instances lacking.
- *Empowering healthcare consumers.* Many policy makers believe that consumers and patients should be prudent managers of their own health and health care. However, consumers need information on the effectiveness, risks, and benefits of alternative treatments if they are to search for and obtain high-value treatments. The current dearth of such information is a substantial obstacle to consumer empowerment.

- *Making health coverage decisions.* Private and public health plans are struggling with an almost daily challenge of learning how their covered populations might benefit—or be harmed by—newly available health services.

This report is a good EBP resource; it includes information about EBP and systematic reviews.

Learning What Works: Infrastructure Required for Comparative Effectiveness Research: Workshop Summary (2011)

With a goal of ensuring that 90% of clinical decisions will be supported by accurate, timely, and up-to-date evidence by 2020, the IOM's report on *Learning What Works* addresses some of the issues that are important in reaching this goal. The purpose of this report is "to explore and assess the infrastructure needed (e.g., skills, workforce, methods, coordination, information networks) to expand the nation's capacity to develop and apply comparative effectiveness information" (2011f, p. xvi). The content includes the need and value of comparative effectiveness research (CER), what needs to be done, required information networks, expertise required, and implementation priorities. The nation needs more trials and studies, systematic reviews, innovative research strategies, and clinical registries to better move what is learned from research into practice. Comparative effectiveness research assists in improving the effectiveness and value of health care. Effectiveness is a critical element that must be considered when research results are evaluated. The IOM identified important themes as this topic was discussed (IOM, 2011f, p. 14):

- Care that is effective and efficient stems from the integrity of the infrastructure for learning.
- Coordinating work and ensuring standards are key components of the evidence infrastructure.
- Learning about effectiveness must continue beyond the transition from testing to practice.
- Timely and dynamic evidence of clinical effectiveness requires bridging research and practice.
- Current infrastructure planning must build for future needs and opportunities.
- Keeping pace with technological innovation compels more than a head-to-head and time-to-time focus.
- Real-time learning depends on health information technology investment.
- Developing and applying tools that foster real-time data analysis is an important element.
- A trained workforce is a vital link in the chain of evidence stewardship.
- Approaches are needed that draw effectively on both public and private capacities.
- Efficiency and effectiveness compel globalizing evidence and localizing decisions.

In addition to the need for more studies and systematic reviews, greater attention should be paid to the use of health informatics (HIT) in practice. There is also a need for more public and private collaboration in support of research. CER should be part of the initiative to transform health care in the United States.

This report also comments on transforming health professions education, highlighting previous IOM reports on health professions education that emphasize a patient-centered health management focus, particularly noting the need for interprofessional teams, from early education through lifelong learning. It provides important information for nurse researchers and for nursing faculty who teach both undergraduate and graduate research courses.

Interprofessional issues have become more and important. The Interprofessional Education Collaborative (IPEC), consisting of the American Association of Colleges of Nursing (AACN), the American Association of Colleges of Osteopathic Medicine (AACOM), the Association of Schools of Public Health (ASPH), the American Association of Colleges of Pharmacy (AACP), the American Dental Education Association, and the American Association of Medical Colleges (AAMC), developed core competencies that should underpin collaborative practice and thus affect interprofessional education at the academic level and interprofessional continuing education (IPEC, 2011). The identified competency domains are:

1. Values/ethics for interprofessional practice
2. Roles/responsibilities
3. Interprofessional communication
4. Teams and teamwork

These domains and their related competencies are based on the IOM reports and competencies already discussed in this part of the book and discussed in more detail later. The significance of this work is twofold. It brought together several of the key healthcare professions to developed a shared vision for healthcare team competencies. It also formulated learning objectives and strategies for integration into curricula. At the same time, the Josiah Macy Foundation (JMF), the ABIM Foundation, and the Robert Wood Johnson Foundation (RWJF), in collaboration with the IPEC, hosted a conference in Washington, D.C., to discuss team-based competencies. The proceedings were published under the title *Team-based Competencies: Building a Shared Foundation for Education and Clinical* Practice (JMF, ABIM, & RWJF, 2011). The outcome of this conference was the development of action strategies. The action strategies are (JMF, ABIM, & RWJF, 2011):

1. Communication and dissemination
2. Development of interprofessional faculty and resources
3. Strengthening of metrics and research
4. Development of new collaborative academic practices and new collaborations with community learning sites
5. Advance policy changes

There has been an increase in calls for proposals for grants to address how to operationalize or implement the educational and practice changes through academic practice partnerships. Part 4 includes more discussion on this topic in relation to nursing education, and Part 5 includes information about teams.

Clinical Practice Guidelines We Can Trust (2011)

Clinical practice guidelines (CPGs) are readily available today. The Agency for Healthcare Research and Quality has a large database of CPGs (more than 2,700) available through its National Guideline Clearinghouse (see http://www.guideline.gov). There are also other sources of guidelines. Nevertheless, even with the availability of so many CPGs, there is still a need to increase their use to improve care. "Research has shown that CPGs have the potential to reduce inappropriate practice variation, enhance translation of research into practice, and improve healthcare quality and safety. CPGs also have had an important influence on development of physician and hospital performance measures. The data gathered from use of such measures have provided consumers with information on the quality of different healthcare providers and, in some instances, provided physicians and hospitals with an economic incentive to improve quality of care" (IOM, 2011b, p. xi).

With the proliferation of research, most practitioners do not have the time or expertise to sift through results so that they can have an impact on clinical decisions. Evidence-based CPGs provide a way to increase evidence-based practice; however, the quality of the CPGs must also be considered. "Certain factors commonly undermine the quality and trustworthiness of CPGs. These include variable quality of individual scientific studies; limitations in systematic reviews (SRs) upon which CPGs are based; lack of transparency of development groups' methodologies (particularly with respect to evidence quality and strength of recommendation appraisals); failure to convene multi-stakeholder, multi-disciplinary guideline development groups, and corresponding non-reconciliation of conflicting guidelines; unmanaged conflicts of interest (COI); and overall failure to use rigorous methodologies in CPG development. Furthermore, evidence supporting clinical decision making and CPG development relevant to subpopulations, such as patients with comorbidities, the socially and economically disadvantaged, and those with rare conditions, is usually absent" (IOM, 2011b, p. 2). The IOM report *Knowing What Works in Health Care* (2008b) alerted the Department of Health and Human Services to the need for a public–private program that would "develop or endorse and promote standards that address the structure, process, reporting, and final products of systematic reviews of comparative effectiveness research and evidence-based clinical practice guidelines" (p. 3). In doing this, the IOM updated its past definition of CPGs to read: "Clinical practice guidelines are statements that include recommendations intended to optimize patient care that are informed by a systematic review of evidence and an assessment of the benefits and harms of alternative care options" (IOM, 2008b, p. 4). It also identified the following guidelines to better ensure the CPG trustworthiness, noting that CPGs should:

- be based on a systematic review of the existing evidence;
- be developed by a knowledgeable, multidisciplinary panel of experts and representatives from key affected groups;
- consider important patient subgroups and patient preferences, as appropriate;
- be based on an explicit and transparent process that minimizes distortions, biases, and conflicts of interest;
- provide a clear explanation of the logical relationships between alternative care options and health outcomes, and provide ratings of both the quality of evidence and the strength of the recommendations; and
- be reconsidered and revised as appropriate when important new evidence warrants modifications of recommendations.

This report includes additional content on CPGs and the need to use them effectively. It is an important resource for students and faculty and nurses about the topic of clinical practice guidelines, which nurses as well as physicians should apply.

Finding What Works in Health Care: Standards for Systematic Reviews (2011)

Finding What Works is the fourth current IOM report focusing on research and evidence-based practice. A published systematic review (SR) of comparative effectiveness research is the most effective tool for ensuring greater application of research in practice, though clearly just having systematic reviews does not mean that practitioners will use them. The report discusses the need for standards to ensure high-quality SRs and identifies what those standards should be. Standards focus on:

- Initiating a systematic review
- Finding and assessing individual studies
- Synthesizing the body of evidence
- Reporting systematic reviews (through publication)

"Organizations establish standards to set performance expectations and to promote accountability for meeting these expectations. For SRs in particular, the principal objective of setting standards is to minimize bias in identifying, selecting, and interpreting evidence" (IOM, 2011c, p. 3). Appendix G describes the standards identified in this report for systematic reviews. SRs are used to develop clinical practice guidelines and thus have a major impact on clinical decisions. SRs focus on comparative effectiveness research (CER), which is "the generation and synthesis of evidence that compares the benefits and harms of alternative methods to prevent, diagnose, treat, and monitor a clinical condition or to improve the delivery of care. The purpose of CER is to assist consumers, clinicians, purchasers, and policy makers to make informed decisions that will improve health care at both the individual and population levels" (IOM, 2011c, p. 42). Thus, there is critical linkage of CER, SRs, and clinical practice guidelines. This report contains important content for research and evidence-based practice.

Healthcare Informatics

Health Literacy, eHealth, and Communication: Putting the Consumer First: Workshop Summary (2009)

With the growing need to improve the quality of care, a study done in 2006 surveyed healthcare opinion leaders to rate the effectiveness of a variety of strategies to improve care (Shea, Shih, & Davis, 2007). The results indicated that 67% thought that accelerating the development and use of health information technology was important. Health informatics (HIT) is viewed as a method for improving quality, safety, and efficiency. HIT should include both electronic health records (EHRs) and personal health records (PHRs). This would provide for greater health information exchange. Adoption rates are still low; health information exchange should include not only hospitals but also other types of healthcare providers, including medical practices and clinics. A survey in 2006 concluded: "According to a Pew Internet and American Life research study, 79 percent of Internet users, or 95 million American adults, have searched online for information on at least one major health topic (Fox, 2006). A more recent Pew survey indicated that adults living with a disability or chronic disease are less likely than others to go online, but once they are online, they are more likely to look for health information (Fox, 2007). Such consumer use of electronic systems for obtaining health information illustrates the potential value of consumer-facing Health IT applications" (IOM, 2009a, p. 7).

The rate of consumer Internet use to find health information has increased further since the publication of this 2009 IOM report. Consumers are looking not only for information but also for information to guide decisions. "Two types of skills are needed for eHealth: general skills and specific skills. General skills apply to a number of different contexts and settings and include traditional literacy (reading, writing, and numeracy), media literacy (media analysis skills), and information literacy (information seeking and understanding). Specific skills include such things as computer literacy (IT skills), health literacy (health knowledge comprehension), and science literacy (science process and outcome)" (IOM, 2009a, p. 12). The critical issues are access to technology and Internet and English proficiency. Greater use of information, and greater availability of effective and reliable information, can help patients prepare for a medical appointment if they understand the information. This report provides many examples of ehealth strategies and their impact on different populations, with a focus on the patient/consumer.

Health IT and Patient Safety: Building Safer Systems for Better Care (2011)

Health IT has not only had an impact on the ease of documentation: It also affects the quality of care and errors. As noted in this report, health IT should maximize patient safety and minimize harm. Research findings are mixed on whether or not health IT actually improves care. Why do we not have better evidence? "Several reasons health IT–related safety data are lacking include the absence of measures and a central repository (or linkages among decentralized repositories) to collect, analyze, and act on information related to safety of this technology. Another impediment to gathering safety data is contractual barriers (e.g., nondisclosure, confidentiality clauses) that can prevent users from sharing information about health IT–related adverse events" (IOM, 2011d, p. S-2). Along with health IT that involves the healthcare provider, the patient and family are using and will use more health IT (for example, monitoring health electronically, personal health records, and a variety of mobile applications). Health IT includes electronic medical records, patient engagement tools, and health information exchanges. Data reported in 2010 (Jha, DesRoches, Kralovec, & Joshi, 2010) note that only 11.9% of U.S hospitals use a comprehensive EHR/EMR; compared with other countries, the United States is behind. Physicians are moving to greater use of EMRs, but the shift is slow: 50.7% use any type of EMR and 10.1% use a fully functional EMR.

The healthcare reform legislation supports greater use of EMRs in all healthcare settings. However, just using health IT does not mean care will always be safe and effective. We need standards, funding, demonstration projects, and monitoring of healthcare outcomes to develop effective use of health IT in the United States.

Nursing

Keeping Patients Safe: Transforming the Work Environment for Nurses (2004)

Although germane to nursing in any healthcare setting, *Keeping Patients Safe* (IOM, 2004b) focuses on acute care. It addresses critical quality and safety issues with an emphasis on nursing care and nurses, particularly the work environment. As the report states, "When we are hospitalized, in a nursing home, or managing a chronic condition in our own homes—at some of our most vulnerable moments—nurses are the healthcare providers we are most likely to encounter, spend the greatest amount of time with, and be dependent upon for our recovery" (IOM, 2004b, p. ix). Following a review of the clinical work environment, the report discusses designs for a work environment in which nurses can provide safer, higher-quality patient care. It explores the nursing shortage, healthcare errors, patient safety risk factors, central role of the nurse in patient safety, and work environment threats to patient safety.

Like earlier quality reports, this report calls for a change from blaming individuals for errors to greater consideration of the many system factors that influence outcomes, such as equipment failures, inadequate staff training, lack of clear supervision and direction, inadequate staffing levels, and so on. Making the necessary improvements will require a transformation of the work environment. It is first important to understand how work is done, so that patient safety measures can be built into the nursing work environment. The report identifies six major concerns for direct care in nursing (IOM, 2004b, pp. 91–100).

1. *Monitoring patient status or surveillance*: According to the report, surveillance is different from assessment. *Surveillance* is defined as "purposeful and *ongoing* acquisition, interpretation, and synthesis of patient data for clinical decision-making" (McCloskey & Bulechek, 2000, p. 629).
2. *Physiologic therapy*. This is the most common visible intervention nurses perform.
3. *Helping patients compensate for loss of function*. Unlicensed assistive personnel (UAPs) perform many related activities under the direction of registered nurses (RNs), but RNs do this as well.
4. *Emotional support*. This is a critical need for patients and their families.
5. *Education for patients and families*. This has become more difficult for practicing nurses to provide because of work conditions and staffing shortages.
6. *Integration and coordination of care*. Patients' needs are complex, and care is complex, two facts that often result in multiple forms of care being provided by multiple providers. There is a high risk of failure in communication and inadequate collaboration, both of which increase the risk of errors. There is a critical need for interprofessional teams.

The report recommends (1) adopting transformational leadership and evidence-based management, (2) maximizing the capability of the workforce, and (3) creating and sustaining cultures of safety. The four key areas discussed in *Keeping Patients Safe* are:

▌ Work design
▌ Safety and the central role of the nurse
▌ Quality
▌ The nursing shortage

The report's recommendations relate to:

▌ Patient safety defenses
▌ The EBP model for safety defenses
▌ Reengineering issues
▌ Use of transformational leadership and EBP management
▌ Maximizing workforce capability through staffing levels
▌ The need for knowledge and skills in clinical decision-making
▌ Interprofessional collaboration

- Work space design (AHRQ promotes EBP hospital design to increase quality and safety)
- Building and creating cultures of safety

The report also recommends:

- Adopting transformational leadership and evidence-based management
- Maximizing the capability of the workforce
- Understanding of work processes so that they can be improved
- Creating and sustaining cultures of safety

These are described in more detail in Appendix H.

Leadership is important in making these changes. This topic should be integrated throughout the curriculum, at both the undergraduate and graduate levels, by focusing on the role that leadership plays in quality improvement (QI). This is a landmark report for nursing; it contains important material for nursing education, staff education, nursing management, direct care nursing, and nursing research. The next IOM report, which was published several years later, also emphasizes the need for leadership.

The Future of Nursing: Leading Change, Advancing Health (2011)

This landmark IOM report on nursing is based on the previous work done by the IOM in the "Quality" series of reports. One of its key messages is that nurses should (I don't like the term "play"—has negative connotation) assume new and expanded roles in a redesigned healthcare system—but to do this there must be greater flexibility in practice based on professional training. Improving nursing education must also be part of this movement. Utilizing forums held across the country, the committee focused on transforming practice, education, and leadership, and the results of those forums led to this report. As the title indicates, nurses need to become leaders of changes that are required to improve health care. The report makes eight important recommendations (2011d, pp. 278–283). How do these relate to changes needed in nursing education, the IOM quality reports, and the five healthcare core competencies? These eight recommendations are discussed below, with commentary in italics.

Recommendation 1: **Remove scope-of-practice barriers.** Advanced practice registered nurses should be able to practice to the full extent of their education and training.

> *APRNs are just as responsible for quality care as any other healthcare provider. We need to ensure that ANP programs integrate the core competencies into the curriculum and contain sufficient content on quality improvement. That content is currently weak in undergraduate programs, so most ANP students have not had much on this topic. They need to understand the national, organizational, individual-practice, and patient implications of quality. APRNs should be leaders in QI wherever they practice.*

Recommendation 2: **Expand opportunities for nurses to lead and diffuse collaborative improvement efforts**. Private and public funders, healthcare organizations, nursing education programs, and nursing associations should expand opportunities for nurses to lead and manage collaborative efforts with physicians and other members of the healthcare team to conduct research and to redesign and improve practice environments and health systems. These entities should also provide opportunities for nurses to diffuse successful practices.

> *None of this will happen if nursing education continues to ignore QI in the curriculum or treat it as a minor subject. Latter parts of this book discuss specific information that is critical to QI. If nurses are prepared, they will have greater opportunities to assume the lead in healthcare organizations regarding care improvement. In addition, each nurse who provides care at the bedside should be the first line of defense for each patient.*

Recommendation 3: **Implement nurse residency programs**. State boards of nursing, accrediting bodies, the federal government, and healthcare organizations should take actions to support nurses' completion of a transition-to-practice program (nurse residency) after they have completed a prelicensure or advanced practice degree program, or when they are transitioning into new clinical practice areas.

> *We have long advocated nurse residency programs. These programs should be based on the IOM's five healthcare core competencies. The difficulty with this recommendation is funding for these programs. Until the funding problem is solved, most residencies will be funded by grants, and may or may not be continued after the grant cycle is completed if the healthcare organization cannot afford to continue the program.*

Recommendation 4: **Increase the proportion of nurses with a baccalaureate degree to 80% by 2020**. Academic nurse leaders across all schools of nursing should work together to increase the proportion of nurses with a baccalaureate degree from 50% to 80% by 2020. These leaders should partner with education accrediting bodies, private and public funders, and employers to ensure funding, monitor progress, and increase the diversity of students and create a workforce that is prepared to meet the demands of diverse populations across the lifespan.

> *More has been done regarding this recommendation than on any of the others, and we are seeing an increased interest in nursing. The economic situation has helped, which may mean that this is a short-term response. In addition, the greater number of expected nurse retirements has not yet happened—but it will. Recruitment of qualified students is of concern. We cannot afford to waste time and energy on students who are entering nursing who may not be successful or fully understand the expectations of the profession. We need to put greater effort*

into recruiting the right match for nursing and finding out more about applicants before acceptance. We need greater ability to assess students at risk and provide program supports to assist them, and also recognize that some should not be accepted into programs and may have to be dropped from programs if they are not successful. We do need to provide supportive services for students, but at some point decisions must be made about who we are sending into practice.

Recommendation 5: Double the number of nurses with a doctorate by 2020. Schools of nursing, with support from private and public funders, academic administrators and university trustees, and accrediting bodies, should double the number of nurses with a doctorate by 2020 to add to the cadre of nurse faculty and researchers, with attention to increasing diversity.

This recommendation may not be so easy to fulfill. We have the PhD in nursing, and now we have the doctor of nursing practice (DNP) degree. The latter is a practice degree, not a research-oriented degree; however, we are finding faculty enrolling in these programs, often with no intention of practice but rather to continue teaching. The DNP is not considered a doctorate by many universities, in the sense that persons with a DNP would not be given tenured positions (which are generally reserved for researchers), but rather clinical positions. It is unclear what the result will be. We will need to increase the percentage at a faster rate per year if we are to meet this goal.

Recommendation 6: Ensure that nurses engage in lifelong learning. Accrediting bodies, schools of nursing, healthcare organizations, and continuing competency educators from multiple health professions should collaborate to ensure that nurses and nursing students and faculty continue their education and engage in lifelong learning to gain the competencies needed to provide care for diverse populations across the lifespan.

Continuing education has long been a part of nursing, but in general it has not been considered worthy of much attention. Some states require continuing education (CE) for relicensure or renewal, but the route to getting CE is really fairly easy. It is also difficult to prove that CE has had any impact on the quality of care. Recently, as noted in this section of this book, there has been some attempt to organize and recommend CE changes by focusing on an interprofessional approach. There is no guarantee that this will result in any more positive impact on care. The typical way RNs get their CE is to go to a conference, but they can also earn the requisite CE credits through online modules, which certainly do not require any interprofessional interaction. Most nurses just do what is convenient, quick, and cheap. In many cases the content has nothing to do with what the nurses do in practice, and there is no requirement to do so. This recommendation is important because improving competency should improve care, but determining if CE accomplishes this is difficult. Currently attendance is a problem unless

CE is required or an employer requires attendance regardless of CE credit. These are critical issues that must be addressed. At the advanced practice level, some specialties (neonatal being one of them) have suggested that the demonstration and documentation of continued competency is important (NANN, 2009). This demonstration can be through portfolio documentation of cases and skills the neonatal nurse practitioner has performed during the year or through simulated experiences (NANN, 2009).

Recommendation 7: **Prepare and enable nurses to lead change to advance health**. Nurses, nursing education programs, and nursing associations should prepare the nursing workforce to assume leadership positions across all levels, while public, private, and governmental healthcare decision-makers should ensure that leadership positions are available to be, and are, filled by nurses.

We must do much more, beginning at the undergraduate level and through graduate programs, to offer courses that engage students in the leadership development process and keep them in it for a lifetime. Schools of nursing need active integration of this type of content and experiences in every course, and need to devise methods that facilitate expansion of learning about and developing leadership.

Recommendation 8: **Build an infrastructure for the collection and analysis of interprofessional healthcare workforce data**. The National Health Care Workforce Commission, with oversight from the Government Accountability Office and the Health Resources and Services Administration (HRSA), should lead a collaborative effort to improve research and the collection and analysis of data on healthcare workforce requirements. The Workforce Commission and the HRSA should collaborate with state licensing boards, state nursing workforce centers, and the Department of Labor in this effort to ensure that the data are timely and publicly accessible.

This recommendation is in the implementation stage, with the designation of a national workforce commission that is part of healthcare reform legislation of 2010. This has relevance for nursing education, as it will provide a resource for projections of need.

This report is a rich source of information for faculty and for students, both undergraduate and graduate. Either the sections or the entire report can be assigned for examination and discussion. It has relevance for courses such as transition or introduction to professional nursing, leadership and management, health policy, trends in health care and the profession, education, and research. All students should be aware of this report and its implications. We do not know what impact the report will have in the long term, but asking students to evaluate progress is also an effective learning experience.

It is important to recognize that *The Future of Nursing* report is part of a series of IOM reports on quality care. The critical reports that examined the problems in health care and set up a process for monitoring and improving care are the most important parts of this series. This report on nursing focuses primarily on regulation, degrees and number of nurses with certain degrees, and the need for nursing leadership in improving care. However, combining this report with the earlier IOM reports as the framework make *The Future of Nursing* more relevant to the delivery of health care. To focus only on the nursing report is to miss the major message of the need for change, why we have this need, and how we can meet the need.

Best Practices for Better Health Care: Examples

After addressing general concerns about healthcare quality, the IOM turned to looking at best practices to discover and demonstrate effective approaches to improving care. The following IOM reports focus on several examples of best practice.

Hospital-Based Emergency Care: At the Breaking Point (2007)

The emergency care system is described as "overburdened, underfunded, and highly fragmented" (IOM, 2007f, p. 1). The report points out that emergency departments cannot handle the load and often must send patients to other hospitals; it also notes that the disaster response system needs improvement. This report is the first of a series on emergency care that includes *Emergency Care for Children: Growing Pains* (IOM, 2007d); *Emergency Medical Services at the Crossroads* (IOM, 2006a); and a follow-up workshop, *Future of Emergency Care* (IOM, 2007e). The report concentrates on:

- The role and impact of the emergency department within the larger hospital and healthcare system
- Patient flow and information technology (IT)
- Workforce issues across multiple disciplines
- Patient safety and the quality and efficiency of emergency care service
- Basic, clinical, and health services research relevant to emergency care
- Special challenges of emergency care in rural settings

Emergency Care for Children: Growing Pains (2007)

Children who receive emergency medical services (EMS) have unique medical needs, and the family has a major role in child emergency care. Physiological differences from adults, safety, the higher risk for errors in treating children, and special communication needs are all matters of concern. "The emergency and trauma care system is highly fragmented, with little coordination among pre-hospital emergency medical services, hospital services, and public health. Use of emergency departments (EDs) has grown considerably even as many EDs have closed, contributing to crowded conditions in those that remain open. Ambulance diversion has become a daily occurrence in many cities around the country" (IOM, 2007d, p. 1).

This report is a good resource for students studying pediatric care and for staff who provide pediatric emergency services. It focuses on:

▮ The role of pediatric emergency services as an integrated component of the overall health system
▮ System-wide pediatric emergency care planning, preparedness, coordination, and funding
▮ Pediatric training in professional education
▮ Research in pediatric emergency care

Emergency Medical Services at the Crossroads (2006)

"EMS encompasses the initial stages of the emergency care continuum. It includes emergency calls to 9-1-1; dispatch of emergency personnel to the scene of an illness or trauma; and triage, treatment, and transport of patients by ambulance and air medical service. The speed and quality of emergency medical services are critical factors in a patient's ultimate outcome" (IOM, 2006a, p. 1). The current delivery system has some major weaknesses: insufficient coordination, disparities in response times, uncertain quality of care, lack of readiness for disasters, divided professional identity, and limited evidence base. The report discusses needs and strategies for improvement.

Future of Emergency Care (2007)

Unlike the other IOM reports, this is a summary of a series of workshops held across the United States to discuss three other reports: *Emergency Medical Services at the Crossroads* (IOM, 2006a); *Hospital-Based Emergency Care: At the Breaking Point* (IOM, 2007f); and *Emergency Care for Children: Growing Pains* (IOM, 2007d). The emergency system is a critical part of the healthcare system. It provides emergency care and serves as an entry point into the healthcare system for hospitalization and referral to ambulatory care such as clinics and physician offices. However, the system is in trouble; it is highly fragmented, overburdened, and underfunded. The reports find multiple problems in emergency care: overcrowding, lack of coordination, workforce shortages, variability in the quality of care, lack of effective disaster preparedness, limited research to support evidence-based practice, and limited services for children requiring emergency care.

Preventing Childhood Obesity: Health in the Balance (2005)

The epidemic of childhood obesity is a critical pediatric health problem with long-term implications for the health of adults. This report notes that obesity affects boys and girls in all areas of the country, across all socioeconomic strata, and across all ethnic groups, with African Americans, Hispanics, and Native American children experiencing a higher level of obesity.

"Childhood obesity involves immediate and long-term risks to physical health. For children born in the United States in 2000, the lifetime risk of being diagnosed with diabetes at some point in their lives is estimated at 30% for boys and 40% for girls if obesity rates level off. Young people are also at risk of developing serious psychosocial burdens related to being obese in a society that stigmatizes this condition. There are also considerable economic costs. The national healthcare expenditures related to obesity and overweight adults alone have been estimated to range from approximately $98 billion to $129 billion after adjusting for inflation and converting estimates to 2004 dollars" (IOM, 2005a, p. 2). Goals of obesity prevention in children and youth include (p. 4):

For the *population* of children and youth:

■ Reduction in the incidence of childhood and adolescent obesity
■ Reduction in the prevalence of childhood and adolescent obesity
■ Reduction of mean-population body mass index (BMI) levels
■ Improvement in the proportion of children meeting Dietary Guidelines for Americans
■ Improvement in the proportion of children meeting physical activity guidelines
■ Achieving physical, psychological, and cognitive growth and developmental goals

For *individual* children and youth:

■ A healthy weight trajectory, as defined by the Centers for Disease Control and Prevention (CDC) BMI charts
■ A healthful diet (quality and quantity)
■ Appropriate amounts and types of physical activity
■ Achieving physical, psychosocial, and cognitive growth and developmental goals

Because it may take a number of years to achieve and sustain these goals, intermediate goals are needed to assess progress toward reduction of obesity through policy and system changes. Examples include:

■ Increased number of children who safely walk and bike to school
■ Improved access to and affordability of fruits and vegetables for low-income populations
■ Increased availability and use of community recreational facilities
■ Increased play and physical activity opportunities
■ Increased number of new industry products and advertising messages that promote energy balance at a healthy weight
■ Increased availability and affordability of healthful foods and beverages at supermarkets, grocery stores, and farmers' markets located within walking distance of the communities they serve
■ Changes in institutional and environmental policies that promote energy balance

Quality through Collaboration: The Future of Rural Health (2005)

Quality through Collaboration (IOM, 2005b) addresses the critical quality care issues of rural areas, which represent 20% of the U.S. population. These diverse populations are found in all regions of the country, and represent vulnerable healthcare populations. Rural areas have the same healthcare quality challenges as other areas, but they also face some circumstances that make it more difficult to achieve quality care. Some major healthcare services are lacking or limited, such as emergency medical services, mental health and substance abuse services, and oral health care. There is a shortage of healthcare providers in all areas of the country, but deficits in rural areas are greater in overall numbers and in specialty providers. Rural populations tend to be older than urban populations and experience higher rates of limitations in daily activities as a result of chronic conditions.

"Rural populations exhibit poorer health behaviors (for example, higher rates of smoking and obesity and lower rates of exercise) relative to urban populations, although there is variability in health behaviors among rural populations" (IOM, 2005b, p. 3). We also need to improve the data collected about health in rural areas, compile evidence to improve care in rural areas, increase education about evidence-based practice, and formulate quality improvement measures for rural areas. The five healthcare professions core competencies discussed in Part 6 certainly apply to care in rural areas, but should also be viewed from the perspective of rural healthcare needs. There is no doubt that we need more rural healthcare providers and healthcare organizations to reduce travel time to provide appropriate, affordable, and effective health care across the life span. Both personal and population health programs are essential to improve health.

The Office of Rural Health Policy (ORHP) is a part of the Department of Health and Human Services (HHS), Health Resources and Services Administration (HRSA). It promotes better healthcare service in rural areas. Its website, http://ruralhealth.hrsa.gov/, describes ORHP activities. This report is particularly relevant to schools of nursing located in rural areas or using clinical agencies in rural areas, though all students need to understand rural healthcare needs.

Improving the Quality of Health Care for Mental and Substance-Use Conditions (2006)

"Millions of Americans today receive health care for mental or substance-use problems and illnesses. These conditions are the leading cause of combined disability and death among women and the second highest among men. Effective treatments exist and continually improve; however, as with general health care, deficiencies in care delivery prevent many from receiving appropriate treatments" (IOM, 2006c, p. 1). We need to ensure that the healthcare system provides care for these vulnerable populations so that (p. 2):

- Individual patient preferences, needs, and values prevail in the face of residual stigma, discrimination, and coercion into treatment.
- The necessary infrastructure exists to produce scientific evidence more quickly and promote its application in patient care.
- Multiple providers' care of the same patient is coordinated.
- Emerging information technology related to health care benefits people with mental or substance-use problems and illnesses.
- The healthcare workforce has the education, training, and capacity to deliver high-quality care for mental and substance-use conditions.

- Government programs, employers, and other group purchasers of health care for mental and substance-use conditions use their dollars in ways that support the delivery of high-quality care.
- Research funds are used to support studies that have direct clinical and policy relevance and that are focused on discovering and testing therapeutic advances.

We have effective treatments for many mental health problems, but these services have to be made accessible and affordable. Some mental health problems require long-term care, and this care also must be accessible, effective, and affordable. In addition, we need to deal with the persistent issue of stigma. There has been greater emphasis on research that examines the interplay between genetic, environmental, biologic, and psychosocial factors in brain function, but much more remains to be done. Mental health and substance-abuse care is not always at the level it should be, and poor care can lead to more serious problems. Mental health needs are frequently associated with other medical conditions; for example, people hospitalized with a myocardial infarction are found to also have a greater risk (one in five) for major depression. Substance abuse leads to multiple biological illnesses, to mental illness, and to sociological problems (abuse, crime, loss of job, limited education, divorce, single parenting, and more). This care must meet all of the requirements for quality care as addressed in the *Quality Chasm* series, such as the six aims of high-quality health care and the ten rules for the 21st century. (The rules are discussed further in Part 5.) This report is a valuable resource for psychiatric-mental health (behavioral) content and clinical experiences.

From Cancer Patient to Cancer Survivor: Lost in Transition (2006)

Cancer care in the past concentrated mostly on acute care, but now many patients are living longer with cancer. Care for survivors who now are considered to have a chronic illness becomes even more important. This has required new approaches to help the 10 million American cancer survivors. "The transition from active treatment to post-treatment care is critical to long-term health. If care is not planned and coordinated, cancer survivors are left without knowledge of their heightened risks and a follow-up plan of action" (IOM, 2006b, p. 1). The aims of the report are to (IOM, 2006b, p. 2):

- Raise awareness of the medical, functional, and psychosocial consequences of cancer and its treatment
- Define quality health care for cancer survivors and identify strategies to achieve it
- Improve the quality of life of cancer survivors through policies to ensure access to psychosocial services, fair employment practices, and health insurance

The focus is on cancer survivorship, which is a "distinct phase of the cancer trajectory which has been relatively neglected in advocacy, education, clinical practice, and research" (IOM, 2006b, p.2). The essential components of survivorship care include (p. 3):

- Prevention of recurrent and new cancers, and of other late effects
- Surveillance for cancer spread, recurrence, or second cancers

- Assessment of medical and psychosocial late effects
- Intervention for consequences of cancer and its treatment: medical problems (lymphedema/sexual dysfunction); symptoms, including pain and fatigue; psychological distress of cancer survivors and their caregivers
- Concerns related to employment, insurance, and disability between specialists and primary care providers to ensure that all survivor health needs are met

This report offers a different perspective on cancer care that is very important to include in content and clinical experiences.

Cancer Care for the Whole Patient: Meeting Psychosocial Health Needs (2007)

The IOM continues to expand its examination of the core elements in the quality framework into specific patient populations and problems, as is noted in reports previously discussed such as emergency care, rural health care, and pediatrics. *Cancer Care for the Whole Patient: Meeting Psychosocial Health Needs* (IOM, 2007c) is another such report. It recommends that all parties that establish or use standards for the quality of cancer care should adopt the following as a guideline. All cancer care should ensure the provision of appropriate psychosocial health services by:

- Facilitating effective communication between patients and care providers
- Identifying each patient's psychosocial health needs
- Designing and implementing a plan that:
  - Links the patient with needed psychosocial services;
  - Coordinates biomedical and psychosocial needs; and
  - Engages and supports patients in managing their illness and health
- Systematically following up on, re-evaluating, and adjusting plans

This report and its recommendations provide an excellent way to meet the need to include psychosocial interventions in nursing education. Some schools of nursing are reducing mental health content, but this ignores the importance of understanding the needs and care for patients in multiple situations that require psychosocial support. "Psychosocial issues have to be a part of routine care, not just in cancer but in any chronic disease" (Young, 2007, p. 750).

Preterm Birth: Causes, Consequences, and Prevention (2007)

The IOM has looked at the problem of preterm births in the United States, which have increased and are particularly connected to racial, ethnic, and socioeconomic disparities. Preterm births increase the risk of mortality and health and development problems. "Complications include acute respiratory, gastrointestinal, immunologic, central nervous system, hearing, and vision problems, as well as longer-term motor, cognitive, visual, hearing, behavioral, social-emotional, health, and growth problems. The birth of a preterm infant can also bring considerable emotional and economic costs to families and have implications for public-sector services, such as health insurance, educational, and other social support systems. The annual societal economic burden associated with preterm birth in the United States was at least $26.2 billion in 2005" (IOM, 2007g, p. 1). We need to know much more about the causes of preterm births and measures to prevent them. This report describes preterm birth priority areas as:

1. Multidisciplinary/interprofessional research centers
2. Priority areas for research
   ▌ Better define the problem of preterm birth with improved data.
   ▌ Improve collection of surveillance and descriptive data in order to better define the nature and scope of the problem of preterm birth.
     a. Improve national data.
     b. Study the economic outcomes for infants born preterm.
   ▌ Conduct clinical and health services research investigations.
   ▌ Examine and improve the clinical treatment of women who deliver preterm, infants born preterm, and the healthcare systems that care for them.
     a. Improve the methods of identifying and treating women at risk for preterm labor.
     b. Study the acute and long-term outcomes for infants born preterm.
     c. Study infertility treatments and institute guidelines to reduce the number of multiple gestations.
     d. Improve the quality of care for women at risk for preterm labor and infants born preterm.
     e. Investigate the impact of the healthcare delivery system on preterm birth.
   ▌ Conduct etiologic and epidemiologic investigations.
   ▌ Examine the potential causes of preterm birth and its distribution in the population.
     a. Investigate the etiologies of preterm birth.
     b. Study the multiple psychosocial, behavioral, and environmental risk factors associated with preterm birth.
     c. Investigate racial-ethnic and socioeconomic disparities in the rates of preterm birth.
3. Informed public policy: Understand the impact of preterm birth on various public programs and how policies can be used to reduce rates of preterm birth.

This report is a good resource for maternal–child and community health providers and facilities, as it identifies content areas, issues for research consideration, and issues related to improvement of services.

Retooling for an Aging America: Building the Healthcare Workforce (2008)

This report (IOM, 2008c) focuses on the needs of the older vulnerable population. With seniors (65 years of age and older) constituting (not sure this change is best choice of words—it is not clear or maybe awkward) approximately 20% of the population and the long-term expectation of this population increasing, they are a critical concern for healthcare services. Medical care has enabled people to live longer. Many are in relatively good health, though chronic illness is a problem. Patients over the age of 75 average three chronic conditions and may take four or more medications.

The healthcare workforce is too small and unprepared for this population with its complex needs, and half of the providers for this population receive very low pay, such as nurse aides. Of older adults who receive care in the home, 90% get help from family and friends, and 80% rely solely on family and friends for care. The report identifies three initiatives to address this problem:

■ Explore ways to broaden the duties and responsibilities of workers at various levels of training.
■ Better prepare informal caregivers to tend to the needs of aging family members and friends.
■ Develop new models of healthcare delivery and payment as old ways sponsored by federal programs such as Medicare prove to be ineffective and inefficient.

Schools of nursing are expanding content on older populations, but much more is needed, along with increased clinical experiences. There are now gerontology centers of excellence, such as the University of Oklahoma College of Nursing Reynolds Center of Geriatric Nursing, that aim to develop greater expertise and competencies in gerontological care, and a greater number of doctoral students are specializing in care for the older adult. Nevertheless, much more is required to improve care and cope with this growing, vulnerable population. The Hartford Institute for Geriatric Nursing is an excellent resource for addressing geriatric nursing. Its mission is to shape the quality of health care of older adults through nursing excellence (see http://hartfordign.org/about), and it emphasizes the values of:

■ Interdisciplinary/interprofessional approaches
■ Quality care
■ Knowledge
■ Respect for older adults and the people who care for them

Relieving Pain in America: A Blueprint for Transforming Prevention, Care, Education, and Research (2011)

Pain management is part of patient-centered care, as noted in earlier IOM reports. "Pain is a universal experience. Common chronic pain conditions affect at least 116 million U.S. adults at a cost of $560–635 billion annually in direct medical treatment costs and lost productivity. Pain's occurrence, severity, duration, response to treatment, and disabling consequences vary from person to person because pain, like other severe chronic conditions, is much more than a biological phenomenon and has profound emotional and cognitive effects. Pain can be mild and easily handled with over-the-counter medications; it can be acute and recede with treatment; it can be recurrent over months or years; or it can be chronic and debilitating, requiring almost constant attention and accommodation" (2011h, pp. 1–2). We need to improve assessment and treatment of pain. Section 4305 of the 2010 Patient Protection and Affordable Care Act (part of the latest healthcare reform legislation), directs the Department of Health and Human Services to request the IOM to examine pain management and recognize that pain is a major public health problem. This report approaches the problem by identifying specific findings and making associated recommendations to address the issue (IOM, 2011h, pp. 5–13).

Finding 2-1. Pain is a public health problem.

Recommendation 2-1. Improve the collection and reporting of data on pain.

Finding 2-2. More consistent data on pain are needed.

Recommendation 2-2. Create a comprehensive population health-level strategy for pain prevention, treatment, management, and research.

Finding 2-3. A population-based strategy for reducing pain and its consequences is needed.

Finding 3-1. Pain care must be tailored to each person's experience.

Recommendation 3-1. Promote and enable self-management of pain.

Finding 3-2. Significant barriers to adequate pain care exist.

Recommendation 3-2. Develop strategies for reducing barriers to pain care.

Recommendation 3-3. Provide educational opportunities in pain assessment and treatment in primary care.

Recommendation 3-4. Support collaboration between pain specialists and primary care clinicians, including referral to pain centers when appropriate.

Recommendation 3-5. Revise reimbursement policies to foster coordinated and evidence-based care.

Recommendation 3-6. Provide consistent and complete pain assessments.

Finding 4-1. Education is a central part of the necessary cultural transformation of the approach to pain.

Recommendation 4-1. Expand and redesign education programs to transform understanding of pain.

Recommendation 4-2. Increase the number of health professionals with advanced expertise in pain care.

Finding 5-1. Research to translate theoretical advances into effective therapies for pain is a continuing need.

Recommendation 5-1. Designate a lead institute at the National Institutes of Health responsible for moving pain research forward and increase the support for and scope of the Pain Consortium.

Recommendation 5-2. Improve the process for developing new agents for pain control.

Recommendation 5-3. Increase support for interdisciplinary/interprofessional research in pain.

Recommendation 5-4. Increase the conduct of longitudinal research.

Recommendation 5-5. Increase the training of pain researchers.

Pain management is a critical element of nursing care, and nursing education should include more on this problem in all types of programs and degrees. This report provides an overview of the problem and describes recommendations or strategies to improve pain management for patients.

Healthcare Professions Education

Health Professions Education (2003)

Education of health professionals is viewed as a bridge to quality care. The discussion in *Health Professions Education* (IOM, 2003b) centers on the need to have qualified, competent staff to improve health care, and concludes that all health professions education should change to meet the growing demands of current and future healthcare systems. The report clearly states that the goal of health professions education should be outcome-based education. Health care in the United States requires changes to improve healthcare quality and safety, and these changes should consider outcomes.

These recommendations are hardly surprising. However, the report makes it clear that health professions education has not kept current with healthcare needs, evidence-based practice, technology, diversity changes, and leadership requirements—shortcomings that put healthcare profession education even further behind in light of newer recommendations. *Essentials of Baccalaureate Education for Professional Nursing Practice* (AACN, 2008c) reflects the importance of all of the core competencies recommended in the IOM report. "Yet the current challenges before us are twofold: to determine why the current workforce of baccalaureate-prepared nurses is not fully actualizing the IOM core competencies and to consider ways to strengthen nursing curricula to better educate nurses" (Long, 2003, pp. 259–260). The five core competencies recommended for implementation by all organizations involved in the education of healthcare professionals are (IOM, 2003b, pp. 49–63):

▌ Provide patient-centered care; focus on the patient rather than the disease or the clinician.
▌ Work in interprofessional teams; use the best healthcare professionals for the needs of the patient and work together to accomplish effective patient care outcomes.
▌ Employ evidence-based practice; integrate best research results, clinical expertise, and patient values to make patient care decisions.
▌ Apply quality improvement (QI) measures and make them effective.
▌ Use informatics; apply it to reduction of errors, management of knowledge and information, decision-making, and communication.

Health Professions Education outlines some strategies to build these competencies. These are found in Appendix I. The integration of the core competencies in the curriculum is discussed in Part 4, and the core competencies are discussed in more detail in Part 5, along with related teaching-learning strategies.

A Summary of the February 2010 Forum on the Future of Nursing Education (2010)

This report focuses on nursing education and was incorporated into *The Future of Nursing. Leading Change, Advancing Health* (IOM, 2011d). Forums were held in several locations to get input from the nursing community, mostly from nursing faculty. The key topics are: what to teach; how to teach; and where to teach. Exemplars are provided in the content, which were forum presentations used to stimulate discussion. Testimony from a variety of nursing leaders and other professionals is also provided. This report provides background for the information on nursing education included in T*he Future of Nursing*. Examples of some of the content items are (2010b, p. x):

▮ The new basics in nursing education are collaboration within the profession and across other health professions, communication, and systems thinking.

▮ Nurses, particularly nurse educators, need to keep up with a rapidly changing knowledge base and new technologies throughout their careers to ensure a well-educated workforce.

▮ Care for older adults, increasingly occurring outside of acute care settings, will be a large and growing component of nursing in the future, and the nursing education system needs to prepare educators and practitioners for that reality.

▮ The nation will face serious consequences if the number of nursing educators is not adequate to develop a more diverse nursing workforce adequate in both number and competencies to meet the needs of diverse populations across the lifespan.

▮ Technology—such as that used in high-fidelity simulations—that fosters problem-solving and critical thinking skills in nurses is essential for nursing education to produce sufficient numbers of competent, well-educated nurses.

▮ Resources and partnerships available in the community should be used to prepare nurses who can serve their communities.

▮ Articulation agreements and education consortiums among different kinds of institutions can provide multiple entry points and continued opportunities for progression through an educational and career ladder.

▮ In addition to necessary skill sets, nursing education needs to provide students with the ability to mature as professionals and to continue learning throughout their careers.

Not only was this content considered for *The Future of Nursing report,* but in reviewing *Educating Nurses. A Call for Radical Transformation* (Benner, Sutphen, Leonard, & Day, 2010), one can also see similar themes.

Redesigning Continuing Education in the Health Professions (2010)

It is not surprising that, after addressing the issue of healthcare profession education from the perspective of degree programs, the IOM would then turn to the issue of lifelong learning for healthcare professionals. It is also significant that, just as with *Healthcare Professions Education,* the IOM addresses all healthcare professions in one report. In one paragraph, it describes the key concerns: "Continuing education (CE) is the process by which health professionals keep up to date with the latest knowledge and advances in health care. However, the CE 'system,' as it is structured today, is so deeply flawed that it cannot properly support the development of health professionals. CE has become structured around health professional participation instead of performance improvement. This has left health professionals unprepared to perform at the highest levels consistently, putting into question whether the public is receiving care of the highest possibly quality and safety" (2010a, p. ix). If CE is used effectively, the healthcare workforce can be strengthened and retooled, something that is critical to improve the quality of care. This report discusses the need for effective CE, the scientific foundations of CE, regulations and financing, and design and implementation of a new CE approach. The report provides useful information about current and possible future approaches to providing CE; this is of particular interest to those who are actively involved in continuing education programs. Another important topic is measurement of the effectiveness of CE, something that has long been difficult to deal with effectively. There is extensive discussion about the issue of licensure and CE requirements, which are not consistent either within all professions or across professions. Accreditation of CE programs is also described, and the report recognizes the need for consistent accreditation standards across professions and states.

Several options for designing a new model for CE are described, but the report recommends that a public–private institute for CE professional development (CPD) be created. This recommendation has been made to the Secretary of the Department of Health and Human Services. Consideration should be given to content, regulation, financing, and the development and strengthening of a scientific basis for the practice of CPD. The system should be based on the IOM-recommended five healthcare profession core competencies. To accomplish this will require greater interprofessional collaboration. "Imagine a healthcare system with the ability to rapidly adapt to the needs of patients, health professionals, and institutions through a shared commitment to CPD and high quality patient care. Imagine a healthcare system in which everyone is a learner, supported on the arc of professional development with knowledge of tailored learning goals, the tools to meet and surpass those goals, and a community of other learners with whom to share the process. A comprehensive CPD system would transform this vision of professional learning into reality" (IOM, 2010a, p. 111).

Implications of the IOM Reports for Clinical Care

Taken together, the IOM reports summarized in the first part of this book have many implications for clinical care in the United States. This final section examines the success of two ongoing, clinically oriented initiatives that have been influenced by and reflect many of these reports: the Transforming Care at the Bedside (TCAB) initiative and the National Database of Nursing Quality Indicators (NDNQI) program. The section concludes with a brief discussion on the degree of improvement in U.S. health care and the influence of the existing and future IOM reports.

Transforming Care at the Bedside (TCAB)

Improving healthcare quality and safety requires active participation from nursing—we provide care 24/7. The push to improve the quality of care comes at a critical time for nursing, one of a growing shortage of personnel, and we have great need to make major improvements in nursing education. This is not the best time to deal with a serious problem like quality of care, but the response cannot be delayed. We need to be innovative. There is more to nursing than just filling positions. What can be done to transform care and make nursing more effective and efficient? We are witnessing a major technological explosion in health care, and we should make it work for us. The IOM has shown us that we—all healthcare professionals—need to work as teams. We need to recognize the value of the evidence we use to support our care decisions. We need more nursing research to solve real clinical problems. We need more quality improvement initiatives that include active nursing participation. Some priority setting is also required so that our efforts will be efficient and effective.

Transforming Care at the Bedside (TCAB) began formally in 2003 with funding and support from the Robert Wood Johnson Foundation (RWJF) and the Institute for *Healthcare Improvement* (IHI, 2008e). This is a collaborative effort to redesign the work environment of nurses and to involve nurses directly in that transformation. TCAB relates to the IOM report *Keeping Patients Safe* (2004b) and now to *The Future of Nursing* report (IOM, 2011d). TCAB uses a QI approach that engages front-line staff and unit managers. In this initiative, staff and unit managers drive problem identification for improvement. Medical–surgical units in acute care were chosen as the first pilots in the initiative. Three hospitals were included in the initial phase, and now many more are running pilots. TCAB is based on four main components (IHI, 2011):

- Safe and reliable care
- Vitality and teamwork
- Patient-centered care
- Value-added care processes

Embedded within TCAB is the language of the *Quality Chasm* series, including the overall goal of care improvement and quality care. TCAB includes the following "tests of change" (Martin, et al., 2007, p. 445):

- Work redesign includes staff that do the work in the healthcare organization where work happens and as it happens (this includes departmental leadership).

- Improvement efforts are centered on a patient's or employee's need.
- Support from executive leadership is critical.
- First test with a small sample, learn, and then spread to a larger scope.
- Teach as you go because, once done, the approach will have to apply to other problems.
- Make it happen tomorrow.

The TCAB process uses deep dive or total immersion into a problem area to explore, brainstorm, and prioritize. Staff members are asked this question: "If you could create the perfect patient and staff experience, what would it look like? Consider the key design themes in guiding your thoughts and ideas. If you find yourself focusing on current problems, push your mind to think of a solution or another way to design it" (Martin et al., 2007, p. 445). The process then follows these steps:

1. Clarify the current state by observations. Include those involved.
2. Understand the root problem to be solved.
3. Select a process to focus on.
4. Design a prototype (Plan, Do, Check, Act or PDSA).
5. Begin small and rapidly move and test.
6. Identify failures quickly and reject them.
7. Determine possible improvements and quickly broaden the test of change.
8. Determine definite "just-do-its" and quickly implement them.

The TCAB framework can be found at http://www.ihi.org/offerings/Initiatives/PastStrategicInitiatives/TCAB/Pages/Framework.aspx

How can information about TCAB be applied to nursing education? Ask students to use the same process, beginning with asking them the same question. Build deep-dive experiences into simulation activities and clinical experiences. When students observe a problem, ask them to use this process. If students are in a TCAB pilot hospital, make sure they know about the projects and results. The TCAB toolkit provides details about the process that TCAB teams use, examples of successes, and a PowerPoint slide presentation. This is a great teaching tool for leadership and management courses at the undergraduate level, for graduate students such as Clinical Nurse Leader students and Clinical Nurse Specialist students, and for staff education to prepare staff to use TCAB. The TCAB website is a rich source of content and examples for faculty, students, and staff.

In an integrative review, Ridley (2008) appraised studies of the relationship between nurse education level and patient safety, assessing the current state of science over a 20-year period. The Agency for Healthcare Research and Quality Patient Safety Indicators were used to measure outcomes, and included the following (AHRQ, 2006):

- Complications of anesthesia
- Death in low-mortality drug-related groups
- Decubitus ulcer

- Failure to rescue
- Foreign body left during procedure
- Iatrogenic pneumothorax
- Selected infections due to medical care
- Postoperative hip infection
- Postoperative hemorrhage or hematoma
- Postoperative physiologic and metabolic derangements
- Postoperative respiratory failure
- Postoperative pulmonary embolism or deep vein thrombosis
- Postoperative sepsis
- Postoperative wound dehiscence
- Accidental puncture or laceration
- Transfusion reaction
- Birth trauma, injury to neonate
- Obstetric trauma, vaginal with instrument
- Obstetric trauma, vaginal without instrument
- Obstetric trauma, cesarean delivery

The review covers 24 studies. It concludes that there is evidence that increased RNs and skill mix improve patient safety, leading to fewer adverse patient outcomes sensitive to nursing care, but there is "virtually nonexistent" evidence thus far about the breakdown of nurse education level (Ridley, 2008, p. 156). Further research is required, as well as examination of the relationship of competence to patient safety. TCAB examines a variety of point-of-care practice issues.

Nursing Data on Quality Care: NDNQI

In 1994, the American Nurses Association (ANA) began an investigation of the impact of workforce restructuring and redesign on the safety and quality of patient care in acute care settings. ANA wanted to "explore the nature and strength of the linkages between nursing care and patient outcomes by identifying nursing quality indicators" (Pollard, Mitra, & Mendelson, 1996, p. 1). A system was designed to educate nurses, consumers, and policy-makers about nursing's contributions in the acute care setting, focusing on monitoring the quality of nursing care. Patients come into the acute care setting primarily because they need 24/7 care, which is the focus of nursing. This early study made it clear that there was a lack of data about nursing and outcomes and nursing-sensitive indicators. Old methods of collecting data were not nursing specific. This project identified 10 "nursing-sensitive indicators" that reflected characteristics of the nursing workforce, nursing processes, or patient outcomes. Today, the NDNQI's "nursing-sensitive indicators reflect the structure, process and outcomes of nursing care. The structure of nursing care focuses on the supply of nursing staff, the skill level of the nursing staff, and the education/certification of nursing staff. *Process* indicators measure aspects of nursing care such as assessment, intervention, and RN job satisfaction. Patient *outcomes* that are determined to be nursing sensitive are those indicators that improve if there is a greater quantity or quality of nursing care (e.g., pressure ulcers, falls, IV infiltrations). Some patient outcomes are more highly related to other aspects of institutional care, such as medical decisions and institutional policies (e.g., frequency of primary C-sections, cardiac failure) and are not considered 'nursing-sensitive'" (NDNQI, 2011, website https://www.nursingquality.org/FAQPage.aspx).

After the 1994 survey, the ANA in collaboration with seven state nurses' associations conducted a pilot to determine whether it was possible to collect data on the indicators from a large number of sites. After this pilot, in 1998 the ANA established the National Database of Nursing Quality Indicators (NDNQI). More than 1500 hospitals participate in this database, providing "each nurse the opportunity to review the evidence, evaluate their practice, and determine what improvements can be made" (Montalvo & Dunton, 2007, p. 3; NDNQI, 2010). The participating hospitals submit their nursing-sensitive indicator data to the NDNQI database. The following are examples of the indicators:

▮ Patient falls/injury falls
▮ Pressure ulcers:
    ▮ Hospital-acquired
    ▮ Unit-acquired
▮ Physical/sexual assault
▮ Pain assessment/intervention/reassessment cycle
▮ Peripheral IV infiltration
▮ Physical restraints
▮ Healthcare-associated infections:
    ▮ Catheter-associated UTI
    ▮ Central-line-associated bloodstream infection
    ▮ Ventilator-associated pneumonia
▮ Staff mix:
    ▮ Registered nurses (RNs)
    ▮ Licensed practical/vocational nurses (LPN/LVNs)
    ▮ Unlicensed assistive personnel (UAPs)
▮ Nursing care hours provided per patient day
▮ Nurse turnover:
    ▮ Total
    ▮ Adapted National Quality Forum (NQF) voluntary
    ▮ Magnet controllable
▮ RN education/certification
▮ RN survey:
    ▮ Practice Environment Scales option
    ▮ Job Satisfaction Scales option
    ▮ Job Satisfaction Scales–Short Form option

The data are now available for research and analysis of nursing-specific quality care issues. Participation in the NDNQI meets the Centers for Medicare and Medicaid

Services (CMS) requirement for a hospital to participate in a systematic clinical database registry for nursing-sensitive care. Some states require this monitoring, though it is not yet required nationally.

In nursing programs, students learn how to provide safe care through didactic content, simulation and laboratory experiences, and clinical/practicum experiences. It is very important that as this learning occurs, students associate care with the need to protect the patient and provide quality care. How might this information about the NDNQI be used with students? What do we need to discuss with students to help them recognize the important role nurses may assume in the QI process?

1. What are the indicators?
2. How are data collected and from whom?
3. What are the characteristics of the nursing-sensitive indicators, nursing workforce, nursing processes, and patient outcomes?
4. What is the value of the data for practice and improvement?
5. How does NDNQI relate to quality improvement in the IOM *Quality Chasm* series?
6. How does NDNQI relate to the new CMS ruling on hospital-acquired complications (HACs)?
7. How does NDNQI relate to the IOM healthcare professions core competencies?

If local hospitals are participating in NDNQI, faculty should ask the staff involved to speak to students about the database and the process. How has use of the NDNQI affected care? This program provides a real-life example of the role of nurses in QI. Students can go to the NDNQI website at http://www.nursingquality.org/ and explore the FAQs. There is an online course on pressure ulcers. Students can also visit the ANA website on NDNQI for additional information: http://www.nursingworld.org/ MainMenuCategories/ThePracticeofProfessionalNursing/PatientSafetyQuality/Research-Measurement/The-National-Database.aspx and at https://www.nursingquality.org/ FAQPage.aspx

An example of a response to the need to prepare all healthcare professionals at all levels in QI is the1998 Veterans Health Administration (VA) initiative that created the VA Quality Scholars Fellowship. This program focuses on improving health care through scholarship (VAQS, 2012). The two-year fellowship was completed after a medical residency. The fellows' work called for collaboration with leadership administrative leaders such as the medical center director, quality management officer, and academic leadership in a medical school. The program emphasized public health and public, business, or health administration (VAQS, 2012). These areas are congruent with the national movement to improve health outcomes by examining patient safety and implementing quality improvement. A key element of this fellowship is provision of a senior academic mentor to guide the fellow toward a career in health services or quality improvement research or practice (VAQS, 2012). The program has expanded in recent years to include nursing leadership, and now incorporates the QSEN (Quality, Safety, Education for Nurses) competencies (QSEN, 2012). Now, senior nurse mentors work with the senior medical school mentors and incorporate interprofessional work. The number of VA fellowship centers is expanding.

Have We Improved Health Care?

One has to ask whether health care in the United States has improved since publication of the first edition of this book in 2007 or even since publication of the first IOM *Quality Chasm* report in 1999. "We all know what we want our healthcare system to deliver: the right care for every patient every time. As the Institute of Medicine has defined it, high-quality care is care that is safe, effective, efficient, patient-centered, timely, and equitable. And with continuing medical progress, the potential for care that is even better in all of these dimensions is increasingly possible. Increasingly, we are finding that high quality means care that is personalized, prevention-oriented, and patient-centered, based on evidence about the benefits and costs for each particular patient. This is the direction of twenty-first century biomedical science, science that is marked by new approaches in the lab like genomics, or nanotechnology, or next-generation information technology and more personalized medicine. These new sciences are only just beginning to have an impact on patient care, but they hold tremendous potential. We also know that there are large gaps, even a chasm, between our goal of high-quality care for every patient every time and what our healthcare system delivers. We have the potential for the best health care in the world—and in so many ways we achieve it, every day, thanks to the talent and commitment and hard work of health professionals, and researchers and product developers, and so many people who work every day to improve the health of Americans. But too often and in too many ways, these dedicated people—who amount to the world's greatest asset for improving public health—are frustrated in their efforts to achieve the goal of closing the gap" (CMS, 2007).

Given the extensive initiative to examine healthcare quality and availability of recommendations for change, where are we today? In April 2008 the IOM announced a two-day public meeting titled "Engineering a Learning Healthcare System: A Look at the Future" (IOM, 2008a). Several issues motivated the IOM to conduct this public forum eight years after the publication of *To Err Is Human* (IOM, 1999):

- Health care is substantially underperforming on most dimensions: effectiveness, appropriateness, safety, cost, efficiency, and value.
- Increasing complexity in health care is likely to intensify current problems unless reform efforts go far beyond financing, to foster significant changes in the culture, practice, and delivery of health care.
- Extensive administrative and clinical data collected in healthcare settings are substantially unused, although these data could provide new insights on the effectiveness of healthcare interventions and systems of care.
- If the effectiveness of health care is to keep pace with the opportunities offered by diagnostic and treatment innovation, system design and information technology

must be structured to assure application of the best evidence, continuous learning, and research insights as a natural byproduct of the care process.

▍ In effect, the nation needs to engineer the development of a learning healthcare system—one structured to keep the patient constantly in focus, while continually improving quality, safety, knowledge, and value in health care.

▍ Striking transformations have occurred through systems and process engineering in service and manufacturing sectors (for example, banking, airline safety, and automobile manufacturing).

▍ Despite the obvious differences that exist in the dynamics of mechanical versus biological and social systems, the current challenges in health care compel an entirely fresh view of the organization, structure, and function of the delivery and monitoring processes in health care.

▍ Meeting the challenges in health care offers the engineering sciences an opportunity to test, learn, and refine approaches to understanding and improving innovation in complex adaptive systems.

Looking at this list of topics, one can clearly identify the key IOM issues: patient-centered care; effective, efficient, timely care; quality improvement and the need for evidence; informatics; diversity and disparity; and more. The first quality report was published in 1999; there were still major problems in 2008, and they continue today. We have much more work to do.

Other data indicate that the United States continues to have major quality care problems. Fineberg, who is the president of the IOM, stated that "a successful health system has three attributes: healthy people, meaning a population that attains the highest level of health possible; superior care, meaning care that is effective, safe, timely, patient-centered, equitable, and efficient; and fairness, meaning that treatment is applied without discrimination or disparities to all individuals and families, regardless of age, group identity, or place, and that the system is fair to the health professions, institutions, and businesses supporting and delivering care" (2012, p. 1020). Dr. Fineberg notes the following as indicators of the status of healthcare delivery system and individuals' health in the United States:

▍ In 2009, 26 countries had a longer life expectancy than the United States (OECD, 2011).

▍ In 2010, when countries were assessed for quality, access, efficiency, and equity, the United States was ranked last (Davis, Schoen, & Stremikis, 2010).

▍ The United States ranks highest in health expenditure (OECD Health Data, 2011).

Summary

The major IOM reports from the Quality Healthcare Initiative (*Quality Chasm* series) provide important data and recommendations that will help to improve healthcare

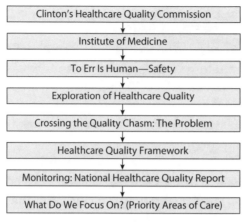

FIGURE 1-1 Development of the *Quality Chasm* Series

quality and safety nationally, if applied. The reports begin with a critical examination of healthcare safety and quality, and proceed to:

1. Develop frameworks and terminology for data analysis, action plans, and reporting mechanisms.
2. Define the role of leadership, particularly the role of government.
3. Explore critical issues related to public health and diversity.
4. Specify the priorities of quality improvement initiatives.
5. Analyze the nursing workplace.
6. Examine health professions education and identify core competencies for all health professions.

Though published separately, the IOM reports do not stand alone; rather, each expands on previous reports in the quality care series. Terminology is consistent from one report to another. This interconnectedness makes it important to understand the general information in each report, how the reports relate, and the recommendations and their implications for nursing and health care. Figure 1-1 describes the development of the *Quality Chasm* series.

Part 2

Implications of Healthcare Reform

The Obama Administration and Healthcare Reform

Not too long after the election of Barack Obama as president in 2008 and the beginning of his administration in 2009, one heard the term "perfect storm" applied to the next phase of U.S. health care. However, this phrase implies a perspective that could have serious negative consequences, not the strong confluence of factors that could contribute to major improvements in the nation's healthcare system. This confluence presents an opportunity for significant and comprehensive reform that has not been available for many years. Accordingly, in 2009 there was an intense nationwide expectation of change that closely matched the need for such change. The Obama administration's initial response was to identify key healthcare principles that would guide its healthcare reform decision-making (http://www.healthcare.gov/):

- Protect families' financial health
- Make health coverage affordable
- Aim for universality
- Provide portability of coverage
- Guarantee choice
- Improve patient safety and quality of care
- Maintain long-term fiscal sustainability

We are no doubt in a healthcare crisis, one that has been going on for some time. Enthoven (2008) comments that "health care drained the federal budget of more than $1 trillion this year. . . . If present trends continue, in ten years the number will almost double" (p. WK9). He goes on to make clear that the only way to avert this increase in cost is to change the way health care is organized. We have been in this place for some time; that is, unable to make the changes in health care that we need. Today, we have even greater evidence of the need for change:

- The IOM *Quality Chasm* series describes a dysfunctional, fragmented healthcare system that is not yielding positive outcomes, either in cost or in quality.
- A growing number of citizens do not have healthcare coverage, and others have inadequate coverage.
- An increasing number of people must deal with chronic illnesses and the complexity of care attendant to those conditions.
- We have a growing shortage of healthcare providers—nurses and others.
- We have an aging population that will require more healthcare services.
- The cost of care is still rising rapidly—for the government, for employers, and for individuals.
- We have serious disparities in healthcare delivery and outcomes.
- We need to expand health promotion and prevention across all populations.
- We have the ability to provide high-quality care, given the advances in pharmaceuticals, technology, and other capabilities, and yet too often we fail to do so. In some cases these opportunities have increased the cost of care.

President Obama's move for healthcare reform was hardly the first on this topic. Senator Daschle provides an overview of the very long history of attempts and failures to reform health care—going back to the development of healthcare reimbursement in the early 20th century to later increased federal government roles through Medicare and Medicaid (Daschle, Lambrew, & Greenberger, 2008). His description is useful in assisting us to better understand healthcare issues. As Daschle notes, we have not been successful: "Our system is fundamentally broken, and decades of failed incremental measures have proven that we need a comprehensive approach to fix it" (Daschle, Lambrew, & Greenberger, 2008, p. xiv). He even describes the efforts as the "tortuous history of health reform" (p. 45). Why have we not succeeded in improving the system? Daschle believes the traditional legislative process cannot deliver the changes we need: It has failed many times to do so even when the broad framework of a plan is acceptable, which is described as "a public-private hybrid that preserves our private system within a strengthened public framework" (Daschle, Lambrew, & Greenberger, 2008, p. 107).

The IOM Report on the Department of Health and Human Services

As was mentioned, a number of issues and initiatives have come together at the same time. One of these is a report published by the IOM, *HHS in the 21st Century: Charting a New Course for a Healthier America* (2009b). As is true for some of the other IOM reports, this particular IOM report was initiated in response to a congressional request, in this case the Congressional Committee on Oversight and Government Reform (Chairman Henry Waxman), on June 20, 2007. The letter requesting the IOM to undertake this task identifies several key questions (IOM, 2009b, p. 162):

- What are the missions of the Department of Health and Human Services (HHS) and its individual agencies, and how do these missions relate to the challenges confronting us?
- How effectively are the agencies organized to achieve their mission?
- Could the missions of individual HHS agencies be consolidated or realigned to make them more effective?
- What recommendations would the IOM make to the Congress and HHS to improve the focus of individual agencies, enhance their accountability, and improve their efficiency?
- What recommendations would the IOM make to more effectively integrate promotion of public health and control of healthcare costs across the department?

The IOM committee did not recommend major reorganization of HHS, but rather used an approach that would transform the department. The recommendations focused on five key areas.

1. Define a 21st-century vision.
2. Foster adaptability and alignment.
3. Increase effectiveness and efficiency of the U.S. healthcare system.
4. Strengthen the HHS and U.S. public health and health care workforces.
5. Improve accountability and decision-making.

Why should nurses care about a report that examines the HHS? First, it is important to recognize that the HHS is the largest federal government agency, based on budget. It has an impact on every American. Its activities are extremely broad and conducted through the work of its multiple agencies, which is also one of its problems. Through this department flow decisions related to health and human services resources (Health Resources and Services Administration), healthcare education, funding for research (grants, the National Institutes of Health), healthcare quality (Agency for Healthcare Research and Quality), the Food and Drug Administration (FDA), the Indian Health Service (IHS), the Substance Abuse and Mental Health Services Administration (SAMHSA), the Centers for Disease Control and Prevention (CDC), and the highly important Centers for Medicare and Medicaid Services (CMS). Just reviewing these agencies within the department indicates the impact HHS has on the entire nation. Nursing is involved in all of these areas—affecting our education, practice, and research. We also need to be more involved in the changes in the HHS department and in healthcare reform.

The scope of the HHS responsibilities and its challenges is very large and significant. The report recommendations are connected to previous IOM reports in the

Quality Chasm series: quality, evidence-based practice, patient-centered care, healthcare informatics; workforce issues; the need for more research; the integrative public health agenda; diversity and disparity; aging population; increase in chronic illness; the need for health promotion and prevention; and more. The HHS needs to reframe itself and to do so in light of the current and future needs that have become clearer since 1999 with the publication of *To Err Is Human*.

The current strategic plan for HHS is for 2010–2015. The plan is available on the HHS website (http://www.hhs.gov), where it is updated periodically. The goals are:

1. Transform health care
2. Advance scientific knowledge and innovation
3. Advance health, safety, and well-being of the American people
4. Increase efficiency, transparency, and accountability of HHS
5. Strengthen the nation's health and human services infrastructure and workforce

The HHS is also charged with implementing parts of the American Recovery and Reinvestment Act of 2009 (ARRA) related to healthcare costs, payments, and health information technology, as well as awarding funding to meet the law's requirements, measure program performance and ensure program integrity, and inform the public of results. Many aspects of the legislation will be implemented over time.

Healthcare Legislation 2010

In 2010, the Patient Protection and Affordable Care Act (Pub. L. No. 11-148) and the Health Care and Education Reconciliation Act (Pub. L. No. 111-152) were passed, initiating the current movement in healthcare reform. In June 2012, the U. S. Supreme Court upheld the constitutionality of most of their provisions. When one reads these laws, it is easy to see the influence of the IOM reports on health care. Nurses need to know about the new provisions and their implications for nursing. The laws support nursing in many ways, such as funding for workforce development, nurse-managed clinics, home care, quality improvement strategies, community-based collaboration, better quality, accessible mental health care, wellness and preventive services, health promotion, primary care, and more. Students typically think of healthcare reform as only health insurance law focusing on reimbursement and access to insurance. This is far too limited a view: nurses need to understand the all aspects of these laws and recognize their relevance to practice. HHS has established a website (http://www.healthcare.gov/) to provide both information about the law and current information about the implementation of healthcare reform.

Part 3

Connecting the IOM Reports to Nursing Standards

Introduction

Nursing as a profession has its standards and its code of ethics. Both are important topics in nursing curricula, mostly in undergraduate programs, though they should also be incorporated into graduate course content. There is a relationship between what the IOM has been doing in its efforts to improve care and the nursing standards and the code of ethics. The following provides an overview of this relationship, in an effort to assist faculty in connecting these important professional statements in the discussion about the need to improve the healthcare system and how this improvement might be done. As will be noted in more detail in later parts of this book, the IOM strongly supports the integration of its five healthcare professions core competencies in all healthcare professions education. Standards are a part of QI, and this includes professional standards.

Nursing's Social Policy Statement: The Essence of the Profession (ANA, 2010)

The social policy statement of the American Nurses Association (ANA) recognizes that nursing has an obligation to the public or the community (ANA, 2010b). These social concerns influence how we practice and our authority to practice.

Social Concerns in Health Care and Nursing: Relevance to IOM Reports

The following lists the social concerns that the profession must be cognizant of, and for which nursing professionals must provide leadership. These areas are identified with their related IOM core competency (ANA, 2010b, pp. 4–5):

- Organization, delivery, and financing of quality health care (relates to IOM core competencies on quality improvement, informatics, evidence-based practice)
- Provision for the public's health (relates to IOM core competencies on patient-centered care, teamwork)
- Expansion of nursing and healthcare knowledge and appropriate application of technology (relates to IOM core competencies on evidence-based practice, informatics)
- Expansion of healthcare resources and health policy (relates to IOM core competency on quality improvement)
- Definitive planning for healthcare policy and regulation (relates to IOM core competencies on patient-centered care, quality improvement, teamwork)
- Duties under extreme conditions (relates to IOM core competency on patient-centered care)

We as nurses have a social responsibility and a social contract with our patients, whether they be individuals, families, or communities. This contract implies two partners. Patient-centered care is central, though this term is not used in the ANA social policy statement. The other core competencies (quality improvement, interprofessional teams, informatics, and evidence-based practice) are all interwoven into the social context in which the practice takes place, and are required for professional nursing to be effective.

Professional collaboration is discussed in the social policy statement, describing collaboration as "true partnership, valuing expertise, power, and respect on all sides and recognizing and accepting separate and combined spheres of activity and responsibility. Collaboration includes mutual safeguarding of the legitimate interests of each party and commonality of goals that is recognized by all parties" (ANA, 2010b, p.7). Faculty need to do more to prepare students for this type of collaboration, and faculty also need to model this type of collaboration. We must emphasize the positive in other healthcare professions: Rather than telling our negative stories of how we are victims, we need to tell stories of effective collaboration and how to make it better. Our social contract says we must do this as a profession.

Scope and Standards of Practice (ANA, 2010)

The professional standards (ANA, 2010c) go hand-in-hand with the social policy statement (ANA, 2010b).

Definition of Nursing's Relationship to Patient-Centered Care

The definition of nursing can be connected to the IOM quality initiative. "Nursing is the protection, promotion, and optimization of health and abilities, prevention of illness and injury, alleviation of suffering through the diagnosis and treatment of human response, and advocacy in the care of individuals, families, communities, and populations" (ANA 2010b, p. 3). To meet this definition, nurses must be competent. *Competency* is "an expected level of performance that integrates knowledge, skills, abilities, and judgment" (ANA, 2010c, p. 12). The IOM core competencies are designed for all healthcare professions, including nursing. The competencies are the basic starting point and do not negate the need for individual professional competencies. As we develop our curricula and courses, then, we must ensure that these competencies are included. To meet nursing profession standards, we must require these competencies.

Tenets of Nursing Practice Relationship to the IOM Five Healthcare Professions Core Competencies

The standards are based on tenets characteristic of nursing practice (ANA, 2010c, p. 4):

1. Nursing practice is individualized *(relates to IOM core competencies of patient-centered care, evidence-based practice, quality improvement)*.
2. Nurses coordinate care by establishing partnerships *(relates to IOM core competencies of patient-centered care, interprofessional teamwork, informatics, quality improvement)*.
3. Caring is central to the practice of the registered nurse *(relates IOM core competency of patient-centered care)*.
4. Registered nurses use the nursing process to plan and provide individualized care to their healthcare consumers *(relates to IOM core competencies of patient-centered care, interprofessional teamwork)*.
5. A strong link exists between the professional work environment and the registered nurse's ability to provide quality health care and achieve optimal outcomes *(relates to IOM core competencies of quality improvement, informatics)*.

In its Model of Professional Nursing Practice Regulation (ANA, 2010c), the ANA integrates key elements that are also found in the IOM quality series of reports and recommendations. We need quality care that is safe for both the patient and the employee, as workplace environment and safety are also critical concerns, and care should be based on the best evidence possible. Figure 3-1 illustrates this model.

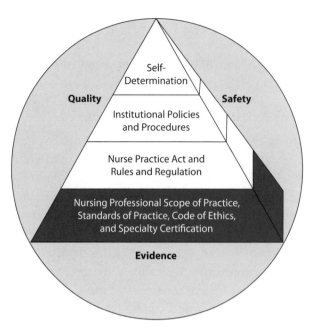

FIGURE 3-1 The ANA Model of Professional Nursing Practice Regulation

Scope and Standards of Nursing Practice (ANA, 2010)

The nursing professional standards (ANA, 2010c) are critical content for all nursing students and are best incorporated in every course to remind students of the standards and how they can be applied. One can even ask students, as they plan patient care, not only to consider the five core competencies but also to identify how each of the standards applies to the patient; alternatively, after faculty identify the standard focus for the day, the student can then be asked to review that standard and describe how it applies. This is the only way students will begin to see relevance in the standards. Just having students read the standards is not enough, though it is still important. The words have to come alive and take on real-life meaning to students.

Students also need to understand the two categories of standards. The Standards of Nursing Practice "describe the competent level of nursing care as demonstrated by the critical thinking model known as the nursing process" (ANA, 2010c, p. 9). These standards are (ANA, 2010c, pp. 9–10).

- *Standard 1.* Assessment
- *Standard 2.* Diagnosis
- *Standard 3.* Outcomes Identification
- *Standard 4.* Planning
- *Standard 5.* Implementation (5A—Coordination of Care; 5B—Health Teaching and Health Promotion; 5C—Consultation; 5D—Prescriptive Authority and Treatment [5D applies only to advanced practice registered nurses])
- *Standard 6.* Evaluation

The second category of standards are the Standards of Professional Performance, which describe "a competent level of behavior in the professional role, including activities related to ethics, education, evidence-based practice and research, quality of practice, communication, leadership, collaboration, professional practice evaluation, resource utilization, and environmental health" (ANA, 2010c, p. 10). All of these issues are related to the IOM work on quality improvement.

Guide to the Code of Ethics for Nurses: Interpretation and Application (ANA, 2010)

Guide to the Code of Ethics for Nurses (ANA, 2010a) is the third of the critical nursing publications from the ANA that form a framework for the practice of nursing. The social policy statement and the standards require an ethical professional approach to health care. The code, which is "the profession's public expression of those values, duties, and commitments" (ANA, 2010a, p. xiii), includes nine provisions. Related IOM competencies are identified for each provision:

- *Provision 1*: The nurse, in all professional relationships, practices with compassion and respect for the inherent dignity, worth, and uniqueness of every individual, unrestricted by considerations of social or economic status, personal attributes, or the nature of health problems *(relates to IOM core competency of patient-centered care, which includes diversity concerns)*.
- *Provision 2*: The nurse's primary commitment is to the patient, whether an individual, family, group, or community *(relates to IOM core competency of patient-centered care)*.
- *Provision 3*: The nurse promotes, advocates for, and strives to protect the health, safety, and rights of patients *(relates to IOM core competencies of patient-centered care, quality improvement)*.
- *Provision 4*: The nurse is responsible and accountable for individual nursing practice and determines the appropriate delegation of tasks consistent with the nurse's obligation to provide optimum patient care *(relates to IOM core competencies of patient-centered care, interprofessional teamwork)*.
- *Provision 5*: The nurse owes the same duties to self as to others, including the responsibility to preserve integrity and safety, to maintain competence, and to continue personal and professional growth *(relates to IOM core competency of quality improvement)*.
- *Provision 6*: The nurse participates in establishing, maintaining, and improving healthcare environments and conditions of employment conducive to the provision of quality health care and consistent with the values of the profession through individual and collective action *(relates to IOM core competencies of quality improvement, interprofessional teamwork, evidence-based practice, use of informatics)*.

- *Provision 7*: The nurse participates in the advancement of the profession through contributions to practice, education, administration, and knowledge development *(relates to IOM core competencies of quality improvement, evidence-based practice/ evidence-based management)*.
- *Provision 8*: The nurse collaborates with other health professionals and the public in promoting community, national, and international efforts to meet health needs *(relates to IOM core competencies of patient-centered care, interprofessional teamwork)*.
- *Provision 9*: The profession of nursing, as represented by associations and their members, is responsible for articulating nursing values, for maintaining the integrity of the profession and its practice, and for shaping social policy *(relates to IOM core competency of quality improvement)*.

Trossman (2011) discusses the role of the nurse ethicist, something students should know about. The nurse ethicist teaches about ethics, provides formal ethics consults, and discusses ethical concerns with nurses informally. Every nurse makes ethical decisions every day, even if it is just to decide who gets care first. This does not mean that there is always an ethical conflict in these decisions. Faculty need to discuss with students how to integrate the code of ethics into daily practice.

Combining the social policy statement, the standards of practice, and the code of ethics with the IOM's in-depth work on the healthcare system, quality improvement, and the core competencies required for improvement provides the student with a strong framework within which to develop as a professional. As noted in the *Future of Nursing*, "By virtue of its numbers and adaptive capacity, the nursing profession has the potential to effect wide-ranging changes in the health care system. Nurses' regular, close proximity to patients and scientific understanding of care processes across the continuum of care give them a unique ability to act as partners with other health professionals and to lead in the improvement and redesign of the health care system and its many practice environments, including hospitals, schools, homes, retail health clinics, long-term care facilities, battlefields, and community and public health centers. Nurses thus are poised to help bridge the gap between coverage and access, to coordinate increasingly complex care for a wide range of patients, to fulfill their potential as primary care providers to the full extent of their education and training, and to enable the full economic value of their contributions across practice settings to be realized. In addition, a promising field of evidence links nursing care to high quality care of patients, including protecting their safety" (IOM, 2011d, p. S-3).

Part 4

Nursing Education and the IOM Reports:

Critical Issues and the Implications for the Curriculum

Introduction

Clearly there is momentum in healthcare organizations (HCOs) and in government to improve health care in the United States. It is not enough to reform just healthcare systems; we need safety and quality strategies to resolve problems in clinical settings and strategies for government and local communities. The IOM report on health professions education identifies the core competences for health professions, which are based on the *Quality Chasm* series. A barrier between practice and education may undermine care, jeopardize care quality, and leave nursing trailing other health professions that do recognize the importance of all the IOM reports and the core competencies and use them to guide decisions about curriculum and clinical learning experiences. New graduates entering the job market who are not prepared for the new quality improvement (QI) environment require additional—and costly—orientation and training and will not be able to meet the call in *The Future of Nursing report* (IOM, 2011d) to provide leadership in the drive to improve care. New graduates may experience frustration at being left behind by their peers, and this increases attrition and affects productivity and quality of care.

Students need to understand and apply the content and recommendations from the IOM reports. This means that faculty must be familiar with the content and incorporate it into curricula, simulation, and clinical nursing experiences. Consider the following questions and their impact on nursing education, curricula, and clinical application:

- What is the safety problem?
- What types of errors occur?
- What methods are used to analyze errors to prevent further errors?
- How does a nurse affect patient safety?
- Does the educational environment support a blame-free culture when students make errors?
- What are HCOs, government, insurers, and professional organizations doing to improve care? Is it working?
- What is quality care?
- How is quality care assessed? What is the status? What needs improvement?
- What are the six improvement aims, and how do they apply to nursing practice?
- Do students recognize the importance of self-evaluation, near misses, and surveillance in their practice?
- What are some of the new methods used to improve care, such as use of Plan-Do-Study-Act (PDSA), rapid response teams, coping with workarounds, improving handoffs, and other issues and methods?
- How does a nurse affect quality care?
- What is the framework for the National Healthcare Quality Report? Where can a nurse access the annual report? Why are the report and its data important?
- How might quality data be used in nursing research to improve nursing curricula and clinical experiences?

- What role does leadership play in improving care? How does this relate to nursing as a profession and to an individual nurse? How do we prepare students to be leaders?
- What are the critical issues in the report on workplace environment and nursing care? How might this information be used to improve nursing care? What are the implications for nursing education?
- What has the nursing profession, such as the American Nurses Association (ANA) and nursing specialty organizations, done to improve care?
- Are students able to meet the core health professions education competencies (patient-centered care, interprofessional teams, evidence-based practice, quality improvement, and informatics)? How do we prepare them to do so?
- What changes have been made to increase interprofessional educational experiences?
- What is the concern about diversity in health care? How might this be changed?
- What impact do diversity and disparities have on a nurse and practice?
- What is the impact of disparity on healthcare delivery?
- What are the priority areas of care? How might they be incorporated into curricula? How are they used in assessing and improving care?
- What are the major issues related to public health? Why is this important? How does *Healthy People 2020* (www.healthypeople.gov) serve as a critical resource?
- What is the role of evidence-based practice (EBP)? How can we continually improve and expand nursing research?
- Why is understanding of the change process important?
- How much content and experience related to informatics and medical technology are included in curricula?
- How can we increase teamwork and team experiences?

These are only a few of the questions we should be asking. This part of the book looks at some of the general issues of concern in nursing education in relationship to the IOM reports, and Part 5 expands the discussion to specific implications for the nursing curriculum.

Where Is Nursing Education in Relation to the IOM Reports?

The IOM report *To Err Is Human* concluded that healthcare professions education is in need of major change: "Clinical education simply has not kept pace with or been responsive enough to shifting patient demographics and desires, changing health system expectations, evolving practice requirements and staffing arrangements, new information, a focus on improving quality, or new technologies" (IOM, 1999, p. 1). The report recommended a shift to competency-based education, which is not new to nursing even though not every nursing education program is competency based today. We need to make learning outcomes explicit, to provide learning opportunities so that students can meet competencies, and use standard assessments to determine competencies. This perspective is expanded in the later IOM report on healthcare professions education (IOM, 2003b), which identifies the five healthcare professions core competencies.

Improvement in health care goes hand-in-hand with improved health professions education (IOM, 2003b). The IOM reports indicate that much has to be done; however, the reports will not mean anything to nursing education unless the recommendations and findings are integrated into educational systems. There is a "quality chasm" between the "ivory tower" of healthcare education and the healthcare system. The later IOM reports clearly show that the gaps in education are still present several years after the first reports were published. The passage from *To Err Is Human* cited earlier is repeated in subsequent IOM reports: "Education for health professions is in need of a major overhaul. Clinical education simply has not kept pace . . ." (IOM, 1999, cited in IOM, 2003b, p. 1).

When Porter-O'Grady addressed an American Academy of Nursing (AAN) leadership conference in November 2004, he stated, "We are never going to combat the nursing shortage with increasing numbers because we have the wrong people doing the wrong things" (Porter-O'Grady, 2005). Likewise, nursing faculty may be teaching the wrong things and emphasizing the wrong skills. This is a challenge for all schools of nursing; they must critically examine what is taught and how it contributes to the education of safe practitioners. Many questions remain unanswered.

Is it still necessary to teach a foundation course to ease students into their clinical skills or to teach health assessment as a separate nursing course? Similar courses are also taught in allied health, medical school, and other health-related disciplines. Health and physical assessment could be taught across disciplines if health professions faculty and administrators would stop arguing about head counts and who gets the tuition dollar and instead work out a business model that dispenses with these antiquated rules. This content could be modularized and taught mostly in a virtual mode with simulation lab sessions. If competency-based evaluation is the objective, once the skill is mastered the student moves on.

Today, many textbook publishers, who have the financial resources to develop sophisticated graphics, audios, and simulations that can be used for content such as health assessment and pharmacology, offer many excellent online materials. Why should nursing education reinvent or try to develop new material? Why not collaborate with other health professions educators, businesses, and publishers? With this material, skills could then be reinforced in the simulation lab and clinical settings. What should be emphasized in either classroom or clinical settings? Critical thinking and clinical reasoning and judgment, rationales behind decisions, and evidence-based practice should get more emphasis. How more content can be added to the curriculum is a legitimate question. Much more must be done to integrate content and use new teaching-learning strategies. It is far more instructive to ask other questions:

▌ Why do faculty feel as if they must try to teach everything?
▌ What is covered? What is repeated and why?

- Have we been routinely updating content?
- What really has to be covered? (nice-to-know versus need-to-know)
- Are schools driven by what individual faculty members want to present rather than what is really required to practice?
- When are we going overboard and losing focus?
- When should faculty expect students to master the content and then work with students to apply that knowledge (critical thinking and clinical reasoning and judgment, EBP, and so on)?
- How can clinical rotations be enhanced so that they optimize learning experiences?

Many faculty complain that not enough time is devoted to clinical experiences without first considering when faculty last evaluated how clinical time was actually used. Faculty should be willing to step back from the way things have always been done and consider new approaches to clinical experiences. It may be more effective to use clinical facilities for several intensive weeks rather than to intersperse clinical with classroom experiences. This may offer students a better chance to see the results of their care planning and continuity of care and to gain the competencies that make them feel more confident. "Visiting" clinical settings has not proven helpful. Students need to spend extended time there to better understand the work environment, professionalism, the complexities of patient care, and the trajectory of illness and healthcare services to understand care outcomes. It is difficult to cultivate more team experiences in only a few hours—often just two days a week that are not even full days.

McBride (2005) suggests that to achieve our goal, nursing education must recognize that health care's paradigm has shifted; the IOM reports show that informatics must be at the core of healthcare systems. She goes on to say, "The emphasis on the nursing process and the nurse–patient relationship may have inadvertently made us less prepared for today's emphasis on outcomes and the obligation we have to transform our work settings into learning organizations. We need to examine our pride in relationship and the need for greater focus on the work setting as a learning organization; from *do no harm* as an individual responsibility to safety as a system concern; from caregiving that is time- and place-bound to caregiving with time and place limitations removed; from focus of care that emphasizes patient compliance to focus on care that emphasizes best practices; from workarounds being the norm to crucial conversations being the norm; from decision-making based on training and experience to evidence-based decision-making; from organizations that encourage professional silos to organizations that encourage interprofessional collaboration; from seeking cost reductions to continuously decreasing waste; from emphasis on discharge planning to emphasis on lifestyle change" (p. 22).

These are some of the more general nursing education issues related to quality, many of which are discussed in more detail in Part 5. It is critical for nursing faculty to respond effectively to these IOM reports and consult with their counterparts in practice to arrive at measures that will improve care through more effective teaching and learning. This material could be added to the admittedly bulging curriculum in the same way that American Association of Colleges of Nursing (AACN) essentials are incorporated. Once educators agree that this is essential content and it appears in our licensure exams, it will be integrated; however, there are different methods for including this content and experience. This also calls for a careful examination of what is currently being taught, with consideration of how the curriculum can fit into a quality framework. For example, a course called Health II that includes content on immune disorders could include cancer as an example of a failure of the immune system. The genetic aspects would be taught with additional coverage of the quality indicators and EBP that are most appropriate for one or two sample cases. Faculty and students could work through the cases using computerized physician order entry (CPOE) and the electronic medical record (EMR) process. This could be done with computer screen shots in the classroom to demonstrate how errors might occur, or to show how override systems stop certain drugs from being ordered beyond normal limits or to prevent a potential interaction with another drug. This case experience would emphasize technology integration, informatics, quality, care needs, and the uniform language of the discipline all in one learning experience. This is not really adding content; it is merely presenting it so that students acquire not only information about a problem but also insight into how that information is applied. Much more teaching could be centered on case-based, problem-based learning. One need not teach about every disease, though frequently efforts are made to do this. If several diseases are used as examples, it will allow more time to include other content such as cultural values and beliefs. For example, discuss diet alterations necessary in cancer treatment with an understanding of Muslim dietary beliefs (patient-centered care), the effects of age and living conditions on health promotion for the individual and family from a team approach (interprofessional care), the impact of healthcare costs and coverage or reimbursement of services, and safety and QI, presenting evidence to support the plan (EBP). This moves the lecture from a laundry list to an application of knowledge, provides students with an up-to-date framework for learning that can then be applied to other diseases, and incorporates critical new concepts into the curriculum.

Critical New Education Reports

Like the IOM, nursing education recognizes the need for competency-based education and is moving in this direction. The IOM core competencies are not unknown to nursing education either, although we need to do much more to incorporate them. This section offers some examples of how nursing is responding to issues raised by the IOM reports.

The Essentials of Baccalaureate Nursing Education (2008)

The American Association of Colleges of Nursing published a new version of *The Essentials of Baccalaureate Education for Professional Nursing Practice* in 2008. The first paragraph highlights the five IOM healthcare professions core competencies. The text presents background information about nursing education, the discipline of nursing, assumptions, baccalaureate generalist nurse roles, preparation, and the components of *Essentials* (AACN, 2008c):

I. Liberal Education for Baccalaureate Generalist Nursing Practice
II. Basic Organizational and Systems Leadership for Quality Care and Patient Safety
III. Scholarship for Evidence-Based Practice
IV. Information Management and Application of Patient Care Technology
V. Healthcare Policy, Finance, and Regulatory Environments
VI. Interprofessional Communication and Collaboration for Improving Patient Health Outcomes
VII. Clinical Prevention and Population Health
VIII. Professionalism and Professional Values
IX. Baccalaureate Generalist Nursing Practice

It is clear from the baccalaureate *Essentials* that the IOM content, recommendations, and terminology are prevalent in this updated version, which sets the standard for Bachelor of Science in Nursing (BSN) programs across the United States.

A New Agenda for Higher Education: Shaping the Mind for Practice (2008)

In 2008, the Carnegie Foundation published a review of the current status of higher education in the United States and proposed changes (Sullivan & Rosen, 2008). It concludes that higher education must emphasize practical reasoning: reasoning directed toward actions and figuring out what to do as contrasted with figuring out how the facts stand. This review also stresses the need for responsible judgment (Sullivan & Rosen, 2008). This new agenda for higher education is relevant to prerequisite courses for students in BSN programs. This approach would be suitable for those prenursing students who often struggle when they come from prenursing courses into a nursing program that expects practical reasoning. The report also emphasizes the need to use cases as a teaching strategy to support more practical reasoning, thereby involving students in critical learning, blending knowledge, skill, and appropriate attitude in response to unique situations that require expert judgment. Professional practice at its best is a prime exemplar of practical reasoning.

Educating Nurses: A Call for Radical Transformation (2010)

Greater changes in nursing education may result from the national nursing education report spearheaded by Patricia Benner of the Carnegie Foundation for the Advancement of Teaching, along with Sutphen, Leonard, and Day (2010). This study was part of the Carnegie Foundation's commitment to studying how higher education contributes to building professional understanding, skills, and integrity. The comparative studies that were included in their Preparation for the Professions Program (PPP) focused on clergy, engineering, law, medicine, nursing, and teaching. This nursing study report is believed by many nursing experts, including Dr. Benner, who believe that this nursing study provides us "evidence" to support excellence in teaching-learning. According to Sullivan and Rosen

(2008), authors of the larger interprofessional report on higher education, professional schools are where professional values are defined and applied and exemplars are used to teach. The Benner et al. study is the first study since the Goldmark report (Goldmark, 1923) to examine nursing professional education in such depth. The IOM report suggests that teaching a practice discipline requires time for experiential teaching-learning.

Use of exemplars and cases is crucial. According to Benner et al. (2010), students are educated in academic silos, but practice and the emphasis on patient safety indicate the need to eliminate this "wall," to move away from the academic silo. In a presentation, Benner (2007) suggests that teaching a practice requires "situated cognition-thinking-in-action (the logic of practice); situated teaching and learning (readiness); reflection on particular cases and situations; and development of ethical comportment (in dispositions and actions, not just beliefs and decisions)." She calls for three intense apprenticeships: not the old form of using students as free labor, but in-depth immersion for the purpose of acquiring knowledge and skills while changing attitudes. The three apprenticeships may be intertwined (Benner, Sutphen, Leonard, & Day, 2010).

- The first is cognitive and theoretical and focuses on teaching "nurse think" or intellectual training. This is not the place for inordinate teaching of taxonomies and disease classifications, but rather the practical reasoning of how to apply knowledge.
- The second is skills based; it teaches clinical reasoning and judgment, which is more in-depth than critical thinking. Benner refers to this as a time of "situated learning" using strong clinical faculty. The model is one of coaching the student. Use of simulation with a level of uncertainty built in will help students achieve and integrate clinical knowledge.
- The third is focused on social roles or moral and ethical behavior. This is aimed at integrating knowledge of the underpinnings of the discipline's values, ethics, and social roles.

Benner and her co-authors give examples of ethical concerns from a student's perspective: meeting the patient as a person; preserving dignity and personhood of the patient; responding to substandard practice; advocating for patients; and engaging fully in learning to do 'good' nursing practice. Students reported that standardized tests and a compilation of skills did not really get at the heart of the knowledge and application they needed for the practice setting. The survey results revealed that there is a disconnect between most teaching and what students need to learn. Benner recommended such measures as the following:

1. Redesign the curriculum for classroom teaching to enhance the cognitive apprenticeship:
   - Teach for engagement and problem-solving.
   - Do not organize classroom teaching around catalogues and taxonomies.
   - Confine taxonomies to assigned reading and web-based instruction.

What would be the effects?

▮ More nurse educators prepared at the doctoral level in nursing and the natural sciences, social sciences, and humanities

▮ Nursing education faculty trained in the natural sciences, social sciences, and humanities co-teach courses

2. Strengthen the cognitive apprenticeship by adding natural and social sciences and humanities relevant to nursing practice:
   ▮ Background natural sciences, including chemistry, microbiology, physics, and genetics
   ▮ Social sciences and humanities relevant to nursing practice, including:
     ▮ Relational skills
     ▮ Coping with illness
     ▮ Psychosocial epidemiology
     ▮ Patient education and counseling skills
     ▮ Communication across cultures and classes
     ▮ Organizational and healthcare services research
     ▮ Healthcare policy
     ▮ Social impact on health

3. Upgrade cognitive apprenticeship and better integration with others:
   ▮ This is best accomplished in both the clinical and classroom settings.
   ▮ Resist the pressure to separate the teaching of the three apprenticeships.

What would be the effects?

▮ Faculty development for more integrative teaching

▮ Emphasis on integrative teaching in the classroom, clinical and skills lab using case studies, simulation in the classroom

▮ Use of web-based teaching by expert teachers

4. Whether in the classroom, a simulation, or the clinical, reflect on these three questions:
   ▮ How does the pedagogy in the learning setting guide the student's approach to the patient and clinical practice?
   ▮ Can the student imaginatively access and rehearse for practice situations?
   ▮ What is the student's relationship to the patient? To the teacher? To other students?

What would be the effects?

▮ All Associate Degree Nursing (ADN) programs should be required to affiliate with baccalaureate programs in nursing to create a seamless transition between the ADN program and the baccalaureate program.

■ The current science and general education prerequisites and introduction to nursing classes should be included in and limited to two years in the programs of study at the community-college level. This will mean that some ADN courses will have to be transferred to the upper-division program in the last two years of the nursing program leading to a baccalaureate degree.

The Carnegie Foundation study on nursing education identifies characteristics of teaching excellence that support the three apprenticeships (Benner, Sutphen, Leonard, & Day, 2010):

■ Have a clear vision of what kind of nurse they would like to graduate.
■ Place their students in a collaborative nursing role.
■ Ask students questions about what is at stake for the patient; what the patient is experiencing; and what the next step is for the patient.
■ Highlight what is salient about a case or a situation and what is an appropriate response.
■ Seamlessly integrate the three apprenticeships to teach how to be a nurse in terms of ethical comportment; knowledge of the humanities, sciences, and social sciences; and practice skills.
■ Engage in dialogue with students to explore their thoughts.

These are achieved through signature pedagogies:

■ *Coaching*, in which faculty draw out what the student knows in a bonded clinical situation.
■ *Simulation*, where students use cases, manikins that represent patients, or equipment common to a particular clinical situation that allows them to practice certain skills over and over. The IOM also recommends simulation to improve quality of care.
■ *Role modeling*, used in classroom, laboratory, and settings to enhance learning and allow students to view care from different perspectives.
■ *Preclinical preparation*, requiring students to come to clinicals prepared.
■ *Postclinical conference*, which provides an excellent opportunity to guide students in reflection on their practice and discuss commonalities across student clinical experiences.
■ *Articulating experiential learning*, which consists of assisting students to expand their learning from experiences.

Many of these strategies can be used with students and for staff education. Examples are discussed in Part 5. This report should be read by all nursing faculty and used in nursing education graduate courses.

The Carnegie nursing study concludes that nurses are undereducated for the demands and complexity of their practice. Nursing educators too often provide an encyclopedic introduction to the discipline that often amounts to a superficial gloss of a complex, layered practice. However, students need a deep understanding of nursing science and background knowledge of natural and social sciences and humanities. Students are often not taught in enough depth and are not taught how to use the knowledge presented in the classroom in practice. Practitioners need rich opportunities to continue to learn, develop their practice, and articulate it as both individual nurses and members of a healthcare team. Nursing has also paid too little attention to the three professional apprenticeships in continuing education. Too many healthcare organizations currently devote their continuing education primarily to teaching nurses to use new technologies and keeping them apprised of new regulations, both of which are necessary but not sufficient for nurses to reflect on and develop clinical knowledge (Benner, Sutphen, Leonard, & Day, 2010).

Graduate *Essentials* from American Association of Colleges of Nursing

The AACN *Essentials* document on master's-level education and doctoral education also includes content related to the IOM quality series of reports (2011; 2006). The master's-level *Essentials* (2011) focuses on:

I. Background for Practice from Sciences and Humanities
II. Organizational and Systems Leadership
III. Quality Improvement and Safety
IV. Translating and Integrating Scholarship into Practice
V. Informatics and Healthcare Technologies
VI. Health Policy and Advocacy
VII. Interprofessional Collaboration for Improving Patient and Population Health Outcomes
VIII. Clinical Prevention and Population Health for Improving Health
IX. Master's-Level Nursing Practice

IOM focus terms, such as *quality improvement, informatics, interprofessional, and evidence-based practice,* are clearly noted in *Essentials*, and they are also included in the *Essentials* version for doctor of nursing practice (2006).

The key issue is that the IOM work on quality in health care and the core competencies must be considered for all types of nursing degrees. Does the curriculum include the needed content, and are the teaching-learning strategies effective in engaging the student in the learning process so that competencies are attained? With the increased emphasis on the need for more nursing leadership in *The Future of Nursing* report, all graduate programs should review their inclusion of this critical content and need for related learning opportunities for students in all nursing programs.

General Nursing Education Issues and Changes

The Faculty Shortage: Some Possible Solutions

We need more faculty with PhDs, but we are unlikely to reach the number we say we need even with the mandate in *The Future of Nursing* report (IOM, 2011d). Just as with the shortage in practice, if we fixate on the numbers we will regret it in the long term. Most likely, for some time we will always have a mix of PhD faculty and faculty with master's degrees. Faculty with doctorates often want to pursue research (in spite of funding difficulties) and not teach, particularly undergraduate courses and clinical segments, yet nursing education needs more faculty with PhDs to help increase enrollment and decrease the nursing shortage long term. Will increasing the number of faculty with PhDs solve the faculty shortage—a shortage of faculty who teach nursing students? Clearly, we need a multifaceted solution to the faculty shortage. There are other approaches to the problem beyond more PhDs. Here are some alternatives to consider.

DNPs and Teaching

We introduced the Doctor of Nursing Practice (DNP) degree, but this role was envisioned to be a practice role. There is also some question in some universities as to whether DNPs would be in the tenure track. We need to consider how DNPs might assist with clinical teaching, particularly at the undergraduate level, while recognizing that the DNP was designed to be a practice role rather than a faculty role. This may be a problem. There is an increase in faculty with master's degrees entering DNP programs, even though they have no plans to practice and do not plan on serving as APRNs. Will this confuse the issue more?

Distance Education

Some schools are increasing their distance-learning course offerings, even offering entire programs online. Retired or soon-to-retire faculty members may be a potential resource for these programs and courses; many retirees may want to continue teaching but not full time. Schools of nursing should be identifying faculty they want to keep and, before retirement, begin to train them in online education. This method offers retirees flexibility, as they can teach anywhere they can access the Internet. This keeps valuable experts in the teaching pool longer. In addition, schools can employ experts who live in other areas, as they are not restricted to face-to-face teaching; this could particularly benefit schools in rural areas that have difficulties attracting faculty.

Increasing distance education may help to resolve some of the issues with attracting faculty, as noted earlier, and adequate classroom space. It does not resolve the problems with finding appropriate clinical sites or obtaining effective preceptors. In addition, some schools of nursing are rapidly increasing enrollment in distance-education programs and may be compromising quality education: too many students in distance-learning courses; faculty not prepared to teach in this format and/or weak in the subject matter; inadequate supervision of precepted experiences from a distance; admitting students who may not be qualified, and the use of "cookbook" courses that are so standardized that faculty who teach the courses have no input into the courses. This problem area is particularly noted in graduate programs and RN-BSN programs. Expanding distance learning requires nursing education to ensure that quality education is the primary goal, not the number of students.

Joint Appointments

Joint appointments with clinical staff are another method to increase faculty. This has been problematic in some states, where regulations determine who can teach and what degrees are required. In the end, nursing loses out when clinical faculty do not have a sound, current clinical background, but clinical staff can be taught about education. This is actually easier than getting faculty that have not cared for patients in many years current with clinical practice. Globally, more schools of nursing use practicing nurses as preceptors for students than we do in the United States. Regulatory barriers make this difficult to change. Active, planned mentorship is critical for these faculty. For example, in other countries nursing staff who want to teach must successfully complete a year-long course, meeting weekly and covering critical education content. They are then mentored and supervised by a faculty member for at least a year, and longer if needed. During this time, the faculty member visits the staff during a given clinical when students are present, reviews all graded assignments before they are returned to students, and then evaluates the staff member before he or she is offered a permanent teaching part-time position. However, even once clinical staff are fully approved to teach, they are always supervised by a full-time faculty member who coordinates the clinical course.

Part-Time Faculty

All disciplines, including nursing, are making greater use of part-time faculty. Part-time faculty typically spend more of their time teaching, but this is changing; more of them are getting involved in research, service, integration, and synthesis (Creech, 2008). There are disadvantages with part-time faculty, such as difficulty in keeping them informed about curriculum and policies; commitment to the school and process; communication problems; and so on. Schools must consider these issues and be proactive in responding to them.

Nursing Education Master's Programs

We also see some growth in master's programs in nursing education. These programs must reflect present and future changes in education: online teaching, online student teaching opportunities, greater use of technology and simulation, and developing clinical reasoning and judgment in practicum experiences. We need to prepare our future faculty to facilitate active learning, and include content on the IOM core competencies and implications for nursing education as well as the Benner report on nursing education. If DNP graduates are going to teach, they too should be expected to take education courses, and this should also be true for students pursuing the PhD in nursing.

Faculty Retention Issues

Faculty salaries are not competitive with practice salaries. Support services for faculty are also critical when they have less time to "play secretary." Efficient IT support and instructional design staff, among many other things, all add to productivity and quality education. All these services require funding at a time of economic constraints.

Faculty morale is low, and burnout is widespread. One reason that faculty retention is not worse is that many nurses find teaching easier than practice, particularly if they have been out of the practice arena for a long time and they want to stay employed and connected to health care. Workloads are often not equitable among faculty. Research is praised as the most important activity, though many in research struggle a great deal with funding and ensuring that studies are productive and make an impact. Less recognition is given to those who teach, even when teaching is the primary goal of the school. Education is a business, and money is the driver that sets an institution's priorities.

Innovation in Nursing Education: Some Approaches

We need to step outside our comfort zone, think outside the box, and overall do whatever we need to do to come up with more creative, effective methods to cultivate and retain faculty. This will require a serious revision of how nursing education relates to nursing practice, to close the gap between the two. We do not advocate returning to diploma schools, but we do need to bring teaching in the clinical setting closer to practice. We must try new approaches, make better use of our colleagues in practice to help with teaching, and change regulations that block us from making innovative changes in clinicals (such as using simulation and preceptors). Maybe we can adapt some elements of medical education to nursing education. Medical faculty are usually part of the clinical setting; students and residents participate fully in the care process. We are reluctant to do this, based on our history with hospitals and given our aversion to saying that any medical-education approach might be helpful to us. This fear, however, may be keeping us from making serious, effective changes.

Dedicated education units (DEUs) are used in some areas of the country. In these cases, schools of nursing use consistent units in hospitals for clinicals. Faculty have a greater role on the unit as members of the team, and this in turn enhances student learning because students are viewed more as part of the team, in same manner as medical students. These units are good examples of academic practice partnerships. We need greater innovations in academic partnerships (Finkelman & Kenner, 2008). (See http://championnursing.org/solution/dedicated-education-unit-increasing-educational-capacity-and-improving-clinical-education for more information on DEUs.)

If we offer more theory and didactic content early in the nursing program, we can put students into clinicals in more immersion-type experiences: five days a week for a long period with a few seminars. If this sounds like medical school, it certainly is similar. Having students in clinicals for one or two days a week, with long gaps in between, does not facilitate student clinical learning. They miss seeing the trajectory of illness and care, viewing patient outcomes, developing clinical reasoning and judgment, and working on a healthcare team to reach outcomes.

We must stop using old methods to resolve issues and recognize that we must take risks to move forward. In the practice arena, we are accustomed to the pressure to assess problems and risk and then make decisions. If the wrong decision is made, then the goal is to learn from it. In nursing education today, budget issues drive decisions, and there is more use of business principles. "Business" is a bad word in nursing education—just try saying that the student who passes boards is the "product" of nursing education. We need to make many changes:

▮ Transform nursing education to better fit with practice.

▮ Look at curricula and make a better fit with practice and the real world, using data from these reports and their recommendations.

▮ Increase interactive learning. We are losing the students who are bored in the classroom, if they even come to class. Interactive learning requires fewer lectures and more case-based and problem-based learning, in which students take more responsibility for their own learning and develop clinical reasoning and judgment throughout the curriculum. It also requires more creativity from faculty.

▮ Use more technology effectively in teaching-learning. However, remember that content, teaching-learning strategies, and learning outcomes should drive the use of technology—online courses, simulations, use of personal digital assistants (PDAs), podcasts, learning communities in the form of blogs, the use of Twitter to engage students, and iPads, and so on; technology does not drive our teaching experiences.

▮ Accept that we cannot teach everything; teach what we need to, including how students can find information for themselves (knowledge management).

▮ Design our curricula so they can be adjusted easily to changing needs. Our complex curriculum processes are unproductive, limit innovation, impair timely change, and block effective improvement.

▮ Revamp clinical experiences; be reasonable about what we cannot teach and teach what we need to. We tend to stick with the same methods (simple-to-complex, every student needs the same clinical experience, and so on). Some schools are using 12-hour shifts. This requires some evaluation: Can students really work for 12-hours and learn for this extended time? Are we limiting their learning and risking an increase in errors? Can faculty reasonably work for 12 hours supervising and facilitating learning for a group of 8 to 10 students? Consider the growing data regarding the impact of long working hours on staff. (See Part 5 for further information.) Some schools are converting a large percentage of clinical time to simulated experiences. The rationale is that practice in a safe environment fosters better use of the clinical agencies, as students are better prepared to provide care for real patients. Obviously, simulation also helps ease the number of hours a school must use in already overburdened clinical institutions. Making this change typically involves consideration of state board of nursing requirements, which may limit the number of hours that can be used for simulation, as discussed later in this book.

- Include more experiences that allow students to understand the trajectory of illness and health from admission to hospital to home, and the roles and communication of the team.
- Involve practicing nurses in clinical teaching and bring nursing faculty back into the clinical setting so they and students are part of the care team and not visitors. This will require less switching of clinical sites for students and reduce the hours required for orientation at each new clinical setting.
- Adhere to standards: We too lapse into the numbers game when admitting students to fill slots and feel that we must graduate a certain number. If a student really cannot meet requirements, do we find ways around this problem to meet our numbers, or do we acknowledge that some students are just not cut out for nursing (though we may not know this when they are admitted)? We need to get better at identifying unqualified students before we admit them. Do we have the resources, such as faculty, clinical sites, and preceptors, to cover increasing numbers of students? If we do not, we will soon find ourselves with major problems regarding workload, lack of faculty, and the quality of our program.
- Include students and clinicians in our decisions about nursing education. The truth is that nursing education exists because the healthcare system needs nurses. If hospitals or other healthcare organizations (HCOs) decided tomorrow that they did not need nurses, schools of nursing would cease to exist. Schools of nursing must listen to and be responsive to the needs of HCOs. Student feedback is important—not only the evaluation forms they complete but also their narrative concerns. We should also garner feedback from our graduates as they begin to practice or practice at a more advanced level.

Nurse Externships and Residencies

There is a clear need to consider the needs of students and new graduates from different perspectives: nurse externships and residencies have been used in the past and have resurfaced. These programs help new graduates transition to practice and offer a host of opportunities to expand their competencies. Nurse externship programs typically are developed by hospitals and other HCOs for nursing students and are offered during the summer between the junior and senior year. Sometimes a school of nursing is involved. Students are employed and get some additional educational opportunities during the externship. The student role varies from state to state based on state board of nursing guidelines for employment of student nurses. Nurse externships should reflect IOM recommendations such as the core competencies and a greater emphasis on quality improvement.

This is also true of nurse residencies, which take place after graduation and can range from several months to one year in length. The longer programs provide more time for the new graduate to transition to practice. Nurse residencies may be organized by a healthcare organization or in collaboration with a school of nursing. Effective residencies should offer graduated patient care responsibilities, additional educational experiences and competency development, professional socialization, and support for the critical transition during the first postgraduation year. These programs, too, should incorporate the recommendations and core competencies from the IOM.

In 2002, the AACN partnered with some HCOs to pilot standardized postbaccalaureate residency programs (IOM, 2004b). This ongoing AACN program is only for BSN graduates, but given the large number of associate degree (AD) graduates, we should also consider their transition to practice. If only BSN graduates can take advantage of residencies, this may imply that AD graduates do not need a residency, which is not the case. Through residency programs one can then encourage AD graduates to continue their education. Nurse residencies that are not AACN residencies tend to accept all types of graduates if they meet the program's specific admission and employment requirements.

The National Council of State Boards of Nursing (NCSBN) has examined the transition-to-practice problem. A model addressing transition to practice is found in Figure 4-1. The NCSBN model for nurse residency program integrates the IOM core competencies.

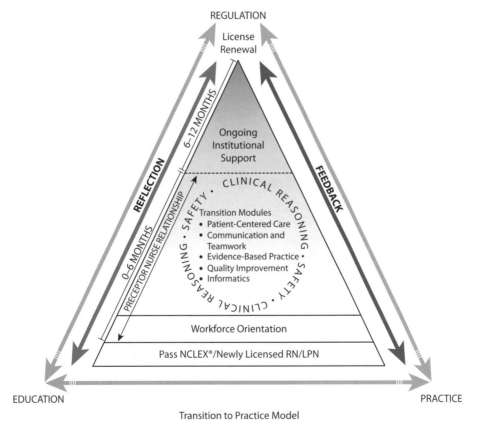

Transition to Practice Model

Source: National Council of State Boards of Nursing. Reprinted with permission. Retrieved from https://www.ncsbn.org/363.htm

FIGURE 4-1 Transition to Practice Model

Simulation: An Expanding Pathway to Learning

Simulation as a Teaching Strategy

Simulation is intended "to replicate some or nearly all of the essential aspects of a clinical situation so that the situation may be more readily understood and managed when it occurs for real in clinical practice" (Morton, 1995, p. 76). Use of human patient simulation is as increasing as a critical teaching strategy. Using planned scenarios, students can experience many different clinical situations: "to work with authentic problems, synthesize data, make clinical decision, and reflect on their practice" (Jeffries, 2007, p. ix). Simulation can be used to learn about errors and reduce errors (IOM, 1999). This is learning without risk in a controlled, predictable, safe environment (Wachter, 2007). According to Beyea and Kobokovich (2004, pp. 738, 741), students can:

▮ Experience preprogrammed rare events;
▮ Repeat procedures and experiences;
▮ Learn by making errors that do not harm an actual patient;
▮ Observe different outcomes of a situation that stem from the actions chosen; and
▮ Practice teamwork, debriefing, and team interactions.

Nehring, Ellis, and Lashely (2001) describe similar advantages of using simulation:

▮ Visualize and observe the physiological effects on the human body.
▮ Observe effects of medications.
▮ Practice in a safe environment; seeing the consequences when wrong decisions are made.
▮ Enhance prior learning.
▮ Improve student confidence, decision-making, and critical thinking (including clinical reasoning and judgment).
▮ Provide opportunities for self-study.
▮ Use structured experiences.
▮ Involve undergraduate and graduate students.
▮ Allow evaluation of the student's competencies.

Other considerations when assessing the use of simulation are that it offers (Issenberg et al., 2005):

▮ Repetitive practice;
▮ Curriculum integration;
▮ Range of difficulty level;

- Multiple learning strategies;
- Clinical variation;
- Controlled environment;
- Individualized learning; and
- Defined outcomes.

Simulation should include more than just crisis or emergency situations. It should present common patient situations that students may encounter. Simulation does not stand alone as a teaching strategy; it should be integrated with other strategies. Faculty need training and time to develop learning experiences. It is important to emphasize the complete process because students may focus on a specific situation or single procedure rather than on patient-centered care.

This is an expensive teaching tool; the cost of equipment, supplies, space and space renovation, faculty training, and faculty planning is significant. The goal is to design and implement simulation that is effective and efficient. Using simulation in addition to clinical experiences enhances the clinical learning for students, who will be better prepared and more confident when they enter the clinical environment (Beyea & Kobokovich, 2004).

When students participate in clinical experiences, they confront the tension between academic ideals and clinical reality. Clinical experiences must dispel the unrealistic notion that there is only one right way (Meyer & Xu, 2005). Students in clinical settings may be frustrated and confused when they see staff using different approaches. Simulation is a good time to discuss how and when one might do something differently and still apply clinical reasoning and judgment. Faculty must consider that some students will find it stressful to think that nurses are not meeting the ideal. Benner's novice-to-expert model helps to explain this experience (2001). Simulation experiences provide many opportunities for working with students to overcome a "procedure approach" to nursing and examine the "ideal" in light of reasoned practice. Simulation should emphasize patient-centered care using clinical reasoning and judgment and also integrate quality care, teamwork, evidence-based practice, and use of informatics such as use of EMRs.

Regulation and Use of Simulation

Many nursing programs that want to use simulation are questioning the barrier of regulation. Some state regulations limit the hours or the percentage of clinical time for which simulation may be used. Given (1) the evidence that simulation is an effective teaching method, (2) the IOM's strong support for the use of simulation to improve quality, and (3) the shortage of clinical experiences, regulations that limit the use of effective teaching strategies such as simulation ought to be changed. Nehring (2008) reviewed state board regulations on this issue. There is no doubt that technology has greatly expanded the capability of equipment that can be used for teaching, and most likely this will only improve. Forty-four states plus the District of Columbia and Puerto Rico (88.5%) responded to Nehring's survey. Many states are currently reviewing their regulations on the use of simulation and have made changes. There is more funding for simulation research and program development, which is additional evidence of the importance and effectiveness of simulation. At the same time, faculty need to consider:

I Development time for effective simulations;
I Integration of simulation throughout the curriculum—not just in the first nursing course—and creation of a clear implementation plan;
I Educating faculty about the use of simulation;
I Equipment purchase, which requires careful consideration of products that best meet desired purposes and costs;
I Space for simulation;
I Faculty preparation and teaching time and lab staff;
I Student orientation to simulation; and
I Evaluation of outcomes.

To obtain more resources, many schools will have to cooperate with their clinical partners, who are also turning to simulation for orientation and staff training. Simulation should incorporate the five core healthcare professions competencies as identified by the IOM reports. The National League for Nursing's Simulation Innovation Resource Center (SIRC) is an example of the expansion in this area and the resources that are available to faculty (http://sirc.nln.org).

NLN Centers of Excellence

Another implication of the IOM reports is a greater need for national recognition of excellence in nursing education. The National League for Nursing (NLN) established one method to identify outstanding schools of nursing through its Centers for Excellence in Nursing Education program, established in 2003 (http://www.nln.org). This program recognizes schools of nursing that demonstrate sustained, evidence-based, and substantive innovation in one of three ways: (1) enhanced student learning and professional development, (2) ongoing faculty development, or (3) advanced nursing education research. Each is critical, but to advance nursing education, a school will have to excel in more than one area. The goals of the NLN recognition program are (2011):

I Identify and reward those schools that excel in creating environments that enhance student learning and professional development, promote the pedagogical expertise of faculty, or advance the science of nursing education.
I Identify and reward healthcare organizations that promote academic progression of their nurses.

- Encourage research in nursing education.
- Facilitate discussions among faculty, students, program graduates, and employers about excellence in nursing education and how to promote it.
- Encourage academic-practice partnerships.
- Encourage the development of innovative schools that attract and retain highly qualified students and faculty.
- Facilitate positive changes that reform nursing education based on the application of evidence gleaned from research in practice and education.
- Influence the development of public policies that benefit nursing education, support nursing education research, and promote excellence in nursing education.

Distance Education or Online Learning

Online education is a offered in many schools today. How it is used, the quality of the courses, and how the outcomes are evaluated are important concerns. Students are more and more involved in information technology (IT) and expect schools and faculty to use it. Some programs blend online education with face-to-face education either in the classroom or in the clinical, or have developed distance-education opportunities more fully. As long as quality education is maintained, these innovative web-based programs yield advantages for nursing programs and students. Students may be better able to adjust their school schedule to personal needs if they can "attend" class when it fits their schedule. In hybrid courses, students still have face-to-face contact with faculty in periodic meetings, seminars, and conferences, or in clinicals. Scheduling and use of space for classes is simplified. However, students must accept more responsibility for their own learning. Online courses provide more opportunities for interactive learning (as opposed to lecture-based learning) by using cases, interactive gaming techniques, and much more, but this does require financial, design, and technology resources, and faculty commitment to alter teaching approaches and move to a facilitator role. However, this method of teaching does not require less faculty time; in fact, in many cases it requires more time. This has not often been considered in faculty assignments and workload.

Another concern is the use of "cookbook" courses. These are courses that are developed by a faculty expert and maybe an instructional design specialist—and then (at least in some instances) faculty are told to use the course as is. What does this do to faculty buy-in? What effect does this have on faculty creativity when faculty members can no longer develop a course based on an approved syllabus that meshes with their teaching style? Will faculty be committed to this type of course, or just go through the motions to get through it? A standardized expert-developed course with instructional design guidance can be positively implemented if it is considered a course master plan that can then be adapted to a particular faculty member's expertise. This type of use is no different from when faculty in the face-to-face environment share course materials and the new faculty teaching the course adapt the materials according to their own teaching styles.

A third choice is to provide technology service and training about online teaching and then have faculty develop their own courses just as they do for face-to-face courses. This keeps the faculty in the role of developing and facilitating learning rather than using work done by others that may not sync with the faculty member's approach or knowledge base.

Questions do remain about which method of course delivery constitutes a better pedagogy: online, hybrid or blended, or face-to-face? Other questions include: Can all nursing content be effectively taught online? How do we effectively handle clinical and preceptor experiences online—or can we? There are problems with this approach that will have a direct impact on the quality of nursing education.

Increasing Need for Interprofessional Education

An important step in answering IOM's call for better collaboration was the 2005 conference "Transforming Health Professional Education," led by Joint Commission Resources and cosponsored by organizations representing nursing, medical, pharmacy, health administration education, and some healthcare organizations. The goal of this conference was to begin an interprofessional dialogue to improve health professions education by discussing topics such as what should be redesigned, what models of change exist, and how to create a learning continuum. One clear theme was the need for more interprofessional education (IPE). Since this conference, several key reports have been published focusing on IPE.

Nurse educators need to assume a major role by actively pursuing opportunities to improve and get involved in more IPE. Healthcare professions students should be included in clinical activities such as attending teams, grand rounds presentations, specialty weekly conferences, patient rounds, and any clinical activity where patient care is discussed. More interprofessional courses are needed. Some might focus only on interprofessional work teams, with content such as advantages and disadvantages of working together; roles and scope of practice; improvement of collaboration, coordination, and communication; impact on the patient; leadership and followership; and impact on safety and quality. Additional teaching-learning strategies are discussed in Part 5.

Getting nursing, medical, pharmacy, physical therapy, allied health, and any other health professions students who may be located in the academic center into a course that asks them to learn about teams and openly discuss these issues would be a significant first step. Other courses might concentrate on cases, health assessment, or quality improvement; or simulation labs might be used so that teams of students are provided with opportunities to respond to simulated scenarios and debrief afterward, but this should not exclude having profession-specific simulation experiences. An interprofessional course might focus on quality improvement with teams of students that select a care-quality problem, analyze it, develop resolutions, and then determine how outcomes would be evaluated. This type of course would naturally include many of the issues described earlier, where students explore what it means to be on an inter-professional team. Here they would experience this fully as they work to reach an outcome. The critical element is that these learning activities must provide opportunities for active student interaction. Just putting the students in a course together is not effective interprofessional education.

IPE is even more important today with the increasing emphasis on interprofessional collaborative teams (Barnsteiner et al., 2007). Teamwork and collaboration are not intuitive, nor is the ability to teach interprofessional teamwork. We have operated in our silos, separate from other healthcare professionals, for a very long time. To make changes in education so that more IPE is used will require determined effort. "Challenges include course scheduling, matching course content, faculty interest and expertise in IPE, a culture of valuing shared learning among faculty and students, and institutional policies for sharing course credit among schools" (Mitchell et al., 2006, as cited in Barnsteiner et al., 2007, p. 144).

Schools and faculty that have tried IPE have faced obstacles such as finding other healthcare professionals to teach; regulatory standards that do not allow non-nurses to teach in nursing programs; lack of respect between healthcare professions and faculty, which students inevitably sense; and differing college schedules within the same university that make it difficult to arrange interprofessional courses. It is difficult enough to make changes in one system, and even more so in multiple systems. The following criteria are recommended to develop effective IPE (Barnsteiner et al., 2007, p. 149):

1. An explicit philosophy of IPE that permeates the organization—well-known, observable, and measurable
2. Faculty from the different professions co-creating the learning experiences
3. Students having integrated and experiential opportunities to learn collaboration and teamwork and how they relate to delivery of quality care
4. IPE learning experiences embedded in the curricula and part of the required caseload for students
5. Competence demonstrated by students with a single set of interprofessional competencies such as those promoted by IOM
6. Organizational infrastructure that fosters IPE, such as faculty time to develop IPE options, incentive systems for faculty to engage in IPE, and integrated activities across schools and professions for students and faculty

The development of interprofessional education has been greater outside the United States. The World Health Organization, recognizing the importance of interprofessional teams in health care, published an extensive report on interprofessional education,

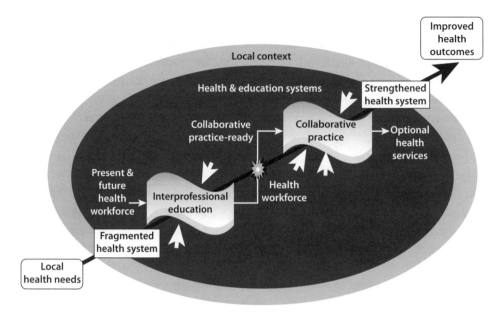

Source: Reprinted with permission from: World Health Organization (WHO), (Framework for Action on Interprofessional Education & Collaboration Practice Goneve: World Health Organization)

F I G U R E   4 - 2   Framework for Action on Interprofessional Education and Collaborative Practice

as described in Figure 4-2 (2010). This report was then used as the framework for a report on the same topic in the United States (Interprofessional Professional Education Collaborative, 2011). Figure 4-2 describes the framework for action on interprofessional education and collaborative practice, describing the connections.

The reports discuss three types of professional competencies. There are certainly individual professional competencies, such as competencies that pertain only to nursing or only to medicine; however, there are also some competencies that are common to all. The third type of competencies pertains to interprofessional collaboration.

Figure 4-3 illustrates how the IOM healthcare professions core competencies relate to the interpersonal collaborative competencies.

The interprofessional competencies, which are discussed in detail in the report, pertain to four focus areas (Interprofessional Professional Education Collaborative, 2011).

1. Values/ethics for interprofessional practice
2. Roles/responsibilities
3. Interprofessional communication
4. Teams and teamwork

Table 4-1 provides some examples of current literature on this important topic. This literature is increasing as more healthcare professional programs integrate IPE into their curricula and learning experiences.

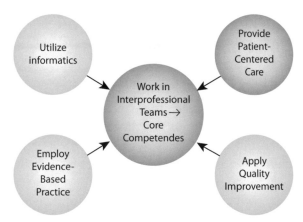

Source: © 2011 Interprofessional Education Collaborative (American Association of Colleges of Nursing, American Association of Colleges of Osteopathic Medicine, American Association of Colleges of Pharmacy, American Dental Education Association, Association of American Medical Colleges, and Association of Schools of Public Health). May be reproduced and distributed according to the terms set forth in this document.

F I G U R E   4 - 3   Interprofessional Teamwork and the IOM Core Competencies

T A B L E   4 - 1   Sample Literature on Interprofessional Teams and Education

Barnsteiner, J., Disch, J., Hall, L., Mayer, D., & Moore, S. (2007). Promoting interprofessional education. *Nursing Outlook, 55, 144–150.*

Barton, S., Patterson, S., Pimlott, J., Sommerfeldt, S., & Stayko, P. (2011). Creating interprofessional clinical learning units: Developing an acute-care model. *Nurse Education in Practice, 38*(7), 273–277.

Bennett, P. N., Gum, L., Lindeman, I., Lawn, S., McAllister, S., Richards, J., Kelton, M., & Ward, H. (2011). Faculty perceptions of interprofessional education. *Nurse Education Today, 31*(6), 571–576.

Bratton, C., Chavin, K., & Baliga, P. (2011). Racial disparities in organ donation and why. *Current Opinion in Organ Transplantation, 16,* 243–249.

Bridges, D., et al. (2011). Interprofessional collaboration: Three best practice models of interprofessional education. *Medical Education Online,* 16.

Carr, D., King, J., Reisling, D., & Shea, R. (2011). Comparison of communication outcomes in traditional versus simulation strategies in nursing and medical students. *Nursing Education Perspectives, 32*(5), 323–327.

Gerrie, V., Barnett, L., H., & Susan, H. (2011). Featured article: Use of the standardized patient to clarify interdisciplinary team roles. *Clinical Simulation in Nursing, 7*(5), e169–e173.

Interprofessional Professional Education Collaborative (IPEC). (2011). *Core competencies for interprofessional collaborative practice.* (Collaborative of AACN, American Association of Colleges of Osteopathic Medicine, American Association of Colleges of Pharmacy, American Dental Education Association, Association of American Medical Colleges, and Association of Schools of Public Health). Retrieved from www.aacn.nche.edu/education-resources/IPECReport.pdf

Li, Y., Glance, L., Yin, J., & Mukamel, D. (2011). Racial disparities in rehospitalization among Medicare patients in skilled nursing facilities. *American Journal of Public Health, 101*(5), 875–882.

Reeves, S. (2009). An overview of continuing interprofessional education. *Journal of Continuing Education in the Health Professions, 29*(3), 142–146.

Remington, T., Foulk, M., & Williams, B. (2006). Evaluation evidence for interprofessional education. *American Journal of Pharmaceutical Education, 70*(3), 66.

Tschannen, D., Keenan, G., Aebersold, M., Kocan, M., Lundy, F., & Averhart, V. (2011). Implications of nurse-physician relations: Report of a successful intervention. *Nursing Economic$, 29*(3), 127–135.

World Health Organization. (2010). *Framework for action on interprofessional education and collaborative practice.* Retrieved from http://www.who.int/hrh/resources/framework_action/en/index.html

The Nursing Curriculum and Integration of the IOM Core Competencies

Reviewing and Updating Nursing Curricula

Nursing educators must find a shorter, more focused method for curriculum review and update. In most nursing programs this process can take years. With the constant changes in knowledge and the power to access knowledge quickly, taking years to accomplish curriculum revision updates will not serve students, their future employers, or patients well. Early in the review process, it is important to make the curriculum something the faculty own and thus feel committed to implementing. There can be no sacred content that cannot be touched. Nurse educators cannot simply continue adding content, so they must show greater flexibility and willingness to consider methods that would improve how content is organized and increase student interactivity in the learning process. Barriers that make faculty think they cannot add more content include:

- Repeated content (for example, students have taken pathophysiology, yet this content is repeated in adult health contexts such as with cardiac disease or diabetes content)
- Thinking that everything must be covered in class, particularly in lectures, instead of expecting students to come to class prepared to apply content to cases and examples
- Faculty adding content that is not officially approved and thus increasing content that may not be needed (and that other faculty may not even know was taught)
- Too much dependence on lecture; this method does not engage students and increases pressure on faculty to add more and more content
- Inadequate review of textbooks when reading assignments are made (students cannot distinguish "nice to know" from "need to know," which makes reading assignments too long)
- Too little expectation that students retain and apply knowledge from previous courses
- Little or ineffective use of simulation
- Ignoring principles of adult education
- Limited use of online methods to cover content that can then be applied in the classroom, seminars, or practica, or used as stand-alone courses
- Lack of innovative methods for integrating online materials
- Designing courses around a specific textbook, making it difficult to change to better, more up-to-date textbooks

In most cases, the need is not to add large amounts of content, but rather to reconfigure content, apply it differently, develop different teaching-learning strategies, describe exemplars, and so on. Curricula do not always consider the real status or multiple dimensions of health care, partly because these data have not been easy to access or even to isolate. Data collected are often related to a single institution, a geographic region, or a specific disease entity, and do not reflect a national perspective. Sometimes faculty prefer to do it the way it is usually done—maybe changing some terminology, but still concentrating on the same healthcare issues.

We now have greater access to data that should improve our curricula and teaching strategies. There is no doubt that nurses today are inundated with crucial information. Textbooks are important, but learning should not end there. Faculty and students can benefit from critical updates about important aspects of health care and needed improvements. This should be true on the undergraduate level as well as the graduate level. The Internet has opened doors to information that once was either unavailable or difficult to find. This book provides resources that can be used to improve courses and update curricula to better integrate the IOM content and recommendations as well as other quality improvement initiatives.

Schools of nursing do not change easily or quickly. Some faculty may not see the connection between the IOM reports and education and may view the reports as related only to the practice area. Faculty who do wish to change the curriculum to include this material find that doing so is often not easy. In addition to the typical, cumbersome, lengthy curriculum process, curriculum changes often involve issues of academic freedom, need for classroom time for more content, and faculty workloads, and then overlook how essential this content is to nurses. The key for success today is to make change happen more quickly and effectively so that students are prepared to provide quality care; keeping up with new healthcare concerns is critical. A curriculum revision process that allows for change as need arises is imperative. Sources such as the National Healthcare Quality Report, IOM reports, and *Healthy People 2020* provide more direction to the review and change process. Schools of nursing that choose not to do this will not produce the best-qualified front-line practitioners. Nurse researchers typically approach research with an open mind receptive to new requirements; nurse educators must do this also.

Integration of IOM Core Competencies into the Nursing Curriculum

Integrating the IOM five healthcare professions core competencies into the nursing curriculum supports the need for nurses to have greater knowledge about the critical healthcare concerns, and also assists them to be more competent leaders in the healthcare delivery system. Figures 4-4 through 4-9 provide examples of how the competencies can be integrated into typical nursing courses, and specific content that is relevant to each competency.

Some of this content may already be in your curriculum, but the curriculum should be reviewed to ensure that it is and to identify what might still be missing. This information applies to both undergraduate and graduate programs, though clearly graduate programs approach content from a more advanced perspective. It is also critical to

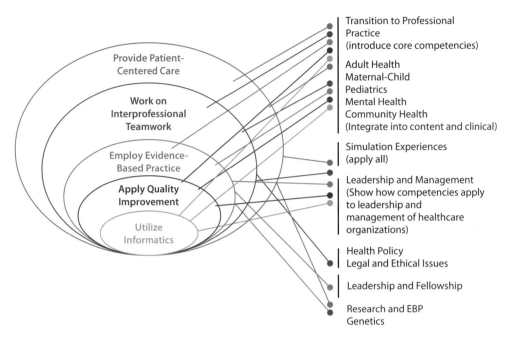

F I G U R E   4 - 4   IOM Five Core Competencies: Where Does Content Belong?

F I G U R E   4 - 5   Content Related to Patient-Centered Care

```
                  Work on Interprofessional Teamwork

    o   Definition of interprofessional team and  implementation
    o   Teamwork
    o   Team leadership
    o   Followership
    o   Care coordination
    o   Collaboration
    o   Team communication
    o   Patient's role on the team
    o   Team planning
    o   Delegation
    o   Transformational leadership
    o   Conflict and conflict resolution
    o   Methods to improve communication (such as Situation-
        Background-Assessment-Recommendation [SBAR])
    o   Types of teams used to resolve specific issues (such as
        rapid response teams)
```

Copyright © Anita Finkelman 2012.

F I G U R E 4 - 6 Content Related to Interprofessional Teamwork

```
                  Employ Evidence-Based Practice

    o   Definition of EBP and implications
    o   EBP relationship to research and QI
    o   Research process
    o   Types of evidence
    o   EBP process
    o   EBP models
    o   Identifying, retrieving, and reviewing EBP and research
        literature
    o   Statistics
    o   EBP relationship to policies and procedures; prioritize
        guidelines and protocols/pathways
    o   Evidence-based management (EBM)
```

Copyright © Anita Finkelman 2012

F I G U R E 4 - 7 Content Related to Evidence-Based Practice

Apply Quality Improvement (QI)

o Definition of quality care and QI; implications of definition	o Patient perspective on errors and error disclosure
o Dimensions of quality care	o Incident reports
o Monitoring care	o Legal and ethical issues
o Analyzing data	o Cost of errors (financial and other)
o Standards	o Safety culture
o Joint Commission and accreditation	o Joint Commission annual safety goals
o Benchmarking	o Adverse events and causes
o Risk management	o Sentinel events
o Utilization review/management	o High-risk times for medication errors (students and staff)
o Case management	o Failure to rescue
o Disease management	o Rapid response teams
o Relationship to policies and procedures	o Handoffs
o Staff performance evaluation	o Checklists
o Implications of regulation and licensure	o SBAR (Situation-Background-Assessment-Recommendation)
o Patient outcomes	o Workarounds and implications
o QI roles of nurse	o Failure mode and effects analysis (FMEA)
o Implications of EBP and EBM for QI	o PDSA (Plan-Do-Study-Act)
o Practice guidelines and protocols	o Uses of patient-centered rounds
o Access to care	o National Healthcare Quality Report
o Cost of care and quality	o IOM aims to improve care
o Safety-net hospitals	o National Database of Nursing Quality Indicators (NDNQI)
o Errors	
o The blame game and change to a just culture	
o Root cause analysis	

Copyright © Anita Finkelman 2012.

FIGURE 4-8   Content Related to Quality Improvement

set up a system for annual review and revision, as this content changes quickly. Part 5 discusses teaching-learning strategies, and there is also information on this topic in the digital-only supplementary instructional materials that are included with this book. As has been noted, just putting content in is not enough; we have to seriously appraise our facilitation of learning, where we need much improvement (Benner, Sutphen, Leonard, & Day, 2010).

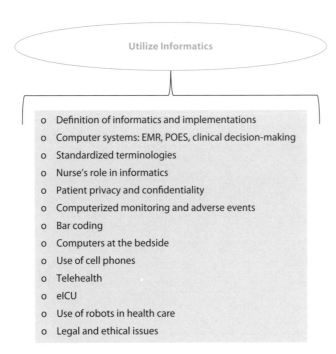

Utilize Informatics

- o Definition of informatics and implementations
- o Computer systems: EMR, POES, clinical decision-making
- o Standardized terminologies
- o Nurse's role in informatics
- o Patient privacy and confidentiality
- o Computerized monitoring and adverse events
- o Bar coding
- o Computers at the bedside
- o Use of cell phones
- o Telehealth
- o eICU
- o Use of robots in health care
- o Legal and ethical issues

Copyright © Anita Finkelman 2012.

FIGURE 4-9 Content Related to Informatics

Summary

The IOM reports have had an impact on nursing education and will continue to influence changes for a long time to come. Nursing education is at a critical point. How we should teach and what we should teach are not always so clear. This part of the book provided some examples of issues and additional reports from different organizations to support the call to consider new approaches to improving the quality of nursing education, so that patient care can be improved through the process of nursing education. This content must be openly discussed among faculty and administration in every nursing program at all levels of education. Further discussion of content, along with teaching-learning strategies related to the five core competencies, are examined in depth in Part 5, as do some of the modules and lesson plans in the digital-only supplementary instructional materials that are included with this book.

Part 5

Incorporating the Core Competencies into Nursing Education

Introduction

The strategies for integrating quality care content and experiences into nursing education are based on the five core competencies found in *Health Professions Education* (IOM, 2003b):

- Provide patient-centered care
- Work in interprofessional teams
- Employ evidence-based practice
- Apply quality improvement
- Utilize informatics

The IOM reports on quality include significant reforms (Tanner, 2003). There has been a shift to a competency-based approach to education for all healthcare professions. The core competencies identified are essential for healthcare professionals to respond effectively to patients' care needs. "It is tempting to say we already do these things (five core competencies). Surely we have been talking about informatics competencies for a long time, and we expect our graduates to be leaders and to work in interdisciplinary [interprofessional] teams. Nursing is, if nothing else, patient-centered. But the competencies advanced by IOM are deep and nuanced, based in evidence and clearly reflective of the major shifts in our patient population and their needs during the past decade. We have been talking about a revolution in nursing education for some time now. Our programs, although perhaps aged to perfection, may no longer be relevant, given the dramatic changes in health care. It is now time to work toward building one bridge over the quality chasm" (Tanner, 2003, p. 432).

As nurse educators, we need to pay attention to the critical concerns about the healthcare delivery system in the United States. From 2007–2009, the system did not improve (Mullin, 2011). The Commonwealth Fund Commission on a High Performance Health System evaluation used 42 indicators related to quality, access, efficiency, equity, and healthy lives, all of which are directly related to the IOM reports on quality. The U.S. score was 64 out of a possible 100. What does this mean? At the first evaluation, in 2006, the score was 67; in 2008, it was 65. The United States is behind the United Kingdom, Canada, Australia, and Germany in improvement of care. It ranked last in a list of 16 countries in number of deaths prevented by timely and effective medical care. Health system efficiency was scored at 53 out of a possible 100. Access to care has decreased. There were, however, some positive changes: for instance, the proportion of home care patients with improved mobility increased from 37% to 47% from 2004 to 2009. Providing the right care to prevent surgical complications improved from 71% in 2004 to 96% in 2009.

Figure 5-1 indicates the connection among the IOM reports in the *Quality Chasm* series and the core competencies. This part of the book discusses content and teaching–learning strategies for each of the five core competencies for healthcare professionals. *Learning IOM* provides a shorter version for students. The files that comprise the

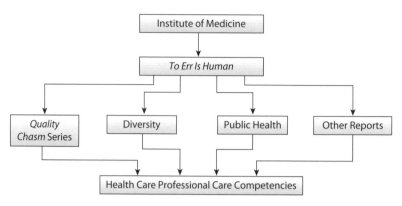

F I G U R E   5 - 1   Development of the IOM Healthcare Core Competencies

teaching–learning PowerPoint and Word documents include module plans for much of this content for faculty and instructor use and planning.

Core Competency: Provide Patient-Centered Care

Identify, respect, and care about patients' differences, values, preferences, and expressed needs; relieve pain and suffering; coordinate continuous care; listen to, clearly inform, communicate with, and educate patients; share decision-making and management; and continuously advocate disease prevention, wellness, and promotion of healthy lifestyles, including a focus on population health.

—IOM, 2003b, p. 4

Patient-centered care (PCC) puts the focus on the patient and family instead of on the health professionals; for example, one approach to emphasize PCC in practice might be to have the health professionals come to the patient instead of moving the patient from room to room to see different specialists. All health professionals should be educated to deliver patient-centered care as members of an interprofessional team, emphasizing evidence-based practice, quality improvement approaches, and informatics (IOM, 2003b). Nursing education must adapt to the changing demographics of the patient population, integrate technologies, and meet critical competencies.

The following content describes some of the issues related to patient-centered care that should be considered in nursing education and staff education to meet this competency.

Decentralized and Fragmented Care

Students experience fragmented care with their patients but may not recognize it; if they do recognize it, they are often frustrated by it. Asking students how it felt when they first entered the healthcare setting as a student—their confusion, inability to understand what was going on, uncertainty as to who staff were and what the expectations were, unclear communication, and so on—can help students better appreciate what patients may be feeling. Many students worry about "drive-through health care." When a test is delayed or postponed because someone did not order it, how does the patient feel and react, and what impact does this have on patient care when the student's well-planned schedule for care is no longer well planned? If we help students recall their own feelings, we can ask, "Well, if you feel this way, how do you think the patient feels?" The goal is to better appreciate the trajectory or course of illness and the continuum of care, including health promotion and illness prevention (Benner, Sutphen, Leonard, & Day, 2010).

Fragmented care exists throughout the healthcare system. Ask students to give examples, and then ask them to think of practical solutions. Iatrogenic injury can be related to fragmented care, and students need to consider how this may occur. Provide specific examples from different healthcare settings, such as acute care, emergency room, ambulatory care, and home care, so that students can gain an understanding of how fragmented care can occur and how the setting and healthcare professionals can influence patient outcomes.

Discuss the implications of decentralization and fragmentation as students learn about the nursing process. This discussion has two sides. Decentralization allows decision-making to be made closer to the patient and reinforces more autonomy at lower levels of an organization, but it can lead to variations in care from unit to unit and fragmentation of services. Consider how plans of care might ensure more decentralization and less fragmentation to improve safety. Give students case scenarios, and then discuss fragmented care, how it can be decreased, and the nurse's role in that effort. This can be done in clinical conferences, in the classroom, in the simulation lab, when students assess their patients and plan care, or when students discuss case studies. This discussion does not require an additional lecture; educators need only be sure that the problem of fragmentation is identified and then woven into critical thinking activities in the classroom, simulation, and clinical experiences.

Changing Our Perspective of the Nursing Assessment

Assessment continues to be an important part of nursing care even while many other nursing activities change. The assessment should be a beginning point for patient-centered care and the first step in the therapeutic nurse–patient relationship (Jones, 2007). Discussing assessment from this perspective with students is important; emphasize its relationship to patient-centered care and the role of data and communication in the care process. It is also important to emphasize that all healthcare professionals, not just nurses, assess patients. This is the ideal time to discuss these other assessments: pertinent topics include how to use these data and the issue of repetitive questions (when are they appropriate and when they are not). Consider how assessment puts the patient in the center.

Self-Management Support

Self-management support is "the systematic provision of education and supportive interventions to increase patients' skills and confidence in managing their health problems, including regular assessment of progress and problems, goal setting, and problem-solving support" (IOM, 2003f, p. 52). Another term for self-management is *self-care*, though the IOM uses *self-management*. Self-management is particularly important in chronic illness, such as diabetes and asthma, and becomes even more complex when patients have multiple problems. Self-management is an appropriate means to assist patients with acute care problems to return to their usual daily functioning as soon as possible; it is also a critical component of care for patients with chronic illnesses. The IOM report *Priority Areas for National Action: Transforming Healthcare Quality* (2003f) lists primarily medical problems as priority concerns. However, the first two priorities are broader in scope: care coordination and self-management. These are very important parts of nursing care, and with the added emphasis on them, nurses should be taking a greater lead in studying and developing self-management interventions for patients and families or significant others.

Self-management should be emphasized throughout the nursing curriculum, at both undergraduate and graduate levels, and in didactic content and clinical experiences (including simulation). Students need to consider self-management for every patient they care for and include the patient and the patient's family in the process; noting that the patient decides if he or she wants family informed, what can be shared, and how family should participate.

Effective self-management support requires collaboration between the patient and all providers involved in the care. Families should also be involved in the process of care. "Healthcare systems can support effective self-management by providing care that builds patient and family skills and confidence, increases patient and family knowledge about the condition, increases provider's knowledge of the needs and preferences of the patient, and supports the patient and family in the psychosocial, as well as medical, responses to the condition" (Institute for Healthcare Improvement [IHI], 2008d). Even patients with acute illnesses can benefit from more effective self-management.

Patient Errors in Self-Management

Students need to understand that although self-management allows patients to be more independent, it can also lead to errors. How can we help patients avoid errors?

Patients at risk for self-management errors include those with multiple chronic problems using multiple medications, and elderly patients trying to practice self-management in their homes. Teach students how to assist patients in using Medisets to administer their medication; how to monitor medication use by patients and caregivers; and how to teach patients and caregivers what to review when they receive their medications, such as drug name and dose. Give students a list of patient orders that include multiple oral medications with complex administration schedules, and ask them to prepare a Mediset based on these orders; they can fill the box with M&Ms in place of the pills.

Put the medications in bottles with and without childproof lids and small-print labels so they can appreciate the many factors (e.g., arthritis, poor eyesight) that affect how a patient practices self-management and how easy it is for a patient to make an error. Use role-play, with students acting as the nurse, the patient, and family members. As they work through the simulation, they will learn better ways to educate patients, prevent errors, and help patients improve their own self-management. Medication reconciliation, which is relevant to self-management, is discussed later.

Disease Management and Patient-Centered Care

Disease management, which involves self-management, can help decrease complications, length of stay, and costs. Patients who can particularly benefit include those who are chronically critically ill. In Long's controlled study (2008), patients on mechanical ventilation for 72 hours or more were included in the sample. Patients were monitored and received disease management interventions from an advanced practice nurse. This coordinated, patient-centered approach improved outcomes. Nurses in the program communicated effectively, showed commitment to good patient outcomes, and understood how to help the patient and family navigate the system. Including disease management in nursing curricula provides excellent examples of care coordination (one of the major priority areas of care), interprofessional teamwork, and patient-centered care. Nurse or patient navigation is being used in some clinical settings to assist patients through their treatment trajectory to meet their health needs, as was mentioned earlier. The nurse navigator works with the patient and family to guide them through the complex healthcare system to ensure better outcomes. Clinical nurse leaders (CNLs) often serve in this role.

The goals of disease management are to improve quality of life, decrease disease progression, and reduce hospitalizations. A nurse call center typically provides services such as monitoring health status; giving patient education and advice; and sharing information from labs, physicians, and pharmacies. Chronic illnesses that are typically monitored include diabetes, heart disease and hypertension, asthma, cancer, depression, renal disease, low back pain, and obesity. Insurers typically develop disease management programs and use case management to control costs. Content on disease management and also case management can be incorporated into community health content and experiences.

Students need to understand that patients with chronic illness need to:

- Understand basic information about their disease. (Even if the patient already has this information, students should confirm patient retention and understanding and be prepared to share or review this information as needed or requested).
- Understand the importance of self-management and development of skills required to effectively self-manage care.
- Recognize the need for ongoing support from members of the practice team, family, friends, and community.

The IHI offers tools to support self-management at http://www.ihi.org/knowledge/Pages/Tools/ToolkitforClinicians.aspx. These tools are great resources for faculty to use in planning learning activities. Examples of the tools are: Quality Compass Benchmarks, Blood Pressure Visual Aid for Patients, Self-Management Support: Patient Planning Worksheet, My Shared Plan, and Group Visit Starter Kit.

Chronic Illness and Self-Management

The number of persons with chronic illnesses has increased, as well as the number of people with more than one chronic illness. Some data on chronic illness includes (Centers for Disease Control and Prevention, 2011):

- Each year, 7 out of 10 deaths among Americans are from chronic diseases. Heart disease, cancer, and stroke account for more than 50% of all deaths each year.
- In 2005, 133 million Americans—almost one out of every two adults—had at least one chronic disease. Nearly half of Americans aged 20–74 have some type of chronic condition.
- Obesity has become a major health concern. One in every three adults is obese, and almost one in five youth between the ages of 6 and 19 is obese (BMI ≥ 95th percentile of the CDC growth chart).
- About one fourth of people with chronic conditions have one or more daily activity limitations.
- Arthritis is the most common cause of disability, with nearly 19 million Americans reporting activity limitations.
- Diabetes continues to be the leading cause of kidney failure, nontraumatic lower-extremity amputations, and blindness among adults.

Why does the United States have these problems with chronic illness? One reason is that with the better treatment available today, people with chronic illnesses live longer; consequently, there are more of them. The United States must improve care provided for those with chronic illness. Many of the IOM priority areas of care, monitored annually in the National Healthcare Quality Report, are chronic illnesses. How are we incorporating content about chronic illness into our curricula, both didactic content and clinical?

Effective management of a chronic illness requires daily management of the illness, and also should include activities to improve health in general. To accomplish this, the person with chronic illness needs to have an understanding of the illness and interventions to achieve self-management. Self-management focuses on care of the body and management of the condition, adapting everyday activities and roles to the condition, and dealing with the emotions arising from having the condition. "Self-management *support* is the care and encouragement provided to people with chronic conditions to help them understand their central role in managing their illness, make informed decisions about care, and engage in healthy behaviors" (IHI, 2008d).

One approach is to use the Chronic Care Model, a patient-centered approach (Wagner, 1998; Improving Chronic Illness Care, 2003). The model emphasizes two principles:

▎ The *community* should have resources and health policies that support care for chronic illnesses.
▎ The *health system* should have healthcare organizations (HCOs) that support self-management, recognizing that the patient is the source of control (patient-centered); a delivery system design that identifies clear roles for staff in relationship to chronic illness care; decision support with evidence-based guidelines integrated into daily practice; and clinical information systems to ensure rapid exchange of information and reminder and feedback systems.

This model is described in Figure 5-2, and at the web site of Improving Chronic Illness Care, http://www.improvingchroniccare.org. This site offers graphics and information that faculty can incorporate into content, cases, and discussions and that students can explore and apply to patients. Staff who care for patients with chronic illness will find the information practical. There are many links to content and application of the model to care issues, including an audiovisual presentation.

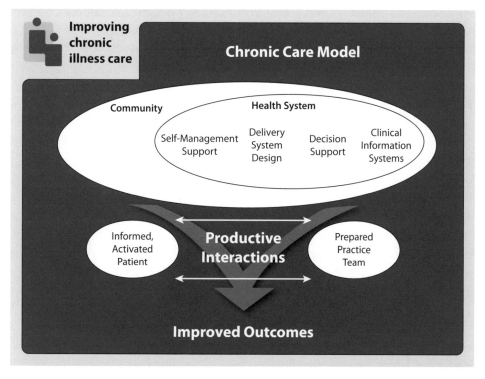

Source: Institute of Healthcare Improvement. *Chronic Conditions*. Retrieved May 26, 2008, from http://www.ihi.org/IHI/Topics/ChronicConditions/AllConditions/Changes/. Reprinted with permission.

F I G U R E 5 - 2 Chronic Care Model

The Improving Chronic Illness Care organization is dedicated to assessing and developing strategies to improve chronic illness care in the United States, and to helping people with chronic illness to lead healthier, quality lives (Improving Chronic Illness Care, 2003). "Over 145 million people—almost half of all Americans—suffer from asthma, depression and other chronic conditions. Over eight percent of the U.S. population has been diagnosed with diabetes. Approximately one third of cases of diabetes are undiagnosed" (Improving Chronic Illness Care, 2011). According to the IOM reports, some of the major issues are:

▌ Healthcare providers who do not have enough time to provide effective care;
▌ Failure to implement established practice guidelines;
▌ Lack of active follow-up to ensure the best outcomes; and
▌ Patients inadequately trained in self-management (a priority area identified by IOM).

(See Teaching–Learning Module 6, Chronic Care Management Model, for more information about chronic illness.)

Self-Management and Diversity

Students need to consider how cultural issues affect self-management. How is the community involved? Students specializing in community health may not concentrate on chronic illness; however, the care for a large number of Americans with at least one chronic condition takes place in the community. Patients from different ethnic groups may respond to chronic illness and to self-management differently. Language affects patients' abilities to understand directions, which is critical to effective self-management. Family roles vary in different cultures, which can influence how families respond and the roles they may or may not assume. The IHI web site includes information on self-management. Health literacy (discussed later) is a critical factor in ensuring quality care in any diversity situation.

Diversity and Disparities in Health Care

Diversity and disparities in health care are critical components of patient-centered care—affecting patient needs and responses, communication, quality, and outcomes throughout the continuum of care. The following content relates to this critical topic. (See Teaching–Learning Module 28, National Healthcare Disparities Monitoring, for more information about healthcare disparities.)

Safety-Net Hospitals

Safety-net hospitals treat poor and underserved patients. Medicaid often reimburses for this care, but many patients may have no way to pay for their care (Reinberg, 2008). Data collected between 2004 and 2006 from 3,665 safety-net and non-safety-net hospitals revealed that the quality of care at safety-net hospitals is below the level of other hospitals (Werner, Goldman, & Dudley, 2008). The results relate directly to healthcare disparities. What do students know about the safety-net system and the needs of vulnerable populations?

These hospitals rely on state and federal funding from Medicaid and other sources. Most are inner-city and teaching hospitals and do not have the funds to improve the quality of care at the same rate as other hospitals. Ironically, though, these hospitals may not receive funding to improve because such funding is often performance-based. Hospitals that receive Medicare and Medicaid Disproportionate Share Hospital (DSH) payments are the hospitals that serve a larger proportion of low-income patients, such as those on Medicaid, and uninsured patients. Though healthcare reform should help reduce this problem, provisions of the current healthcare reform legislation dealing with this issue do not go into effect until 2014.

Quality ratings at hospitals that are described as safety-net hospitals have been variable. McHugh, Kang, and Hasnain-Wynia (2009) note in their study that one has to be careful and consider the criteria used to classify a hospital as a safety-net hospital: "Public or teaching hospitals had lower performance scores on four 'process of care' measures than did private, nonteaching hospitals, but results were mixed for safety-net hospitals identified by the level of uncompensated care they provide." This is a topic that students can explore and then discuss as to its impact on quality care and on nursing.

Reaction to the Shifting Demographics of the Patient Population

Americans are older than ever, living with multiple comorbidities and chronic health needs. The other end of the life span is also at increasing risk, with a population of children who before the age of 10 are experiencing comorbidities such as hypertension, diabetes, and obesity; furthermore, many women are delaying childbearing well into their forties, which may lead to complications during pregnancy and for the newborn. These demographics indicate that long-term health care will require a delivery system capable of handling this growing complexity. Because these are major shifts from the patient pool of the past, healthcare professionals need education that prepares them to intervene in complex health problems in a more efficient, safer way to reach quality outcomes that are also cost-effective.

At the same time, the population is becoming more diverse. Cultural beliefs and values and their relationship to the life span must be integrated into teaching health, yet most programs gloss over cultural competence. The challenge is not to add content, but to integrate content and keep it current with quality care and diversity issues. This will become part of the routine learning experience when students in the clinical setting are expected to include the demographics and cultural backgrounds of their patients in clinical conferences, address them in patient care plans, and incorporate them into written assignments.

An example for students to examine is found in a study by Li, Glance, Yin, and Mukamel (2011). This study considers the impact of racial disparities on rehospitalization among Medicare patients in skilled nursing facilities (SNFs). There was a difference in readmission rates between White patients and Black patients (rehospitalization at

30 days was 14.3% for White patients and 18.6% for Black patients; at 90 days it was 22.1% for White patients and 29.5% for Black patients). The researchers commented that the SNFs that had more Black patients tended to have fewer resources. Students could then relate this back to comments about safety-net hospitals.

Emergency Care and Diversity and Disparities

Emergency care is a critical concern in the United States, as noted in three IOM reports from 2007 discussed in Part 1. A common assumption is that we have this problem because so many uninsured persons use the ER when they do not need urgent care. Actually this is not correct. The uninsured do not come to the ER for a bad cold because they have to pay for this care; someone with insurance coverage has to pay only a copayment for this service (Carmichael, 2008). Carmichael (2008) notes that 17% of people are uninsured, but they account for only 10% to 15% of ER visits. From 2008–2009, though, there was an increase in use of emergency departments (EDs) by the uninsured. However, diversity issues are prevalent in emergency care, and the need for quick, effective communication with patients and families is critical. Accessibility of interpreters is often a barrier in the emergency care delivery system.

"Emergency departments have the only legal mandate in the U.S. healthcare system to provide health care according to the Emergency Medical Treatment and Labor Act (EMTALA). This law ensures that anyone who comes to an emergency department, regardless of their insurance status or ability to pay, must receive a medical screening exam and be stabilized. According to a 2009 American College of Emergency Physicians (ACEP) survey on the U.S. financial crisis, 66 percent of emergency physicians polled have seen an increase of uninsured patients in their emergency departments during the current financial crisis" (ACEP, 2011).

Patients with nonurgent medical conditions may wait longer for care, but once seen, they are treated quickly and released. "Dangerous overcrowding is caused when a lack of hospital resources results in acutely ill patients being 'boarded' in an emergency department because no hospital inpatient beds are available, and ambulances must be diverted to other hospitals. The Centers for Disease Control and Prevention (CDC) classified only 12.1 percent of hospital emergency department visits as nonurgent in 2006" (ACEP, 2011). The IOM reports on emergency services included in Part 1 discuss these issues.

Clinical Trials and Disparities

The current design and administration of clinical trials in the United States underrepresents certain populations (Mozes, 2008). Participation in clinical studies among African Americans, Hispanics, and older Americans is disproportionately low. Mozes's study indicates that the disparities are largely due to reliance on strict sample inclusion or exclusion criteria, the use of lengthy and complicated consent forms available only in English, and a lack of specific information on cost reimbursement for participants. These disparities can skew treatment recommendations based on studies with inequitable representation in their samples. We need to expand clinical trial participation so research results can better reflect all populations.

Evidence-based practice (EBP) includes consideration of diversity (Wessling, 2008). Because many studies do not include racially diverse participants, it is critical to consider similarities or differences in populations when reviewing evidence, to better ensure effective EBP. This content is relevant to nursing research courses and all courses that integrate EBP.

Disparities in Rural Areas

Typically, care for people who live in rural areas is covered in community health content. The rural population often includes multiple ethnic groups, but the rural population as a whole also experiences disparities in health care (*Healthy People 2020*; South Carolina Rural Health Research Center, 2009):

- In rural areas, poverty rates are two to three times higher for minorities than for Whites.
- 13% of rural whites are poor, compared to 34% of African Americans, 25% of Hispanics, and 34% of Native Americans in rural environments.
- Rural residents are less likely than urban residents to receive preventive health services, and rural Hispanics are significantly less likely than rural non-Hispanic Whites to report receiving preventive medical services.
- 20% of nonmetropolitan counties lack mental health services, compared to 5% of metropolitan counties.
- There are 2,157 health professional shortage areas (HPSAs) in rural America, compared to 910 in urban areas.
- Three out of four rural minorities live in HPSAs, versus three out of five rural Whites.
- About 20% of the U.S. population lives in rural areas, but only 10% of physicians practice in rural America.

Much more must be done to improve care in rural areas. Students need this content in their courses, and if possible clinical experiences in rural areas. The latter is particularly important in states that have large rural populations. The National Rural Health Association provides important current information on this topic that can be used in developing courses and for students to explore (http://www.ruralhealthweb.org/go/left/about-rural-health/what-s-different-about-rural-health-care).

Diversity and The Joint Commission

The Joint Commission published a practical guide that healthcare organizations can use to develop and improve programs and services that accommodate the needs of diverse populations (Joint Commission, 2008). The recommendations of this report include:

- ▮ Build a leadership-driven foundation to establish specific organization-wide policies and procedures for better meeting patients' diverse cultural and language needs.
- ▮ Collect and use data to assess community and patient needs and improve current cultural and language services (such as interpreter services, spiritual services, and dietary services).
- ▮ Accommodate the needs of specific populations through a continuous process of targeting culturally competent initiatives to those needs; include staff training and education, patient education, and other strategies that help patients better manage their care.
- ▮ Establish internal and external collaborations with the local community to share information and resources that meet the needs of diverse patients.

The report is available online, along with other Joint Commission resources on diverse patient populations, at http://www.jointcommission.org/Advancing_Effective_Communication/

Workforce Diversity

National League for Nursing (NLN) data for 2005–2006 (March 3, 2008) indicate that the percentage of graduating prelicensed students who are members of racial or ethnic minority groups increased from 2008 to 2009 (NLN, 2009). There was also an increase in the percentage of men. This is good news, but much more remains to be done regarding workforce diversity. An increasing number of grant opportunities are aimed at increasing the mix of ethnic groups among nurses so they can provide more culturally sensitive, appropriate care. Data about the nursing workforce also indicate more diversity. HRSA reports that in 2008, 16.8% of nurses were Asian, Black/African American, American Indian/Alaska Native, and/or Hispanic, which is an increase from 12.2% in 2004 (HRSA, 2010).

The National Healthcare Disparities Report (NHDR)

As mentioned in Part 1, there is a pressing need to monitor healthcare disparities (IOM, 2002). The annual report is available at www.ahrq.gov/qual/qrdr10.htm. The current report focuses on three questions (AHRQ, 2010a, 2010b):
- ▮ What is the status of healthcare quality and disparities in the United States?
- ▮ How have healthcare quality and disparities changed over time?
- ▮ Where is the need to improve healthcare quality and reduce disparities greatest?

Figure 5-3 describes the most current matrix for the report. The matrix has changed since the first IOM report on disparities, which was described in Part 1. The annual report matrix provides an excellent tool for students to understand the issues and to use the annual report data.

Crosscutting Dimensions		Component of Quality Care	Types of Care		
			Preventive Care	Acute Treatment	Chronic Condition Management
EQUITY	VALUE	Effectiveness			
		Safety			
		Timeliness			
		Patient/Family Centeredness			
		Access			
		Efficiency			
		Care Coordination			
		Health Systems Infrastructure Capabilities			

Source: Institute of Medicine. (2010). *Future directions for the National Healthcare Quality and Disparities Reports*. Committee on Future Directions of the National Healthcare Quality and Disparities Reports, Institute of Medicine. Washington, DC: National Academies Press.

F I G U R E   5 - 3   Quality Framework for the 2010 NHQR and NHDR

Since 2003, the Agency for Healthcare Research and Quality (AHRQ) has prepared the NHDR. The annual report analyzes racial, ethnic, socioeconomic, and geographic disparities in health care. The IOM recommendations for this annual report included (IOM, 2002, p. 7):

▌ Analyze racial and ethnic disparities, considering socioeconomic status;
▌ Conduct research to determine how best to measure socioeconomic status as it relates to healthcare access, service use, and quality;
▌ Recognize that access is a critical element of healthcare quality;
▌ Measure high and low use of certain healthcare services (include data state by state);
▌ Work with public and private organizations that provide data to increase standardization; and
▌ Provide AHRQ with resources to compile an annual survey of disparity in health care, the National Healthcare Disparities Report (NHDR).

(See Teaching–Learning Module 28, National Healthcare Disparities Monitoring, for more information about healthcare disparities.)

Cultural Competence

A paper from AACN (2008a) describes background and content that should be considered in baccalaureate programs to facilitate cultural competence. This document complements *Essentials of Baccalaureate Education for Professional Nursing Practice* (AACN, 2008b). The AACN cultural competence toolkit identifies five competencies for culturally competent care and content recommendations. The competencies are (2008a, pp. 2–3).

1. Apply knowledge of social and cultural factors that affect nursing and health care across multiple contexts.
2. Use relevant data sources and best evidence in providing culturally competent care.
3. Promote achievement of safe and quality outcomes of care for diverse populations.
4. Advocate for social justice, including commitment to the health of vulnerable populations and the elimination of health disparities.
5. Participate in continuous cultural competent development.

Disparities can be a difficult topic for faculty and students. Healthcare providers view themselves as caring people who are open. "Discourse on provider bias has been silent in healthcare literature. Medicine and nursing as predominantly White professions have failed to acknowledge the White domination inherent in and perpetuated by its research, clinical, and educational practices" (Byrne, 2000; Feagin & Vera, 1995, as cited in Baldwin, 2003, p. 8). Students need opportunities to discuss these issues in a safe environment—one in which their opinions will not be negatively criticized, but rather will be used to develop professional attitudes and behaviors. For example, students need to understand that many patients mistrust the healthcare system because they have experienced bias from healthcare providers in the past, which affects future encounters. Communication is a critical element, and health literacy also plays a major role in disparities. (Information about health literacy is covered in this section.)

"The process of developing cultural competence is a means of responding effectively to the huge ethnic and racial demographic shifts and changes that are confronting our country's healthcare system. Cultural competence is a defined set of policies, behaviors, attitudes, and practices that enable individuals and organizations to work effectively in cross-cultural situations. Cultural competence is the ability of systems to provide care to patients with diverse values, beliefs, and behaviors, including the tailoring of delivery to meet patients' social, cultural, and linguistic needs" (Salisbury & Byrd, 2006, p. 90). The American Association of Colleges of Nursing (AACN) strongly supports teaching cultural competence in baccalaureate education, as stated in *The Essentials of Baccalaureate Education for Professional Nursing Practice* (AACN, 2008b)—a viewpoint that clearly derives from the IOM reports on diversity and healthcare disparities. Another definition of *cultural competence* is the "attitudes, knowledge, and skills necessary for providing quality care to diverse populations" (California Endowment, 2003, as cited in AACN, 2008b, p. 1). *The Essentials of Masters Education in Nursing* also emphasizes the need for cultural competence in its Essential VIII, which "recognizes that the master's-prepared nurse applies and integrates broad, organizational, client-centered, and *culturally appropriate* concepts in the planning, delivery, management, and evaluation of evidence-based clinical prevention and population care and services to individuals, families, and aggregates/identified populations" (AACN, 2011, p. 5).

Cultural competence must be integrated in the curriculum. This perspective is based on the following assumptions (AACN, 2008b, pp. 2–3; Paasche-Orlow, 2004):

- Liberal education for nurses provides a foundation of intellectual skills and capacities for learning and working with diverse populations and contexts.
- Faculty with requisite attitudes, knowledge, and skills can develop relevant culturally diverse learning experiences.
- Development of cultural competence in students and faculty occurs best in environments supportive of diversity and facilitated by guided experiences with diversity.
- Cultural competence is grounded in the appreciation of the profound influence of culture in people's lives, and the commitment to minimize the negative responses of healthcare providers to these differences.
- Cultural competence results in improved measurable outcomes, which includes the perspectives of those served.

The AACN also provides a toolkit for culturally competent education at www.aacn.nche.edu/education-resources/toolkit.pdf

Campinha-Bacote (2003) developed a cultural competence assessment tool in versions for staff and students. It is based on Campinha-Bacote's volcano model of the process of cultural competence in the delivery of healthcare services, which defines *cultural competence* as "the process in which the healthcare professional continually strives to achieve the ability and availability to effectively work within the cultural context of a client" (Campinha-Bacote, 2008). It is a process of *becoming* culturally competent, not *being* culturally competent. Campinha-Bacote's model of cultural competence views cultural awareness, cultural knowledge, cultural skill, cultural encounters, and cultural desire as the five constructs of cultural competence. The five constructs are:

- *Cultural awareness,* defined as the process of conducting a self-examination of one's own biases toward other cultures and the in-depth exploration of one's cultural and professional background. Cultural awareness also involves being aware of the existence of documented racism and other "isms" in healthcare delivery.
- *Cultural knowledge,* defined as the process in which the healthcare professional seeks and obtains a sound information base regarding the worldviews of different cultural and ethnic groups, as well as biological variations, diseases and health conditions, and variations in drug metabolism found among ethnic groups (biocultural ecology).
- *Cultural skill,* the ability to conduct a cultural assessment to collect relevant cultural data regarding the client's presenting problem, and to accurately conduct a culturally based physical assessment.

- *Cultural encounters,* the process that encourages the healthcare professional to directly engage in face-to-face cultural interactions and other types of encounters with clients from culturally diverse backgrounds in order to modify existing beliefs about a cultural group and to prevent possible stereotyping.
- *Cultural desire,* the motivation of the healthcare professional to "want to"—rather than "have to"—engage in the process of becoming culturally aware, culturally knowledgeable, and culturally skillful and to seek cultural encounters. Cultural desire is the spiritual and pivotal construct of cultural competence that provides the energy source and foundation for the healthcare professional's journey toward cultural competence. This model views cultural competence as a volcano, which symbolically represents cultural desire as stimulating the process of cultural competence. When cultural desire erupts, it powers entry into the process of becoming culturally competent by genuinely seeking cultural encounters, obtaining cultural knowledge, conducting culturally sensitive assessments, and being humble in the process of cultural awareness.

Healthcare Literacy

Healthcare literacy is "the ability to read, understand, and act on healthcare information" (IOM, 2004a, p. 52). Health literacy should be carefully considered in the creation and use of teaching materials for patients and families. In particular, because students teach patients, students need to learn how to assess patient understanding and to make changes as required. Showing students examples of medical forms and information can help them appreciate that the information is not always so easy to understand, even for people whose first language is English!

An investigation of the relationship between health literacy and adherence to clinical outcomes reviewed 44 studies (DeWalt et al., 2004). Some of the findings from this review are:

- People who have low literacy are 1.5 to 3 times more likely to have adverse outcomes than those with higher literacy.
- Medicare enrollees with lower literacy have a greater chance of never having a Pap smear, not getting a mammogram within the past two years, and not receiving influenza and pneumococcal immunizations than those with higher health literacy.
- Lower literacy is associated with increased risk for hospitalization.

Health illiteracy is more common in vulnerable populations such as low-income or racial and ethnic minorities (Ferguson, 2008). Women influence the health of children because they are mostly the caregivers. If women's health literacy is low, this puts these women's children at risk. Pregnant women who do not understand health information can affect the fetus and the infant's health and development after birth (Puchner, 1995; Ferguson, 2008). The major barriers to quality health care associated with health literacy are inabilities to access care, manage illness, and process information (DeWalt & Pignone, 2008).

1. *Accessing care*: Critical issues are obtaining health insurance; finding healthcare providers; and knowing when to seek health care. For example, finding contact information, making appointments, and keeping a record of appointments may all be difficult for someone who cannot read or write.

2. *Managing illness*: Managing illness today, whether acute or chronic illness, can be complex; it may involve complicated prescription recommendations, testing schedules, and appointments with different providers at different places. Patients need to know the right questions to ask, as information is often not freely shared. Healthcare transitions (*handoffs*) are very common; patients move from provider to provider even within the same healthcare organization, increasing the risk of errors but also requiring the patient to adapt to changes and new providers. (Handoffs are discussed later in the content about the quality improvement core competency.)

3. *Processing information*: Patients are presented with informed consents and other documents, often written in a manner they cannot understand, especially under stressful situations. Family members can be very helpful with this type of information. Medical bills can easily overwhelm someone even if the person reads English well; for those who do not, the inability to read and comprehend bills can lead to major problems and stress.

Patient advocacy can make a major difference in helping patients and families who are experiencing health literacy problems. One of the goals of *Healthy People 2020* is to improve consumer health literacy. The Food and Drug Administration has also made changes to regulate drug information and improve health literacy. A good source to illustrate to students the importance of labeling and health literacy is the American College of Physicians Foundation's (2007) white paper on drug container labeling. Limited health literacy leads to higher outpatient medication errors, possible complications, increased costs, and inability to reach positive outcomes.

As noted in the National Assessment of Adult Literacy in the United States, 14% of the population is at the basic literacy level, with 29% below basic, and the ability to use numbers is even lower (National Center for Education Statistics, 2003). Five percent are not literate in English, and with the increasing number of immigrants, this percentage is likely to increase in many areas of the country. "The Joint Commission's accreditation standards underscore the fundamental right and need for patients to receive information—both orally and written—about their care in a way in which they can understand this information" (Joint Commission, 2007, p. 5). Some of the means to improve health literacy identified by The Joint Commission are:

▍ Create patient-centered environments where the patient is involved in decision-making and safety processes;

- Increase awareness and understanding of health literacy;
- Ensure that interpreters are available when needed;
- Develop cultural competence;
- Understand how communication affects quality care;
- Teach consumers how to better access the care they need;
- Review and improve informed consent materials and processes;
- Use a disease management approach to better individualize care and reduce errors;
- Standardize handoffs; and
- Give patients clear information.

Faculty should use these examples in the development of content and teaching–learning strategies to improve student cultural competence, and thus improve patient-centered care competence. (See Teaching–Learning Module 28, National Healthcare Disparities Monitoring, for more information about healthcare disparities.)

Health Literacy and Self-Management

Students need to understand that self-management will not be effective if the patient has a low level of health literacy. Ask the student to explain why. What skills does the patient need to manage his diabetes or her arthritis? Include health literacy problems in case examples related to adult health, pediatrics, mental health, obstetrics, and community/public health. This will help students to appreciate that health literacy issues can arise in all types of situations and can have an important impact on care and outcomes.

Students may have a difficult time appreciating what health literacy means and how it affects patient care. First, ask students to define health literacy. Have them compare the definition of health literacy used in the IOM report with their own. Students may then need assistance imagining the stigma that illiterate patients may feel. Role-play may be useful here. Provide students with information such as an admission form or patient education forms; then ask a student in the role of the nurse to teach a patient, played by another student, about a disease and give the patient the written information. This information could actually be in another language (most hospitals have this information at least in Spanish), which would give the student a more realistic experience. However, even material in English can be a challenge to understand, even to a native speaker. Another student might act as an observer and critique the interaction. Afterward, discuss how the students felt and what was observed. Ask the students how the inability to read or understand prescriptions or discharge instructions might be dangerous. For example, in Spanish *once per day* translates to *una vez por día*. However, the English word *once* is spelled exactly like the Spanish word for *eleven*. So, a Spanish speaker trying to read an English prescription could think that the patient needs the medication 11 times per day. This exercise also ties in with the IOM themes of quality of care, particularly the quality element of patient safety.

Interpreters

If possible, students should work with an interpreter to facilitate communication with a patient. Students can experience the frustration of trying to communicate through a third party, and then discuss how it feels. They need guidance in using interpreters; for example, the student should speak directly to the patient, even though the natural tendency is to speak to the interpreter. This is also a good time to discuss the advantages and disadvantages of depending on family members as interpreters. What might be the impact of a culture in which the husband makes decisions? Would the wife feel comfortable expressing herself, and would the husband try to soften difficult messages? Would it be better to use a native speaker or a language expert to interpret? Discuss the options if no interpreter is available: finding a healthcare provider who speaks the language, working with community groups to help interpret, preparing visual materials that might aid communication, and so on.

Health Literacy and Health Education

It is important to connect health literacy with health education. Give students consent forms, admission forms, and patient rights information, and let them assess their own ability to understand those forms and documents. Ask them what might interfere with reading and understanding what they have read. What would help them understand the documents better? Students have some healthcare background, but what about patients and families who have none? During clinical experiences, ask students how health literacy might affect their teaching of specific assigned patients. This can also be done during pre- and post-conferences. When students develop health education plans for individual patients, families, caregivers, or groups, they should consider assessment of health literacy issues in the assignment. Make sure this assessment is included in the plan of care.

Health Literacy and the Healthcare Delivery System

What is done in a specific healthcare organization to address health literacy? How do health agencies used for clinical experiences respond to health literacy in their patient information and education programs? Students can gather information by observation, interviewing staff, and reviewing written materials and other types of educational materials (such as videos that might be shown to patients). Are interpreters available, and are they used? Is hearing-impaired equipment accessible, and is it used? Look at signs and their effectiveness (for example, the use of color to direct patients). Students can then discuss what they have learned, what could be improved, and how to change the environment so all patients can be understood and can better understand healthcare providers. This content and activities could be part of a leadership and management course; emphasized in content about how healthcare organizations address diversity.

Health Literacy, Nursing Assessment, and Interventions

Students can assess health literacy levels with a population group in their community or an agency and its patients, identifying problems and interventions that might have been taken and outcomes, and consider other types of interventions that might improve health literacy. Health literacy should be part of individual patient assessments. Is health literacy included in the assessments expected of students? How should this assessment be done? Is it part of a healthcare organization's standard assessment forms? Compare assessment forms from different healthcare organizations or different services within an organization.

What is the best way to assess patient health literacy? The typical response would be to identify years of school completed or birth location. However, Rapid Estimate of Adult Literacy in Medicine (REALM), a standardized tool that takes only five minutes to administer, is a more effective method (Baker, 2007).

Pain Management

Pain is a major healthcare problem, with 116 million adults in the United States experiencing common chronic pain conditions, at a conservatively estimated annual cost of $560 to $635 billion (IOM, 2011h). "Pain can be conceptualized as a public health challenge for a number of important reasons having to do with prevalence, seriousness, disparities, vulnerable populations, the utility of population health strategies, and the importance of prevention at both the population and individual levels" (IOM, 2011h, p. 55). In addition, *Healthy People 2020* includes an objective related to pain: Increase the safe and effective treatment of pain. Health literacy is related to pain management. "Problems with understanding medication instructions contribute to the estimated 1.5 million preventable adverse drug events that occur each year" (IOM, 2011h, p. 66). There are also disparities in who receives effective treatment for pain, as discussed in the IOM reports on pain management. Patient education is a critical intervention, and one that directly involves nurses. The IOM notes the important roles that nurses have in providing care for patients with pain, describing pain management as an essential responsibility of nurses. Nurses can also be involved in research to improve care for pain, particularly interprofessional research.

Pain management has long been a part of nursing curricula, though all teaching institutions should review their content and placement of content to ensure that it is as up-to-date as possible. The IOM identified pain management as a critical part of patient-centered care, and published a report on pain (2011h) as discussed in Part 1. This IOM report is an excellent resource for faculty and students, providing background information on pain as well as viewing pain as a public health challenge. The report describes the picture of pain, identifying the many different types of people with pain in an excellent figure (IOM, 2011h, Figure 1-1). The report makes several recommendations:

- **Recommendation 3.1.** Promote and enable self-management of pain.
- **Recommendation 3.2.** Develop strategies for reducing barriers to pain care.
- **Recommendation 3.3.** Provide education opportunities in pain assessment and treatment in primary care.
- **Recommendation 3.4.** Support collaboration between pain specialists and primary care clinicians, including referral to pain centers when appropriate.

- **Recommendation 3.5.** Revise reimbursement policies to foster coordinated and evidence-based pain care.
- **Recommendation 3.6.** Provide consistent and complete pain assessments.

End-of-Life and Palliative Care

End-of-life and palliative care are two topics that are finding their way into more nursing curricula. The IOM includes these topics in its description of patient-centered care, and published a report called *Improving Palliative Care for Cancer: Summary and Recommendations* (2003c). This report is a good resource for faculty and students. According to this IOM report, the healthcare system continues to underrecognize, underdiagnose, and undertreat patients who experience significant suffering from their illness. "Palliative care focuses on addressing the control of pain and other symptoms, as well as psychological, social, and spiritual distress. Six major skill sets comprise complete palliative care" (IOM, 2003c, p. 3):

1. Communication
2. Decision-making
3. Management of complications of treatment and the disease
4. Symptom control
5. Psychosocial care of the dying
6. Care of the dying

Students need to have an understanding of these important aspects of care, the barriers to providing effective care, interventions that can assist patients and families. They also should experience an open dialogue about provider aspects of responses to patients who require this care.

Consumer Perspectives

Staying healthy, getting better, living with illness or disability, and coping with the end of life represent the consumer dimension described in the IOM report on the need to monitor healthcare quality (IOM, 2003f). They are also important parts of nursing care. The consumer perspective may help students remember these elements when working with patients and their families. Ask students to explore what each of the components of the quality framework (discussed in more detail in the quality improvement core competency section in this part) really means in practice. Patients may be asked to talk with students about the implications of these perspectives in their own lives. What do they mean to a person with diabetes, mental illness, or breast cancer, or to a family with a newborn? These perspectives can help students working with individuals, families, or groups in a variety of healthcare settings and in the community have a better appreciation of PCC.

Privacy, Confidentiality, HIPAA

The topics of privacy, confidentiality, and HIPAA relate to patient-centered care and should be introduced early in the curriculum when patient-centered care is introduced.

In addition, the content should be integrated throughout the curriculum. The critical issue is that *the patient makes decisions about his or her health care.* Healthcare providers share their expertise and recommendations, but do not make the decisions; a patient may decide to defer to the healthcare professional, but it should never be assumed that the patient will do so. Student also need to clearly understand all aspects of patient information use and sharing. For example, they should investigate the ramifications of electronic communication within the course: the issue of taking photos with cell phones while in clinical areas and then sharing them through social media networks, as well as telling friends on Facebook, Twitter, and the like about patients they have cared for in enough detail that the agency, patient, and/or staff could be identified. This topic can be expanded to cover electronic (and other) communication throughout the healthcare delivery system.

Patient Advocacy

"There is a growing appreciation of the centrality of patient involvement as a contributor to positive healthcare outcomes and as a catalyst for change in healthcare delivery" (IOM, 2007e, p. 25). It is difficult to discuss patient-centered care without considering patient advocacy. A patient advocate is "the patient navigator, both in its aim to help and guide patients to make well-informed decisions about their health for the best outcomes and in its quest to create more effective systems and policies" (Earp, French, & Gilkey, 2008, p. xv). Earlier sections discussed some of the critical characteristics of patient-centered care as described by IOM. Gerteis, Edgman-Levitan, Daley, and Delbanco (1993) describe dimensions of patient-centered care as:

▪ Respect for patients' values, preferences, and expressed needs
▪ Coordination and integration of care among providers and healthcare institutions
▪ Information, communication, and education tailored to patients' needs
▪ Physical comfort, especially freedom from pain
▪ Emotional support to reduce the fear and worry associated with illness and treatment
▪ Involvement of family and friends in caregiving and decision-making
▪ Planning for transition and continuity to ensure that patients continue to heal after they leave the hospital

The three overarching goals of patient advocacy are patient-centered care, safer medical systems, and increased patient involvement (Gilkey, Earp, & French, 2008). Safety, as highlighted in the IOM reports, is critical, and there is greater need to bring the patient into the safety process (as discussed further regarding the quality improvement core competency). All three patient advocacy goals are related, and patient involvement is necessary for success of advocacy.

Patients have not always been welcomed into the healthcare process. Patients need to be partners in their own care; they have important information to share and must be involved in the decisions. Patient–provider communication plays a key role in meeting all three goals of patient advocacy. Patient advocacy can be described as a continuum (Gilkey, Earp, & French, 2008).

- The *individual level*, which is the central level, emphasizes informing patients. The more patients know about their health and illness, the better they can participate in their care decisions and care.
- The *interpersonal level* supports and empowers patients by connecting them with people who can help them and from whom they can get information. Patient–provider information is important at this level, where providers are concerned not just with biological but also with psychosocial issues and social, cultural, and financial factors that influence health and needs. Family and friends are also important.
- The *organizational and community level*, which transforms the healthcare culture as to where, when, and how care is delivered.
- The last is the *policy level*, where the consumer's voice is translated into policy and law to ensure that patient advocacy is maintained.

The key strategies to meet the three patient advocacy goals are as follows (Earp, French, & Gilkey, 2008, pp. v–vii):

- Understanding what patients are doing now and what providers can do to support them
- Improving providers' ability to communicate and create relationships
- Making consumers' voices heard in policy and law
- Advancing education and professional roles in advocacy
- Transforming hospital and medical school culture (and nursing schools) to support patient- and family-centered care

Nursing should be part of this strategy, particularly this last item. Nurses describe themselves as patient advocates, but in this major publication on patient advocacy there were no nurse authors, and nursing is mentioned only in the beginning of the book. The book is based on a large conference on patient advocacy that was held in 2003 and 2005; it is notable that nursing did not have a leadership role.

Students need to understand patient advocacy, their own role, and strategies to improve advocacy. Patients can help teach students; explain about illness and care experiences; help to create more effective patient teaching materials; and participate on health boards, advisory committees, and other types of health organizations, providing valuable input in each instance. Faculty need to discuss advocacy in relevant content and in clinical experiences. Some students have had patient experiences either of their own or through members of their families. These can be used to discuss the need for patient advocacy.

Patient Etiquette: How Does This Relate to Patient-Centered Care?

Patient etiquette may seem like a strange topic, but it is relevant to patient-centered care. Kahn (2008) discusses the need for etiquette-based medicine, but it seems to get lost in quite a few nursing education programs and experiences. Students need to be taught to treat patients with respect; we cannot assume that they will do this automatically or naturally. This is also part of the nursing profession's image. Kahn provides a checklist and suggests that medical students be taught to use it. It includes items such as: ask permission to enter the room and wait for an answer; introduce yourself, shake hands, sit down, and smile as appropriate; briefly explain your role on the team, or ask patients how they are feeling and how they feel about their illness and the care they have received. This would "[p]ut professionalism and patient satisfaction at the center of the clinical encounter and bring back some of the elements of ritual that have always been an important part of the healing process" (Kahn, 2008, p. 1988). Nursing students need to be reminded to talk with patients and families in a manner that demonstrates respect for the patient and the patient's values and preferences (patient-centered care).

Patient Education

Patient education is a complex process and should be included in all nursing curricula. If a patient does not have enough information, this can affect care. Some areas that require patient education are identified in the IOM reports, such as tobacco, alcohol, high-fat foods, and firearm injuries. Nurses in community settings typically include such topics in community education, but patients in other settings also need similar counseling. Patient education must be culturally sensitive because the meanings of health, illness, and death are not the same everywhere. For example, some Muslim families believe that this plane of life is just one level of existence, and thus resuscitating the patient is not as important as honoring the predestination of life events. The saving of locks of hair or pictures of Indian babies who are dying is not culturally accepted in all families; some believe that these mementos bind the child to this earthly world and do not allow the child to reach the next.

Keeping the patient in the center of care means that we need to consider what the patient feels is important and listen to the patient. Patient, family, or community health education should also address safety issues such as prevention of medication errors, and its relationship to self-management of care. Health literacy must be considered when patient education is planned, implemented, and evaluated.

Family or Caregiver Roles: Family-Centered Care

Patient advocacy and patient-centered care are directly related to family-centered care. "Family-centered care is a partnership approach to the planning, delivery, and evaluation of health care and is grounded in a belief that each participant in a clinical encounter brings valuable experience to the table" (Seyda, Shelton, & DiVenere, 2008, p. 64). One cannot assume that all patients want their families involved, nor can one take for granted what level of involvement there will be and what information may be shared with the family. Patients must be asked about this before steps are taken to communicate with and include the family. The core principles of family-centered care are dignity and respect, information sharing, participation, and collaboration. As with patient-centered care, the overall goal is better outcomes. Family-centered care is "increasingly linked to improved health outcomes, lower healthcare costs, more effective allocation of resources, reduced medical errors and litigation, greater patient, family, and professional satisfaction, increased patient/family self-efficacy/advocacy, and improved medical/health education" (Seyda, Shelton, & DiVenere, 2008, p. 66).

Family-centered care is most likely thought of as relevant only to children's health, but it applies to all patients. The family will naturally be involved in the support of a dying patient, such as hospice care; and in caring for older family members, a growing responsibility in the United States. Families can be very important in preventing errors; they have valuable information for healthcare providers and may observe as care is provided—asking questions, noting differences, and so on. This can lead to fewer errors and improved communication that reduces the likelihood of litigation.

The Patient-Centered Medical Home Model: A New View of Primary Care

The American Academy of Pediatrics (2007) describes the medical home as a model of delivering primary care that is accessible, continuous, comprehensive, family-centered, coordinated, compassionate, and culturally effective. This same model can be applied to adults. The Association of American Medical Colleges (AAMC) also describes the medical home. "Every person should have access to a medical home—a person who serves as a trusted advisor and provider supported by a coordinated team—with whom they have a continuous relationship. The medical home promotes prevention; provides care for most problems and serves as the point of first-contact for that care; coordinates care with other providers and community resources when necessary; integrates care across the health system; and provides care and health education in a culturally competent manner in the context of family and community" (AAMC, 2008).

The medical home model is based on patient-centered care. Individualized care is preventive and manages chronic illness. Same-day appointments and expanded appointment hours are more available; tools like secure e-mail enhance communication; prescriptions are transmitted electronically; and electronic health records (EHRs) are used. Students can explore and learn more about this concept at http://www.medicalhomeinfo.org. What would be the nurse's role, both ANPs and non-ANPs, in this model? Ask students to research information about medical homes and consider how this new model might affect nursing roles and responsibilities.

Patient- and Family-Centered Rounds

Patient- and family-centered rounds lead to greater patient-centered care (Siserhen, Blaszak, Woods, & Smith, 2007). This should be an interprofessional approach. If, however, nursing staff do not attend these rounds—which they should—then nursing can change nursing rounds only. Rounds should also include the patient's family if the patient does not object. Engaging the family is important when the family is a significant part of the patient's life, but in some cases patients may not want family members to hear the information. Students should participate in these important learning opportunities. They demonstrate the impact of care that includes the family, interprofessional teams, communication, coordination, and collaboration. Ask students to reflect on the experience and identify examples from the rounds where these activities were evident. It is also important to prepare students for rounds—communication methods, general process of rounds, and so on. This could be practiced in the simulation lab.

Gerontology

We must recognize that the world's population is aging and that, to provide quality care, we need to educate nurses to meet the special needs of older adults. The IOM recognized the importance of care for the elderly and the chronically ill in the priority areas of care. As noted in *Retooling for an Aging America* (IOM, 2008c), there is a growing need to educate staff so they can effectively care for the older adult. There are greater funding opportunities for research and programs. Gerontology should be integrated into all nursing programs.

Clinical Prevention and Population Health: Curricular Framework for Health Professionals

The *Essentials for Baccalaureate Nursing Education* includes "Clinical Prevention and Population Health" as one of the nine essential curricular areas. The *Essentials for Doctoral Education* also includes this (Maeshiro et al., (2011). The Association for Prevention Teaching and Research (APTR) has resources for faculty for the development of curriculum in relationship to *Healthy People 2020*. Information can be found at http://atpm.org/educationforhealth/index.html. "Going forward, all health professional schools—medicine, nursing, pharmacy, dentistry, and physical therapy, to name a few—can reaffirm the priority of population health and interdisciplinary [interprofessional] learning. Evidence-based thinking approaches in both discipline-specific and public health graduate programs can also gently push students to consider the social determinants in all aspects of their work" (Koh, Nowinski, & Piotrowski, 2011, p. 201). There is need for public health leadership that is responsible, uses social strategy and political will, and has interpersonal skill.

Nursing faculty should use the revised Clinical Prevention and Population Health Curriculum Framework to improve this content in curricula. "The Curriculum Framework provides a structure for organizing curriculum, monitoring curriculum, and communicating within and among professions. It is designed to provide guidelines for student education in the clinical health professions represented on the Healthy People Curriculum Task Force, but can be adapted by other health professions disciplines to suit their needs. The Framework consists of four components" (APTR, 2009):

1. Evidence-based practice
2. Clinical preventive services and health promotion
3. Health systems and health policy
4. Population health and community aspects of practice

The framework includes 19 domains and also teaching methods and materials. The full framework can be obtained from www.aptrweb.org/educationforhealth/

Revised_CPPH_Framework_2009.pdf. The web site for APTR (http://www.aptrweb.org) includes a number of resources for faculty on this topic.

This type of initiative illustrates the impact of the IOM reports, in this case the public health reports. Some of the reports describe the current state of public health and the need for changes. Combining them with the focus on *Healthy People 2020*, we are again reminded of the need to look at our curricula from the perspective of populations and health promotion and prevention for all healthcare professions. (See Teaching–Learning Module 21, *Healthy People 2020*, for more information on that topic.)

Core Competency: Work on Interdisciplinary/ Interprofessional Teams

Cooperate, collaborate, communicate, and integrate care in teams to ensure that care is continuous and reliable (IOM, 2003b, p. 4).

Interprofessional teams work collaboratively and collegially, not in parallel. No health professional plans any aspect of care in isolation; instead, all team members should work together to plan and implement care.

Teamwork

Salmon states, "I must say, I have grown tired of us saying that we are making major strides in collaboration and partnership with others beyond nursing. I worry that we in nursing have fought so hard for our professional identity and autonomy that we see being separate from others as a condition for future success. I see our separateness as antithetical to our most basic professional values. How can we reconcile our commitment to providing the best possible care when we still grapple with the place that nursing assistants, technicians, and others have in relation to our work" (Salmon, 2007, p. 117).

Just as Salmon noted, working in interprofessional teams is a difficult competency to accomplish when we continue to separate all education by professions. We keep healthcare professions separate in most U.S. universities and other types of educational programs. Students are socialized in isolation. This all affects the quality of care. When healthcare providers do not know how to communicate with one another; when we have abusive language and conflict; when we do not understand our different roles and responsibilities and thus do not know how to make the most of what each profession can offer; when we work against each other rather than with each other to provide care; and when we speak different languages or terminologies, we undermine quality, safe care and are unable to provide patient-centered care. The National Council of State Boards of Nursing (NCSBN) reported that "when newly licensed nurses did not work effectively with a healthcare team or did not know when and how to call a patient's physician, they were more likely to report being involved in patient errors" (Smith & Crawford, 2003, as cited in NCSBN, 2005, p. 5). We are going to have to be creative about developing effective strategies to achieve the competency of working in teams.

Every student needs both knowledge and experience working on teams. Schools of nursing typically include some of this content in their courses, though much more is needed, as is more experience in real teamwork. Simulations can model teams so that students can experience teams in a safe learning environment. Students also need guidance and opportunities to discuss team experience. They can be assigned to staff teams and also observe teams on a unit and then discuss their observations. (See Teaching–Learning Module 42, Teams and Quality Improvement, and Module 43, TeamSTEPPS, for more information about teams and QI and TeamSTEPPS.)

Care Coordination

Care coordination or adherence to care coordination must be a topic in all courses and clinical experiences from the very beginning of every nursing program, whether undergraduate or graduate (Craig, Eby, & Whittington, 2011). What are the roles of the nurse and the roles of other team members—nursing staff and other healthcare professionals? How can care coordination be improved? What is the integrator role that some nurses play? What can nurses do to improve interprofessional care coordination? How does this role affect adherence to treatment plans and quality of care? It is vital to ask students specific questions about coordination in clinical settings to stimulate them to use critical thinking and clinical reasoning and judgment and to consider the need for coordination. When students prepare care plans, they should be expected to address care coordination. When they participate in analyzing case studies and in simulations, students should be expected to respond to questions related to care coordination.

Interprofessional Collaborative Teams

Precursors to collaboration are individual clinical competence and mutual trust and respect. Collaboration requires shared understanding of goals and roles, shared decision-making, and conflict management. Students need formal experience with collaboration so that they can receive support and guidance from faculty. They must learn how to have a respectful professional dialogue that considers different perspectives. Students also need to understand that although the history of nursing has fostered permissive, submissive language and actions, these do not constitute effective professional communication (Gordon, 2005).

Transformational Leadership

Transformational leadership is highly regarded today, and the IOM reports (for example, *Leadership by Example*, 2003d) consider it the best leadership approach. This, however, does not mean that it is easy to implement; it is not. Students need to understand leadership and followership and appreciate how they respond both as leaders and as followers. What makes an effective leader and an effective follower?

Most organizations are in a state of perpetual change. It is necessary to engage students in discussions about how they respond to change. They will soon have to step up, take a stand, and be leaders, and this should begin while they are students. What is empowerment, and why is it important to nurses? Shared governance is one approach that may develop a productive work climate. When students are in healthcare organizations for practicum, faculty need to guide students by asking questions about leadership and organizational effectiveness within the organization. How does the organization respond to change? How well does the staff trust leadership? Why would this be important to know before taking a new position? Ask students to consider the need for a close fit between their personal values and the values and mission of the organization. Ask about whistleblowing regulations and the implications if a student decides to be a real agent for change. Leadership content is found in all nursing programs in leadership and management courses, but it should be a critical thread throughout the curriculum and also in graduate curricula. Leadership can be emphasized in any course. In addition, we tend to put leadership and management courses at the end of undergraduate programs and thus miss all the opportunities to apply this content throughout the curriculum.

Allied Health Team Members

Nursing students need to understand the roles of all possible team members, including allied health members. The IOM addressed the issue of the growing number of allied healthcare providers in a workshop in 2011. One of the key issues was defining *allied healthcare providers*. "According to Title 42 of the U.S. Code, an allied health professional is a health professional other than a registered nurse or physician assistant who has a certificate, associate's degree, bachelor's degree, master's degree, doctoral degree, or post-baccalaureate training in a science relating to health care and who shares in the responsibility for the delivery of health care services or related services, including:

- services related to the identification, evaluation, and prevention of diseases and disorders;
- dietary and nutrition services;
- health promotion services;
- rehabilitation services; or
- health system management services."

The definition excludes those with a "degree in medicine, osteopathy, dentistry, veterinary medicine, optometry, podiatric medicine, pharmacy, public health, chiropractic, health administration, clinical psychology, social work, or counseling" (IOM, 2011a, p. 2).

Faculty can ask students to search for information about allied health roles and responsibilities and then discuss how the team works together with different types of providers. When students first go into healthcare settings, faculty should ask students to identify different team members and to observe what they do with patients and their responsibilities as members of the healthcare team.

Communication

Communication is a complex process that is integrated into everything done in healthcare delivery. Aspects that typically cause problems are team communication, written communication, issues of verbal abuse among staff, and patient-clinician communication.

Student Communication Requirements

Clinical documentation and paperwork seem only to increase, and this profusion of paperwork also plagues schools of nursing. Students typically spend much of their time on written assignments. It is often difficult for faculty to step back and ask whether the assignments are helpful and whether they aid learning, meet course objectives, or develop competencies. What is the student perspective on the assignments? Requiring nursing students to write everything down may interfere with their ability to think on their feet, discuss an issue or problem, and use critical thinking and clinical reasoning and judgment. Some written assignments accomplish this, but not all. It is always difficult to give up a course activity after it has become routine, but if schools of nursing are to graduate competent entry-level nurses who can function in an ever-changing healthcare environment, nursing faculty too need to change and be willing to concede that a strategy or learning activity is not yielding expected outcomes.

Team Communication

Team communication is a critical element in meeting patient needs, providing quality care, and reaching effective patient outcomes. It is critically intertwined with healthcare professional roles, ability to work with others, recognition that the team is the best method for reaching required goals, and willingness to compromise, collaborate, and coordinate together. It also has a major impact on errors. (See Teaching–Learning Module 42, Teams and Quality Improvement, and Module 43, TeamSTEPPS, for more information about teams and QI, TeamSTEPPS, and SBAR.)

Written Communication

The team should be an important element of the discussion of communication. Teams do not just communicate orally. It is easy for students to view documentation as something done to communicate nurse to nurse; however, there is much more to written communication. It helps the entire healthcare team to communicate the plan of care, what has been done, and outcomes. Not only is documentation important to all the healthcare providers, but it also provides data for quality improvement and is essential to reimbursement. There are important legal implications of documentation and written communication, particularly when there are problems (though this is typically emphasized in curricula). Students need to see all these implications. A source for further discussion and examples of current documentation issues can be found at http://www.medscape.com/viewarticle/754374?src=ptalk

Verbal Abuse

Communication skills are always important and should be developed throughout the curriculum. A growing concern for nurses is verbal abuse from other staff, physicians, and family members. In fact, verbal abuse is cited as one of the reasons that nursing is such a stressful profession. Students need guidance in how to respond and examples of the strategies that some HCOs are using to prevent verbal abuse. Schools of nursing should also establish a policy of no tolerance of verbal abuse from students, faculty, administrators, or staff.

Patient–Clinician Communication

In 2011, the IOM published a brief report on patient–clinician communication, noting its importance to healthcare delivery, particularly quality care (Paget et al., 2011). Seven basic principles should be integrated into this communication.

1. Mutual respect
2. Harmonized goals
3. A supportive environment
4. Appropriate decision partners
5. The right information
6. Transparency and full disclosure
7. Continuous learning.

The IOM report discusses each of these principles, all of which are important for nurse educators to incorporate into learning experiences.

The Joint Commission notes that "ineffective communication is the most cited category of root causes of sentinel events" (2007, p. 2). Communication is closely connected to healthcare literacy, diversity, and patient education. How do we teach patients, and how do we teach students how to provide patient or family education? Effective patient education has become more and more difficult because of the nursing shortage, patients who may not be able to concentrate, short lengths of stay, and the highly stressful healthcare environment that does not allow much time for staff even to talk with patients and families.

Our old methods of patient teaching most likely need revision. Are we considering the communication principles noted earlier in this part? Are we taking full advantage of technology today? Patients are much more involved in all types of technology that could be used for patient education; for example, patients can download patient discharge information into a handheld computer and take the information with them, or access this information on a web site or through e-mail. The Joint Commission strongly supports effective communications, which must be an organization's priority to protect the safety of patients across the continuum of care (Joint Commission, 2007).

Staffing, Teams, and Quality: Maximizing Workforce Capability

The IOM's previous work *Keeping Patients Safe: Transforming the Work Environment for Nurses* (2004b) suggests that the current nursing shortage is a significant risk to patient safety. This report describes nurses as the glue that holds healthcare organizations together at the point of care. Nurses serve as integrators to determine patient needs and alert other professionals who are not at the bedside or in the community clinics, and should actively use patient surveillance. If a nurse does not provide surveillance for the healthcare team, significant patient data are lost, and often physicians and other professionals may not be alerted to impending care problems. Some of the work must be delegated to others, and some must be transformed by technology; however, this requires careful consideration based on education and expertise. Many consider this report the tipping point that allows nursing's contribution to patient outcomes to be quantified. This report was completed long before *The Future of Nursing* (2011d) report, and it is an important document recognizing the needs of the staff nurse, leadership role of the staff nurse and nurse managers (particularly in relationship to quality care), and the work environment. It is this group of nurses who provide most of the care and will have the greatest impact on the quality of care.

Promoting Safe Staffing Levels: Recruitment and Retention

Improving care is possible only if the problems of recruitment and retention are solved. Staff shortages have an impact on how care is provided and how well it meets standards. Nursing students need help building job-hunting skills, such as interviewing, looking for a positive work environment, writing résumés and query letters, and matching a job to their competencies and personal needs. Schools of nursing could also reduce attrition by making clear to students what they may experience during the first year and cultivating skills such as stress management, assertiveness, and problem-solving. Nurse externships and residencies are used by some healthcare organizations to increase recruitment and retention of new graduates, decrease costs related to orientation and turnover, and increase quality of care.

Design of Work Hours and Risks

"The link between healthcare worker fatigue and adverse events is well documented, with substantial number of studies indicating that the practice of extended work hours contributes to high levels of worker fatigue and reduced productivity" (Joint Commission, 2011, p. 1). Students need information about fatigue and its effects on work: slowed reactions, diminished attention to detail, errors of omission, compromised problem-solving, reduced motivation and decreased vigor for successful completion of required tasks, the circadian rhythm, reactions to working a night shift and how shift work is arranged, adjusting to changing hours, and impact on personal lives. Hughes and Rogers (2004) note that fatigue resulting from an inadequate amount of sleep or insufficient quality of sleep over an extended period can lead to a number of problems, including:

- Lapses in attention and inability to stay focused
- Reduced motivation
- Compromised problem-solving
- Confusion
- Irritability
- Memory lapses
- Impaired communication
- Slowed or faulty information processing and judgment

■ Diminished reaction time

■ Indifference and loss of empathy

The IOM report on nursing (2004b) notes the need to limit the hours of nurses who provide direct patient care to 12 hours in a 24-hour period and 60 hours in a 7-day period. Several studies indicate that errors increase with increased hours worked. Rogers et al. (2004) noted that errors increased threefold when a nurse worked a shift longer than 12.5 hours. Another study of more than 600 nurses indicated that rotating shifts and inadequate sleep patterns increased the risk of errors (Gold et al., 1992).

Kalisch, Begeny, and Anderson (2008) note that consistent scheduling is critical to high-level teamwork and does have an impact on errors. They discuss the work environment today: an environment with staff moving in and out of a unit based on multiple time schedules. Staff on a single unit may work 3-, 6-, 8-, 10-, and 12-hour shifts. This means that many changes occur in each shift, with multiple staff working different hours. This clearly hampers teams and means that patients must cope with multiple staff in a 24-hour period. This type of scheduling increases the risk of errors and affects patient-centered care, teams, and quality improvement.

The ANA also recognizes that staff fatigue has a major impact on errors and the quality of care (2006a; 2006b; 2008). In the past few years, medicine has recognized the impact of fatigue on physician residents and has instituted changes in shifts and hours that reflect the need for sleep during long shifts. Nursing has not done much; in fact, with mandatory overtime, more 12-hour shifts, the nursing shortage in some locations, and high patient acuity, nurses are probably more fatigued today than in the past. This is a good time to introduce students to the multiple factors that can add to staff fatigue, such as mandatory overtime, shifts, and stress. And yet there are schools of nursing where clinical or practicum is configured in 12-hour shifts. Consider the implications: increased student error due to fatigue; inadequate faculty guidance due to faculty and student fatigue; impact on student learning when the student is tired; and the message it sends to students that 12-hour shifts should be the norm.

Discuss how these factors affect the quality of care, the risk of errors, and teamwork to help students recognize the many factors that affect safe care. This can initially be done in the simulation lab and then re-emphasized during clinical experiences. Students need to be realistically prepared for work and should also learn how to prevent fatigue whenever possible.

Mandatory overtime is a growing concern in health care today. What do students know about it? *Keeping Patients Safe* (IOM, 2004b) recommends that nurses not work more than 12 hours in any 23-hour period or more than 60 hours in any 7-day period, emphasizing that 12-hour shifts increase risk of errors and staff injuries. As mentioned earlier, there is increasing concern about 12-hour shifts for undergraduate students. Students can research what their own states are doing about the problem at the ANA web site (http://www.nursingworld.org), search nursing literature, and investigate working conditions in local HCOs. This is an effective discussion topic to connect with staffing, the level of nursing shortage, leadership, management, how HCO administration affects nursing, quality of care, costs of care, health policies, and regulation such as state board of nursing regulations.

Contingent Workers

Healthcare organizations use contingent workers (temporary agency nurses and traveling nurses) to fill empty positions, particularly during shortage periods. This costly solution affects employee morale and probably the quality of care. It is also a growing problem for nursing education. Contingent workers who work alongside students may not be fully aware of the organization's policies, procedures, communication systems, or the nursing program, and may not even be willing to assist with teaching and supporting students. Contingent staff have not had time to become members of the team, which can undermine teamwork and the quality of care. If a practicum requires the use of preceptors, it may be difficult to find enough qualified preceptors who are regular employees. Faculty need to know about the types of staff on units. Schools of nursing need to work with healthcare organizations to determine how best to use available staff as effective preceptors and how to prepare and support preceptors. If contingent nurses must be used as preceptors—and in some cases this cannot be avoided due to the shortage—then faculty, organizations, and regulatory boards must to work together to make the experience safe and effective for students and patients.

Delegation

Teamwork is also a critical component of delegation. This is an important discussion to have with students as they learn about the delegation process and how to apply it. For example, how would surveillance and failure to rescue, topics discussed later, fit in with delegation? Delegation identifies what team members will be doing. We can provide students with cases to explore this. Delegation should also be emphasized in simulations. Delegation is related to all five core competencies. To participate in the delegation process, the patient must understand staff roles and responsibilities; patients can then appreciate why certain staff may be providing certain care. There are some aspects of care that patients may be doing for themselves (self-management) or through family members. Quality improvement should be considered during delegation: ensuring that care is provided as needed and is effective, safe, and efficient to meet outcomes. Informatics is applied both to communicating among team members and to documenting work that is done, which are parts of delegation. EBP and evidence-based management (EBM) provide evidence about what must be done, and may also provide evidence about who can best provide which type of care (intervention) to patients. We need much more research to expand the available data and evidence, but the other EBP elements (patient values and preferences, assessment data, and clinical expertise) should not be ignored. There is a tendency in discussing EBP to focus only on research evidence, and often we do not have enough research evidence. The National Council of State Boards of Nursing provides a description of the delegation decision tree, delegation and nursing assistive personnel, and other information about delegation at https://www.ncsbn.org/1625.htm

Workspace Design and Work Environment

Students probably do not think much about workspace and the work environment, but both are important. Ask students to assess a unit they are on for clinical/practicum: describe the lighting; space; accessibility for patients, families, and staff; nurses' work area; noise; furnishings; flooring (different flooring can affect fatigue, noise, cleanliness, and so on); traffic through the unit; accessibility of supplies and equipment; space for medication preparation and distractions in the space; documentation system and accessibility; space for private discussion and meetings; communication methods (notebooks, computer, bulletin boards, and so on); and space for staff to relax. What is the students' first impression when they step onto the unit? How does the unit atmosphere make them feel? For example, when neonatal intensive care units (NICUs) were traditional open rooms with no noise abatement, most of the nurses felt anxious and tense because of noise and bright lights. When more attention was paid to dimming lights and banning overhead pages, and more units were designed as pods or modules, staff tended to talk softly, were more mindful of noise and lights, and were less tense.

What is a healing environment, and how would one be created and maintained? Ask students how the environment and workspace affect how care is provided and received and how they affect the risk of errors. What could be changed to improve work space and the work environment? What could be done, that is not too costly and complex, to make the unit a better place to deliver and receive care? Students may have many creative ideas.

Learning Organizations

The concept of a learning organization, in which the organization explicitly recognizes the importance of ongoing learning for its staff, is used in many Fortune 500 companies to stay abreast of changes and to encourage retention of staff. This same concept is now used in healthcare organizations and in some schools of nursing as the profession begins to recognize nurses as knowledge workers and knowledge as intellectual capital. Have students consider why it would be important to understand the learning organization and how it might affect the quality of patient care. When students consider accepting a position, why should they assess the learning environment within the organization? How would a learning environment affect teamwork? Is learning an expectation in the HCO? Does the administration support lifelong learning, either financially or with time off? Faculty can help students formulate questions to find out if a healthcare organization is a learning organization. What type of orientation is provided for new staff? Does the hospital offer nurse mentorship, externship, or residency? If so, how long does it last, and what is included in the program? What education is provided, by whom, for whom, and can staff get time off to attend education within the organization? Does the organization cover any fees for academic courses or for continuing education courses? Is cross-training offered when staff members are expected to work in different areas? What is the quality of staff education, and does it meet the needs of the staff and patient care? It is also important to find out how unlicensed assistive personnel (UAPs) are trained. Staff nurses may be expected to provide some training on the job for UAPs, though this is not recommended. New graduates are not usually prepared for this role. Answers to these questions indicate how committed the organization is to staff education and to supporting a learning organization.

Students could assess a healthcare organization to determine whether it is a learning organization; discussing this in the education program will help students appreciate this critical issue when they look for their first job. They should also ask about the organization's attitude toward knowledge and the sharing of information. It is not uncommon for HCOs that are experiencing financial problems to reduce funding for staff education and tuition reimbursement. Share an actual staff education schedule from an HCO for review. Ask them to assess the educational programs offered by an HCO over a particular period. What types of educational methods were used? What was the content of the courses offered? How often were programs or courses offered? Were the programs appropriate to the competencies required in the HCO? Did the schedule meet the needs of staff that work on different shifts? Were instructors qualified? How did the staff rate the quality of education?

The goal is to get students thinking about what is an effective learning environment. Magnet hospitals have high levels of training and education for their staff and are more successful in recruitment and retention. Students also need to explore their own individual responsibility to improve competency. Lifelong learning is critical for any professional nurse today. (See earlier discussion on the continuing education report.) Assigning students to attend a continuing education (CE) program and to critique it is another strategy to help students understand the need for lifelong learning. They can also explore the certification process in a specialty that interests them.

Students experienced in working on a team, delegating, prioritizing, managing conflict, and critical thinking and clinical reasoning and judgment are more successful in their first jobs. Students also need experience recognizing when they need more information and where to find it, such as professional literature, the Internet, government resources, and experts. This acknowledges that learning is a lifelong pursuit. Greater use of preceptors, especially near the end of a nursing program, can help students gain important competencies, confidence, and better understanding of professional roles and teamwork. Faculty need to be aware that some state regulations prohibit substantial precepted hours in nursing programs, and that this can affect quality of education, patient safety, and the nursing shortage.

Nursing Education: What Should Be Done about Interprofessional Education?

Training in Teams: Interprofessional Education (IPE)

To transform nursing education, we need to include interprofessional learning experiences, which will act as a bridge to better professional teamwork. If we expect nurses to communicate with each other and with other healthcare professionals, we must not be afraid to have others teach healthcare content or to have students from different health professions take courses together. Several significant reports have been published recently about interprofessional education (IPE).

Learning should be interprofessional and active. Projects selected for experiences should help to demonstrate the rapid-cycle model, Plan-Do-Study-Act (Langley, Nolan, Norman, Provost, & Nolan, 1996). Content should include core improvement principles and the basics of effective team processes. For interprofessional learning to be effective, barriers must be addressed, such as a common professional language (for example, *patient* versus *client* when the latter is not typically used in healthcare organizations, diagnosis nomenclature such as NANDA); getting different learners together in one place (for example, academic calendars may vary; policies may be obstructive); varying tuition and fee structures; different work standards; differences in age, education, and amount of clinical experience; and the feeling that there is already too much in the curriculum.

Have students from nursing, medicine, respiratory therapy, and any other types of staff that might be involved in a code or cardiac arrest response work together in a simulation, to allow each team member to learn the perspectives of other individuals. Simulating interprofessional experiences, so that each professional student or staff learns his or her role in this type of high-stress, high-risk intervention, helps when the real-life situation arises. Interprofessional schools might organize an annual safety fair for students and faculty. This can highlight safety concerns, current evidence-based practice, and other related issues. Assign students from different healthcare professional schools to teams and ask them to create a poster or display on a facet of safety or quality. This provides an opportunity to plan, research, and implement the project as a team.

Achieving Competence Today (ACT) is a teaching strategy used to address interprofessional team competency. It was designed for interprofessional education focusing on quality, safety, and health systems improvement (Ladden, Bednash, Stevens, & Moore, 2006). ACT students from different healthcare professions work together to address a quality or safety problem in their own practice system. As of 2006, this has been piloted in 12 teaching hospitals with more than 350 learners from 5 different healthcare professions. Composed of four modules, it is a self-directed, web-facilitated, action-learning curriculum for graduate-level interprofessional learners. Students are provided information about "root cause analysis, the Plan-Do-Study-Act (PDSA) cycle, and effort–yield tables to investigate problems that affect everyday practice and job satisfaction" (Ladden, Bednash, Stevens, & Moore, 2006, p. 499). Learners also develop a quality improvement plan (QIP). Ladden et al. comment that the process "brings learners together to do real work and also to learn" (2006, p. 501). "Learners often think of themselves as renters, rather than owners; programs like ACT get them involved and invested in hospital processes" (p. 503).

Team-Based Learning

Team-based learning can be used in the classroom to teach students how to apply knowledge as a team (Michaelsen, Knight, & Fink, 2004). Students first complete an individual quiz on the content for the class session, to stimulate preparation before class, and then complete the same quiz with their team. Thereafter, faculty review the answers with all the teams, comparing responses and asking students for rationales to support their responses. The teams then apply the content to cases. Each step is interactive and offers faculty the opportunity to evaluate the students' clinical reasoning and judgment as well as knowledge. This method is now used in many colleges of medicine and some colleges of nursing. It is not based primarily on lectures—in many cases there is no lecture, or material might be posted online for students to review before class.

Interprofessional Continuing Education

There is greater emphasis today on interprofessional continuing education, or rather the desire to have more of it. The 2010 report *Lifelong Learning in Medicine and Nursing* represents a collaboration between the American Association of Colleges of Nursing and the Association of American Medical Colleges. Structured interprofessional forums, such as team planning, team rounds, meetings, and task groups, are important opportunities to learn about collaboration, interprofessional issues, planning, and communication. These provide opportunities for students to assess situations and learn from them with faculty support, and to develop effective communication skills. The report states: "We envision a continuum of health professional education from admission into a health professional program to retirement that values, exemplifies, and assesses lifelong learning skills; emphasizes interprofessional and team-based education and practice; employs tested, outcomes-based continuing education methods; and links health professional education and delivery of care within the workplace" (p. 3). The recommendations relate to continuing education methods, interprofessional education, lifelong learning, and workplace learning as well as the major stakeholders—education, practice, and regulatory. This report is important and should be reviewed by faculty when they discuss continuing education with both undergraduate and graduate students. Graduate students who are in the education track should pay particular attention to the content.

This report is tied to the IOM report, *Redesigning Continuing Education in the Health Professions* (2010a), though this latter report focuses on all healthcare professions, not just medicine and nursing, and is much more detailed. The message from this report is similar in content to that of the other report, but it includes a strong statement about the status of professional continuing education. "Continuing education (CE) is the process by which health professionals keep up to date with the latest knowledge and advances in health care. However, the CE 'system,' as it is structured today, is so deeply flawed that it cannot properly support the development of health professionals. CE has become structured around health professional participation instead of performance improvement. This has left health professionals unprepared to perform at the highest levels consistently, putting into question whether the public is receiving care of the highest possibly quality and safety" (IOM, 2010a, p. ix).

Core Competency: Employ Evidence-Based Practice

Integrate best research with clinical expertise and patient values for optimum care, and participate in learning and research activities to the extent feasible (IOM, 2003b, p. 4).

Evidence-based practice (EBP) facilitates the use of research findings in practice; however, there is more than one source of evidence. In addition to research evidence, there are patient values and preferences, history and assessment data, and the healthcare provider's expertise. The emphasis should be on evidence; students need to understand how to select an appropriate level of evidence or evaluate expert opinions and research findings. The tendency is just to assume that research is the only type of EBP evidence, when, in fact, there are several types of evidence. Students are fearful of research, but they can embrace a scientific basis for interventions and see the application in practice when provided with sufficient background information about the importance of research findings and their relationship to best practice. (See Teaching–Learning Module 8, Clinical Guidelines, for more information about EBP and QI in the context of clinical guidelines.)

Research

The NIH Common Fund provides some National Institutes of Health funding that would cross NIH institutes. "The broad goal for the IR program, therefore, is to change academic research culture, both in the extramural research community and in the extramural program at the NIH, such that interdisciplinary [interprofessional] approaches are facilitated. The Interdisciplinary Research Program includes initiatives to dissolve academic department boundaries within academic institutions and increase cooperation between institutions, train scientists to cultivate interdisciplinary efforts, and build bridges between the biological sciences and the behavioral and social sciences. Collectively, these efforts are intended to change academic research culture so that interdisciplinary [interprofessional] approaches and team science are a normal mode of conducting research and scientists who pursue these approaches are adequately recognized and rewarded" (NIH Common Fund, 2011). In 2008, the Robert Wood Johnson Foundation (RWJF) invited proposals for an interprofessional nursing quality research initiative to "generate, disseminate, and translate research to improve quality of care" (Robert Wood Johnson Foundation, 2008a). There is a definite trend toward encouraging more interprofessional research whenever this applicable. Nurses need to be involved in quality research and participate in evaluating how nursing care is connected to quality care. The reports recommend expansion of nursing research to increase nursing's understanding of the relationship of patient safety to nursing care, outcomes, and the role of nurses and interprofessional collaborations.

In addition to curriculum changes, funding streams for HCOs are also influenced by the IOM. As noted in the reports, AHRQ should fund research to evaluate how the current regulatory and legal systems facilitate or inhibit the changes needed for the 21st-century healthcare delivery system, and how they can be modified to support healthcare professionals and organizations working to accomplish the six aims identified by the IOM (2001a). This work has yet to be completed. Nursing should be involved so that nursing input can be included; critical issues such as licensure and liability are involved in this recommendation. The multiple-state compact on licensure, which has been instituted in some states, is one example of thinking outside the box.

Any improvement in care requires data, analysis, and practical solutions. Increased clinical research, effectiveness studies, health services research, and outcomes studies are all needed. Nursing is collecting data, but much more must be done in this area (Lamb, Jennings, Mitchell, & Lang, 2004). Collecting data takes time and money, so the process must be as efficient as possible. Data must also be collected systematically or data validity will be suspect. More research should examine the critical factors related to quality, such as staffing, shift hours, workload, control over practice, collaboration, teamwork, and communication.

Nursing education is involved in research. Some schools of nursing are studying these critical quality issues, though more should, as nursing is directly involved in quality of care. One area that requires further exploration is how education affects student performance, and their future performance in the workplace. Other potential areas for nursing research related to quality include:

▐ Fragmentation of care
▐ Errors and error prevention
▐ Safe medication administration
▐ Priority areas of care (IOM)
▐ Impact of medical and information technology
▐ Implementation of the five core competencies in the curriculum and in practice
▐ Prevention of patient falls
▐ Care coordination
▐ Teamwork (including its impact on care and its implementation in education)
▐ Operating room and surgery procedures
▐ Emergency department practices and procedures
▐ Management of diagnostic tests, screening, and information
▐ Intensive care units: adult, neonatal, pediatric
▐ Care of frail elderly (for example, falls, decubiti)
▐ Quality improvement and making changes in practice
▐ Effective use of QI methods such as Plan-Do-Study-Act (PDSA), failure modes and effects analysis (FMEA), checklists, and methods to reduce workarounds and improve handoffs

Evidence-Based Practice

Sigma Theta Tau (2006, p. 3) defines *evidence-based practice* as "integration of best clinical practice, research evidence, nursing expertise, and the values and preferences of the individuals, families, and communities who are served." Some schools of nursing have changed their research courses to an evidence-based methodology, particularly for undergraduate students. In other courses, such as those with practica (for example, pediatrics, adult health, mental health, family-focused, community), it is important that faculty incorporate evidence-based practice throughout the nursing curriculum, both undergraduate and graduate. The Academic Center of Evidence-Based Practice at the University of Texas Health Science Center in San Antonio published *Essential Competencies for Evidence-Based Practice in Nursing* (Stevens, 2009) (the second edition of the competencies can be obtained at http://www.acestar.uthscsa.edu/ebp_compet.asp). This is a useful guide to developing EBP competencies at the undergraduate, master's, and doctoral levels. The competencies are based on the Ace Star Model of Transformation described in Appendix J.

In addition, there is now an Improvement Science Research Network (http://www.ISRN.net) whose purpose is to "advance the scientific foundation for quality improvement, safety, and efficiency through transdisciplinary research addressing healthcare systems, patient-centeredness, and integration of evidence into practice" (Improvement Science Research Network, 2012). This collaborative network has four research priorities, all of which relate to the IOM work on QI and to content in this book:

▌ Coordination and transitions of care
▌ High-performing clinical systems and microsystems approaches to improvement
▌ Evidence-based quality improvement and best practice
▌ Learning organizations and culture of quality and safety

Browsing the Cochrane Collaborative Library (http://www.cochrane.org) or the Joanna Briggs Institute (JBI) (http://www.joannabriggs.edu.au) for systematic reviews and a collection of EBP guidelines will show students the linkages between the science of nursing and the art of delivering care (research to practice). Joanna Briggs Institute has a software program called RAPid (Rapid Assessment Protocol Internet database), part of the JBI's Critical Appraisal Network (http://www.joannabriggs.edu.au/Appraise%20Evidence). This can be integrated into a research course or even a nursing core course to teach students how to judge whether a study or a systematic review provides strong evidence to support a certain intervention. This activity also helps tie together research, EBP, and best practices.

Students learning to support intervention choices should review EBP resources (such as http://www.guideline.gov/) in all clinical courses. Students need to know about systematic reviews that examine multiple primary investigations addressing a particular question, practice guidelines, and how to use computer-based clinical decision support systems. Evidence-based guidelines promote quality of care, and these should be incorporated in all courses. For example, students can review guidelines and consider how the guidelines might affect the care for a specific health problem and population. The AHRQ evidence-based practice centers are important resources for students and faculty. The nursing profession should be actively involved in the development of EBP centers and the evidence-based process, and then ensure that nurses can access information relevant to nursing care.

"In a system that learns from data collected at the point-of-care and applies the lessons to patient care improvement, healthcare professionals will continue to be the key components at the front lines, assessing the needs, directing the approaches, ensuring the integrity of the tracking and quality of outcomes, and leading innovations. However, what these practitioners will need to know and how they learn will change dramatically. Orienting practice around a continually evolving evidence base requires new ways of thinking about how to create and sustain a healthcare workforce that recognizes the role of evidence in decision making and is attuned to lifelong learning" (IOM, 2007g, p. 28). EBP has to be embedded in practice, but to accomplish this it is necessary to embed it into nursing education. This also applies to continuing education (CE). The IOM recommends that healthcare CE should move to a team approach, including physicians, nurses, pharmacists, and when applicable patients, and that CE should include EBP (Davies et al., 2003). This approach would support the IOM competencies of working in interprofessional teams, patient-centered care, EBP, and collaboration.

As noted in Part 1, four major IOM reports relate to research and EBP. These reports can be used as resources for faculty and students. For example, ask students to review the report summaries and comment on several aspects of the report that they found interesting or unexpected. This can be a particularly useful activity in an interprofessional healthcare research course that includes EBP content.

Collaborative Evidence-Based Practice

Nursing is focusing on nursing and EBP, and other healthcare professions are focusing on their own EBP. Certainly each profession has to do this; however, healthcare professions must also work collaboratively in their EBP efforts. With the increased need to use interprofessional teams, teams need to consider EBP for the patient—all aspects of care, keeping the patient in the center of EBP and all elements of EBP (research, clinician expertise, patient preferences and values, and patient history and assessment data). In addition, quality improvement (QI) covers all areas of care, and use of EBP should improve care, again requiring a collaborative effort. When patients are divided into domains or territories by different healthcare professions, then patient-centered care is impossible, risk of errors increases, and quality of care declines. Newhouse (2008, p. 416) comments, "Despite the clear need to work together for a common patient-centered approach, professions tend to approach improvements in care by setting boundaries around their scope-specific activities. Profession-specific patient goals are important, but must also be integrated into unified action."

Shared evidence and collaboration will best meet this goal. Schools of nursing are including more EBP content and experiences in all their programs, and nursing in hospitals tends to focus on nursing EBP; however, this approach puts us back into our silos, disregarding IOM's recommendations and the core competency of greater focus on interprofessional collaborative care. Patient engagement and patient-centered care are central to interprofessional collaborative practice. A new agency, called the Patient-Centered Outcomes Research Institute (PCORI), has been designed to fund research focusing on the production of evidence-based information (PCORI, 2012). This agency is linked with AHRQ in an effort to ensure that evidence-based guidelines are used and adapted for the patient population so that the patient and family understand the treatment plan. The PCORI web site provides information that can be used in teaching (www.pcori.org).

Teaching Research and EBP Online

To appreciate EBP and EBP literature, students need to understand the research process. EBP and research content can be effectively combined in undergraduate and graduate courses on nursing research, and should be integrated throughout the curriculum. Though not all nursing content can be taught effectively online, EBP content certainly can. This content can be made available to students in highly interactive online courses that require students to apply knowledge through readings, audio lectures, handouts, and other interactive resources. Divide students into teams of three or four. Have each student search for a published study, then identify and critique it part by part, such as the statement of problem, purpose research question, hypothesis, and so on. The student should describe each part of the study briefly and critique it by comparing it to content about the research process. The student posts the article and the critique to the team discussion forum, where team members then comment on each other's critiques. It takes at least five discussion assignments to work through the major parts of a research study. During this time, students are reading about the steps in the research process, and they can then apply the content to these assignments. Faculty need to actively participate in the discussion and review of the assignments. This type of assignment could also be done in the classroom. Lecture should be limited if used at all, with students coming to class prepared to discuss the parts of their study that are the focus for the day.

EBP should be more than educators citing studies in various classes. In exercises, students should gather evidence and critically review studies (in much the same way as the research process has been taught in the past), but now students should be asked to determine what level of evidence supports the nursing interventions they implement. Students may work on evidence-based projects instead of a thesis. Where there is an evidence-based practice center, undergraduates can learn how to glean information from the literature and evaluate its credibility, and then write a short report on the process as part of the center's activities.

Ask students to write a patient intervention comparison outcome (PICO) question and to find two separate studies related to the PICO and a related systematic review. It is difficult to find systematic reviews on all PICOs, so some students may end up using a systematic review that does not apply specifically to their PICO question. The purpose of this assignment, which is written and submitted to faculty, is to:

1. Identify a PICO
2. Gain further experience searching the literature
3. Review single studies (identify parts and critique the study)

4. Summarize key points from single studies and clinical implications
5. Identify a systematic review and its parts, critique the review, and discuss how the systematic review is different from a single study

Providing students with a chart can help them complete each stage of the assignment, with sections of the chart pertaining to the sections of a research article. Discussion during this time focuses on implementation of EBP in practice settings. This assignment allows students to learn how a discipline examines evidence, how little evidence there is to support many nursing interventions, the need for more rigorous studies, and the use of computer skills to gather information quickly and condense it into a usable form. Informatics is a critical tool for students as they learn to apply EBP. A sample form for this assignment is available in the instructional materials. Table 5-1 describes information about PICO questions included in an IOM report.

As faculty work to integrate EBP into learning experiences, several key questions are typically considered:

▌ Do we drop all research content on the undergraduate level and just include EBP?
▌ Do we try to teach the same research content and add on EBP?
▌ What research content could we leave out?

There is no course in which EBP cannot be discussed and applied, and EBP should also be an integral part of clinical. We need textbooks that are better suited to a blend of research and EBP. Employers expect that new graduates will come to the workplace with a sound background in EBP. HCOs do not want to absorb the substantial cost to teach this subject, though some are providing education about EBP to staff whose nursing programs did not include it. Nurse educators also have to remember that many

T A B L E 5 - 1 PICO Format for Formulating an Evidence Question

PICO Component	Tips for Building Question	Example
Patient population or problem	"How would I describe this group of patients?" *Balance precision with brevity*	"In patients with heart failure from dilated cardiomyopathy who are in sinus rhythm . . ."
Intervention (a cause, prognostic factor, treatment, etc.)	"Which main intervention is of interest?" *Be specific*	" . . . would adding anticoagulation with warfarin to standard heart failure therapy . . ."
Comparison intervention (if necessary)	"What is the main alternative to be compared with the intervention?" *Be specific*	" . . . when compared with standard therapy alone . . ."
Outcomes	"What do I hope the intervention will accomplish?" "What could this exposure really affect?" *Be specific*	" . . . lead to lower mortality or morbidity from thromboembolism? Is this enough to be worth the increased risk of bleeding?"

Source: Institute of Medicine. (2008). *Knowing what works in healthcare*. Washington, DC: National Academies Press, p. 88. Reprinted with permission.

entering graduate students did not have EBP content in their undergraduate programs. Over time this will change; however, most of these students currently need the same basic information about EBP as prelicensure students.

Evidence-Based Management

EBP also should also be used in management. "Leaders who have staunchly advocated best-evidence application in patient care have been less aggressive in applying the same logic to management decisions" (Pfeffer & Sutton, 2006, as cited in Marshall, 2008, p. 205). "Reports of medical mistakes have splashed across newspapers and magazines in the United States. At the same time, instances of overuse, underuse, and misuse of management tactics and strategies receive far less attention. The sense of urgency associated with improving the quality of medical care does not exist with respect to improving the quality of management decisions. [T]aking a more evidence-based approach would improve the competence of the decision-makers and their motivation to use more scientific methods when making a decision" (Kovner, Fine, & D'Aquila, 2009, p. 53). One of the American Organization of Nurse Executives (AONE) strategic objectives is to "Encourage the utilization of evidence-based management practice and sound research to explore and support the interrelations of technology, facility design and patient care delivery models" (AONE, 2012, p. 2). Students need to understand EBM, which is the "systematic application of the best available evidence to the evaluation of managerial strategies for improving the performance of health services organizations" (Kovner, Fine, & D'Aquila, 2009, p. 56). The steps in the EBM process are similar to those in the EBP process:

1. Formulate the question
2. Acquire the research evidence
3. Assess the quality of the evidence
4. Present the evidence
5. Apply the evidence

As is true with EBP—even more so with EBM—it is not always easy to find management research to use as evidence in decision-making. Leadership and management content and experiences should discuss how EBP relates to management. Students need to know that EBP is not related only to patient care practice; it is also related to management and education.

Core Competency: Apply Quality Improvement

This core competency has come to the forefront due to the ongoing concerns for patient safety and the role of medication errors.

Identify errors and hazards in care; understand and implement basic safety design principles, such as standardization and simplification; continually understand and measure quality of care in terms of structure, process, and outcomes in relation to patient and community needs; and design and test interventions to change processes and systems of care, with the objective of improving quality (IOM, 2003b, p. 4).

The IOM findings on patient safety and error rates have made quality improvement (QI) a vital concern and expanded the need to focus on quality of care in general, not just errors. We need new teaching strategies and course content to ensure continuous quality and to ensure that nurses are prepared to participate actively in the QI process and serve as leaders. Many of the IOM reports on quality have been in existence now for 10 years. Where are we today? "Despite these efforts, quality improvement throughout much of the U.S. healthcare system is still proceeding at a glacial pace. The *National Healthcare Quality Report* by the Agency for Healthcare Research and Quality (AHRQ) revealed that while nearly two-thirds of 179 measures of healthcare quality did show improvement, the median annual rate of change was only 2.3 percent. Several quality measures relating to cancer screening and diabetes management actually worsened during this time" (AHRQ, 2010b). In terms of safety, several new studies have suggested that patients continue to experience high rates of safety problems during hospital stays. "Indeed, one study found adverse events continue to occur in as many as one-third of hospital patients" (Classen et al., 2011, as cited in IOM, 2011g, p. I-2).

Building a Healthcare Quality Framework

Definition of Quality

Quality is not easy to define. The traditional view of quality, which is also found in the IOM reports, focuses on structure, process, and outcomes (Donabedian, 1988), as described in Figure 5-4.

Donabedian's quality model (1980) describes each of the major components as:

- ▪ *Structure*: System characteristics, provider characteristics, and patient characteristics, or the environment in which care is provided
- ▪ *Process*: Technical style and interpersonal style, or the manner in which care is provided
- ▪ *Outcomes*: Clinical end points or results, satisfaction with care, functional status of the patient

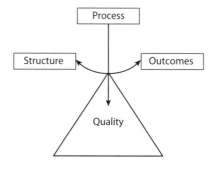

F I G U R E 5 - 4 The Elements of Quality

Discussing quality related to each of these components and how they interact allows students to gain a perspective on the dynamic quality process. The IOM defines *quality care* as "providing patients with appropriate services in a technically competent manner, with good communication, shared decision-making, and cultural sensitivity" (IOM, 2001a, p. 432).

We know we need more content about QI for students in all healthcare professions and more application of this content. If this is done effectively, students will enter their respective professions with greater knowledge of QI, motivation to improve care, and the ability to participate actively in the QI process. The Institute for Healthcare Improvement (IHI) has identified eight domains of core content for QI that still apply today (Batalden, 1998).

- *Health care as a process system*: The interdependent people (patients, families, eligible populations, caregivers), procedures, activities, and technologies of healthcare giving that come together to meet the needs of individuals and communities.
- *Variation and measurement*: The use of measurement to understand the variation of performance in processes and systems.
- *Customer/beneficiary knowledge*: Identification of the person, persons, or groups of persons for whom health care is provided; assessment of their needs and preferences and the relationship of health care to those needs and preferences.
- *Leading, following, and making changes in health care*: Leadership is required for successful QI; however, followership must be included in the process of change. Staff need to understand the roles of leaders and followers.
- *Collaboration*: The knowledge, methods, and skills needed to work effectively in groups (teams), to understand and value the perspectives and responsibilities of others, and the capacity to foster the same in others.
- *Social context and accountability*: An understanding of the social contexts (local, regional, national, global) of health care and the way expectations arise from them, including the financial impact and costs of health care.
- *Developing new, locally useful knowledge*: The recognition of the need for new knowledge in personal daily health professional practice and the skill to develop new knowledge through empiric testing.
- *Professional subject matter*: The health professional knowledge appropriate for a specific discipline and the ability to apply and connect it to all of the other QI domains; core competencies published by professional boards, accreditors (surveyors), and other certifying entities.

Critical Definitions

The IOM reports expanded knowledge about safety and errors, and part of this is identification of key terms. A common language facilitates communication among healthcare professions and improves data collection and analysis. The following terms are relevant to nurses involved in initiatives to reduce errors and improve safety (Chassin & Galvin, 1998; IOM, 1999).

- *Safety.* Freedom from accidental injury.
  Example: The patient leaves the hospital after surgery and a three-day stay with expected outcomes reached and no complications occur.

- *Error.* The failure of a planned action to be completed as intended or the use of a wrong plan to achieve an aim. Errors are directly related to outcomes. There are two types of errors: *error of planning* and *error of execution*. Errors harm the patient, and some may be *preventable adverse events*.
  Example: The patient is given the wrong medication (error of execution).

- *Adverse event.* An injury resulting from a medical intervention, not due to the patient's underlying condition. Not all adverse events are due to errors and not all are preventable. Only investigation and analysis can determine the relationship of an error to an adverse event. When an adverse event is the result of an error, it is considered a *preventable adverse event*.
  Example: The patient is given the wrong medication and experiences a seizure. If the patient does not have a seizure disorder, this is most likely a preventable adverse event, but more must be discovered about the causes. How did the error happen that led to the adverse event? Would this medication error cause a seizure? Are there other possible causes for the seizure?

Examples of causes and types of adverse errors are described in Table 5-2. This information is useful for development of simulations, scenarios, cases, and other learning activities for students.

T A B L E   5 - 2   Clinical Guidelines and Recommendations

Causes of Adverse Events	Types of Adverse Events
Care planning	Anesthesia events
Care process design	Behavioral events
Communication	Criminal events
Continuum of care	Environment-related events
Human factors	Equipment-related events
Information management	Infection-related events
Organization culture	Medication errors
Patient assessment	Medical events
Patient identification	Pediatric events
Patient involvement & education	Surgical events
Physical resources	Transfer-discharge related events
—	Other unanticipated events

Source: WHO Collaborating Centre for Patient Safety Solutions. (2008). Adverse events. Retrieved on November 6, 2008, from http://www.ccforpatientsafety.org/. Reprinted with permission.

▌ *Misuse.* Avoidable complications that prevent patients from receiving full potential benefit of a service.
Example: The patient receives a medication that is not prescribed and conflicts with the patient's allergies; the patient experiences anaphylaxis.

▌ *Overuse.* Potential for harm that exceeds the possible benefit from a service.
Example: An older patient is taking multiple medications, some of which may interact negatively, and the patient's multiple healthcare providers are not aware of the medications prescribed by different specialists.

▌ *Underuse.* Failure to provide a service that would have produced a favorable outcome for the patient.
Example: The patient is not able to get specialty treatment needed for cancer because of the distance from resources, or the patient's insurer will not reimburse for an arthritis medication that could make the patient more mobile.

▌ *Near miss.* Recognition that an event occurred that *might* have led to an adverse event. This means the error almost happened. It is important to understand such errors; they provide valuable information for preventing future actual errors.
Example: The surgical team is preparing for knee surgery. The right knee is prepped, but when a team member checks the records the team member finds out that it is the left knee that requires surgery. An error was prevented, but why was the wrong knee initially prepped?

▌ *Active error.* An error that results from noncompliance with a procedure (Reason, 1990).
Example: A nurse does not check vital signs to confirm the need for a specific medication. The medication is administered when the patient does not need it, and the patient experiences side effects.

▌ *Latent conditions.* Threats not immediately apparent. These indicate problems in the system (Reason, 1990).
Example: Some staff are not familiar with a change in policy, though it is assumed that all are implementing the new policy. An error occurs due to lack of knowledge.

▌ *Sentinel event.* An event that has a drastic negative outcome; unexpected death, serious physical or psychological injury, or serious risk. A root cause analysis of the event is conducted to examine the process, not just the individual staff involved. The goal is not blame but prevention of future events.
Example: The patient commits suicide while in the hospital for treatment.

▌ *Root cause analysis.* An in-depth analysis of an error to assess the event and identify causes and possible solutions. The Joint Commission root cause analysis matrix includes the following dimensions to be assessed (Joint Commission, 2005).
  ▌ Behavioral assessment process (includes assessment of patient risk to self and to others as appropriate)

- Physical assessment process (includes search for contraband)
- Patient identification process, patient observation procedures, care planning process
- Continuum of care
- Staffing levels
- Orientation and training of staff
- Competency assessment and credentialing
- Supervision of staff (includes supervision of physicians in training)
- Communication with patient or family
- Communication among staff members
- Availability of information
- Adequacy of technological support
- Equipment maintenance and management
- Physical environment (includes furnishings, hardware such as bars, hooks, rods, lighting, distractions)
- Security systems and processes
- Medication management (includes selection and procurement, storage, ordering and transcribing, preparing and dispensing, administration, and monitoring)

Not all of these dimensions apply to every event, but each must be considered and then eliminated if not applicable.

Simple Rules for the 21st Century

The *Quality Chasm* (IOM, 2001a) report identifies simple rules that should be considered as care is improved. These are listed in Table 5-3. This table describes current approaches (old rules) compared with new rules for healthcare delivery or a vision of

T A B L E 5 - 3 Simple Rules for the 21st-Century Healthcare System

Current Approach (Old Rule)	New Rule
Care is based primarily on visits.	Care is based on continuous healing relationships.
Professional autonomy drives variability.	Care is customized according to patient needs and values.
Professionals control care.	The patient is the source of control.
Information is a record.	Knowledge is shared and information flows freely.
Decision-making is an individual responsibility.	Decision-making is evidence-based.
Do no harm is an individual responsibility.	Safety is a system property.
Secrecy is necessary.	Transparency is necessary.
The system reacts to needs.	Needs are anticipated.
Cost reduction is sought.	Waste is continuously decreased.
Preference is given to professional roles over the system.	Cooperation among clinicians is a priority.

Source: Institute of Medicine. (2001). *Crossing the Quality Chasm: A New Health System for the 21st Century*. Washington, DC: National Academies Press, p. 67. Reprinted with permission.

U.S. healthcare. How can this information be used with students? The rules represent the philosophical direction of the changes or vision that IOM recommends for the healthcare system. Ask students to consider the following or, in the case of staff, ask them to consider their own professional experiences in light of these rules.

1. Compare the current rule with the new rule.
2. How does each rule apply to nursing practice?
3. What changes are needed to meet each new rule?
4. How does each rule affect interprofessional teamwork?

Faculty need to consider what changes are needed to prepare nurses who understand and practice using the new rules. Entering students can be asked to discuss their perspectives on the rules and then to reflect on them again at the end of the nursing program. Student perspectives should change over time and with educational experiences.

Six Aims

Crossing the Quality Chasm identifies six major improvement aims or goals to be considered and adopted by all healthcare providers, including nursing education. Reviewing these aims (discussed briefly later), one might wonder, "Aren't we doing this already?" Perhaps, but we are not doing it effectively. On one level, these aims are not surprising; they might seem obvious and straightforward to the point of being simple. However, these six aims are imperative (IOM, 2001a, pp. 42–53).

1. *Safe.* Avoid injuries to patients from the care that is intended to help them. The critical elements are as follows:
   ▪ Patients should not have to repeat information as they go through the healthcare system or go from system to system.
   ▪ The healthcare system and process should be seamless and interprofessional.
   ▪ Healthcare providers need the right knowledge about their patients.
   ▪ Patients need to be informed and participate in their own care.
   ▪ When complications occur, patients need to be informed and involved in decision-making.

All of these elements are related to nursing practice. Ask students: *How does this apply to your patient care?*

2. *Effective.* Provide services based on scientific knowledge or EBP to all who could benefit, and refrain from providing services to those who are not likely to benefit (avoid underuse and overuse, respectively). Effective care implies evidence-based health care with integration of best research evidence, clinical expertise, and patient values (Sackett, Rosenberg, & Gray, 1996). Nursing is incorporating evidence-based practice in the clinical setting and needs to apply evidence-based management as well. Nursing education must provide content in this area so that graduates are able to understand and participate in evidence-based practice as HCO staff. The report defines EBP as the

integration of best practice with expertise and patient values. Ask students: *How does this apply to your patient care?*

3. *Patient-centered*. Provide care that is respectful of and responsive to individual patient preferences, needs, and values, and ensure that patient values guide all clinical decisions. The key focus is on the patient's experience of illness and health care. It is quite clear that patients are entering the healthcare system more informed than in the past, due to the easy accessibility of health information. Patients need support in their efforts to be more informed, and nurses have long been advocates of patient education. However, nurses have little time to educate patients or guide them to needed information. This problem must be resolved from both the nursing education and practice perspectives. How are students taught about patient education? Are they provided with education interventions that are easy to apply, or are these proposed interventions unrealistic given the nature of the work environment today? Most schools of nursing would say that patient education is included in their curricula; however, many probably have not reviewed their content and teaching approaches based on the following: Are the patient education methods used today effective given the current healthcare environment (rapid turnover of patients, acuity of patients, staff shortages, and work issues)? Are we making the best use of technology in patient education? Ask students: *Reflect on how you are providing patient-centered care.*

4. *Timely*. Reduce waits and sometimes harmful delays for both patients who receive care and those who give care. Problems with timeliness can lead to physical harm, and even more frequently causes emotional stress. Such problems also affect the patient's trust in the system. Ask students: *How does time affect your patient care delivery and quality?*

5. *Efficient*. Avoid waste, including waste of equipment, supplies, ideas, and energy. Better use of resources reduces costs and makes resources more available to those who need them. *How often do we ask students to consider efficiency in their patient care? Certainly their future employers will do so.*

6. *Equitable*. Provide care that does not vary in quality because of personal characteristics such as gender, ethnicity, geographic location, and socioeconomic status. Access to care and healthcare disparity have become major concerns in the United States. There is increased emphasis on diversity training, but it is not yet clear whether this training improves the situation or which type of approach is the best to take. Ask students: *How does this apply to the patient care you provide?*

Each of the six aims is highly relevant to nursing. They can be incorporated into leadership and management content by discussing implications for nurse managers and for healthcare organizations. Students can be asked to provide examples of application of these aims from what they observe in the healthcare organizations where they are doing clinical. Ask students to determine how each one of the aims affects their assigned patients, as the aims are integrated into the plan of care; how the aims affect an aggregate or population; and what can be done to resolve problems that may block meeting these aims. Using case studies, discussion, and clinical experience will make students more aware of the aims and how they affect care. The aims may conflict at times, and it is important for students to discuss how this might occur and how such conflicts can be resolved. For example, can safe care always be efficient? Some of this discussion will involve ethics and legal issues.

Priority Areas for National Action

The IOM explored the quality of care in detail. The resulting recommendations include regular reports on the status of health care (such as the National Healthcare Quality Report and the National Healthcare Disparities Report), but there is a missing piece. The potential number of healthcare problems and diagnoses is huge. What do we focus on? We cannot improve in every area at once. What is critical? This led to the IOM report on *Priority Areas for National Action* (IOM, 2003f). Three criteria were used to determine the priority areas (IOM, 2003f, p. 4):

▮ *Impact*. The extent of the burden (disability, mortality, and economic costs) that occurs because of a condition, and its effects on patients, families, communities, and societies.

▮ *Improvability*. The extent of the gap between current practice and evidence-based best practice and whether the gap can be closed; particularly focusing on the six national quality aims of safety, effectiveness, patient-centeredness, timeliness, efficiency, and equity.

▮ *Inclusiveness*. The relevance of an area to a broad range of individuals (age, gender, socioeconomic status, ethnicity, or race); generalizability of QI strategies; and the level of change that occurs because of the QI strategies.

The following discussion of the original IOM priority areas of care is based on these three criteria. The list was expected to change as improvement is noted and other problems become more critical. However, each one of these priority areas should be included in curricula. We cannot teach everything, but the priority areas are critical. As the list changes, nursing curricula must be flexible enough to adjust to the need for change in content and experiences of students. These are the IOM priority areas of care identified for the *first* national report on healthcare quality. The first two priority areas—care coordination, self-management and health literacy—apply to all the subsequent priority areas, and most likely will remain on the list. *Healthy People 2020* also relates to these priority areas; there is an effort to integrate the IOM approaches with *Healthy People*. To review current priorities, see the National Healthcare Quality Report at http://www.innovations.ahrq.gov/content.aspx?id=3135

Care Coordination

Clinical integration is defined as "the extent to which patient care services are coordinated across people, functions, activities, and sites over time so as to maximize the value of services delivered to patients" (Shortell, Gillies, & Anderson, 2000, as cited in IOM, 2003f, p. 49). Care coordination is an important aspect of all care. Students at all levels need to understand care coordination and describe the role of nursing in it. In clinical, ask students how care coordination could be improved, and have them participate in coordination in acute care and in the community. As content is presented (such as content related to the priority areas), faculty can approach it from the perspectives of care coordination and self-management. Several reports indicate that interprofessional care is important and ought be to improve. Preparing nursing students to participate as members of interdisciplinary teams is a challenge. It will take time to build relationships with other healthcare faculty so that students get interprofessional experience. Schools of nursing that work toward this goal will excel, and their graduates will be better prepared to practice in the real world.

Self-Management

As is made clear by the emphasis on patient-centered care, patients must be in control of their own health and care. Self-management supports this basic principle.

Self-management includes education and supportive interventions so that patients can participate as actively as possible in managing their health problems. Health literacy is an important component of self-management because it determines how much information the patient can understand and use to manage health. As has been noted, the incidence of chronic illness is growing, and many of the priority areas concern chronic illnesses. Self-management is particularly important to people with chronic illnesses, and therefore is also discussed throughout these pages. (Self-management is discussed in more detail in the patient-centered care core competency section.)

Adequate Pain Control

Pain management is a part of curricula in a variety of nursing courses. Most schools include more than just the use of medications to control pain, and have expanded into alternative pain control methods. Evidence-based practice becomes important as students learn about the varying effectiveness of pain control methods in different patient populations. Students need opportunities to observe or use these alternatives. Pain is now referred to as the fifth vital sign, and The Joint Commission requires an assessment of pain; students need to understand why. (Pain management is discussed in more detail in the patient-centered care core competency section.)

Asthma

Asthma is an important subject for nursing students. It affects all age groups in all settings. As in some other priority areas, students can assess the incidence of asthma in the community; compare these data with state and national data; investigate causes of asthma, and types of treatment and their efficacy; and devise strategies for self-management. Disease management programs for asthma are available. What do students know about disease management programs? Why have these programs improved outcomes? What is the role of nurses in these programs? Preparing and delivering education to the community is also a helpful learning activity. Be sure students appreciate the importance of improved patient outcomes, understand the process, and consider the role of the nurse in improving care.

Obesity

Obesity is a complex challenge. Discuss risk factors, prevention, nutrition, exercise, complications, pharmacology, drug effects on weight, pathophysiology, and treatment and efficacy. Given its health implications and prevalence today, obesity should be discussed in many content areas: nutrition, exercise, pediatrics, pregnancy, adults, community, and mental health.

Major Depression

Mental health courses typically cover depression. Depression affects people in all age groups and all settings. Students may assume that they will encounter patients with depression only in their mental health rotation, but faculty should point out that it strikes many other patients (for example, cancer patients, victims of myocardial infarction, postpartum mothers, and children). Nursing students in clinical experiences in public schools can explore the level of depression and suicide in various age groups. What type of education (for example, self-esteem, stress and coping skills, depression, and suicide) do school students need? At what age? In any setting, nursing students need to understand that depression should be part of a general assessment, not something that is assessed only in behavioral healthcare units or mental health clinics.

Nosocomial Infections

The risk of nosocomial infections is high today. When students are first introduced to handwashing and sterile technique, they need to be told about nosocomial infections: causes, prevention, and the role of nurses, as well as the importance of reducing these infections to improve care. What is the impact of increased nosocomial infections on healthcare delivery, in terms of economics, quality of care, complications, and prolonged hospital stays?

Pregnancy and Childbirth

Pregnancy and childbirth are normally positive, healthy experiences, but when they are not, it affects the mother, the newborn, and other family members. Preventing complications and adverse outcomes for mothers and infants is a critical goal. Tobacco cessation, another priority area, should be part of care for all pregnant women. There are also serious racial and ethnic disparities in this area. Students can explore these issues in their community/public course and then apply the information to their experiences in clinical settings.

Severe and Persistent Mental Illness

Severe and persistent mental illness is not an easy topic for students. They may experience a sense of hopelessness. Nevertheless, students do need to understand serious mental illness, including its impact on the patient, family, and community; types of treatment and their efficacy and side effects; and outcomes to improve care. When students investigate the types of treatment and support services available in the community, it is usually an eye-opener. Discuss the issue of parity and the current status of legislation at the state and national levels. This topic typically involves ethical and legal issues. Do staff have the right to force medications on patients or to use restraints? What patient rights are important, and how are they protected? What is involved in commitment? Why should this "chronic" illness be any different from diabetes or any other chronic illness? Providing some clinical experience with this population is important. Students will encounter patients with severe and persistent mental illness in all settings because such patients do experience other types of medical problems as well.

Stroke

Stroke is covered in nursing curricula, and typically includes the full range of content and settings where patients receive treatment, from emergency room to rehabilitation and home. All curricula should do more in discussing quality of life and disabilities.

Tobacco Dependence

Tobacco use is the "single most preventable cause of disease and death" (IOM, 2003f, p. 89). Students need information about risks, prevention, age groups and why each group might require different strategies to decrease dependence, the dependence process, complications, and methods used to help individuals stop smoking. Students also need to understand the impact of politics and economics on the availability of tobacco.

Cancer Screening

Cancer screening should be evidence based. Students can research the rates of colorectal cancer and cervical cancer in their local community. How do these rates compare with state and national rates? What screening is being done, and by whom? What are the outcomes of the screening efforts? What could be done to improve the outcomes? Students can be given information about the screening for these two types of cancer as well as observe a screening program.

Children with Special Needs

Some schools of nursing offer content or specific courses on the care of children with special needs. Students often encounter children with special needs during clinical experiences in schools or in acute care pediatric settings. These children have complex needs—physical, emotional, family, financial, and so on. Care coordination is an important part of the care for this population. What are the community resources for children with special needs? Are they easy for families to access? What type of help do caregivers need?

Diabetes

Diabetes is a growing problem and an important content area for nursing students. Diabetes affects patients in all age groups and all settings. How does diversity affect the rate of diabetes and care received? Working with diabetes nurse educators or in a diabetes clinic is a helpful learning experience. Involvement with the local chapter of the American Diabetic Association will help students understand the role of consumers in self-advocacy and the resources available in the community. Self-management plays a critical role in this priority area. Patients need effective care coordination that supports effective self-management.

End of Life

More and more information is now available for schools of nursing about end-of–life (EOL) issues. The Hartford Institute for Geriatric Nursing (http://www.hartfordign.org) offers important information that can enhance content and student experiences. Many schools of nursing are also participating in the AACN End-of-Life Nursing Education Consortium (ELNEC), which is furthering the effort to integrate EOL and palliative care into nursing curricula and teach-the-teachers initiatives for continuing education. Hospitals and healthcare facilities are forming palliative care teams in response to patients who want to be allowed to die a natural death and to be provided adequate pain control. Students need these skills to provide comforting care and anticipate family and patient needs in the face of a life-threatening or terminal illness.

Frailty Associated with Old Age

Preventing falls and pressure ulcers, maximizing function, and developing advanced care plans are all key nursing concerns. Information about aging and the needs of the aged population is online at the Hartford Institute for Geriatric Nursing (http://www.hartfordign.org). What type of clinical experience with this population do students have? Many students do not like working with older adults; however, it is important clinical experience, given the size of the aging population. Faculty should examine their own attitudes toward this patient population and toward nurses who work in this specialty. It may not be positive, and they may be sharing it with students, perhaps unconsciously.

Begin by emphasizing fall prevention and skin care throughout the curriculum. Ask students to evaluate their patients' fall risk and skin condition, which must be part of routine care. Healthcare organizations emphasize this with their staff, and The Joint Commission also includes it as an important part of its standards and accreditation surveys. How do students plan to maximize patient function? Students need to be specific and consider individual needs and limitations. Preventing falls and pressure ulcers and maximizing function are also potential problems for nursing research. Some research has been done, but more is needed because nursing care can influence outcomes. As will be discussed later, there is now an economic consequence for HCOs when patients experience falls and other complications during hospitalization; Medicare and Medicaid will not reimburse for hospital-acquired conditions (HACs). Some insurers now also have similar lists.

Advanced care plans must be understood. Students need an opportunity to consider the complex needs of the aging adult and how they personally feel about these needs. The goal is "to provide integrated dignified care for those of advanced age" (IOM, 2003f, p. 47). Care has to be respectful of patient and family wishes, and this is not always easy. It is best to work through these issues as much as possible while a student. Pre- and post-conferences are good places to address them.

Hypertension

Care for hypertension mostly means management of early disease before it progress. Hypertension is typically included in content. Students, however, also need to understand the need for prevention, early detection, and strategies to help newly diagnosed patients. What screening is done in the community, and by whom? Students may participate in screenings. Ask students what could happen if a person is not diagnosed early. What impact does diversity have on the risk for hypertension and care received?

Immunization

Immunization is important for both children and adults. Each year awareness campaigns remind people about the need for immunization. Often nursing students participate in community immunization clinics or drives. Although the United States has done better in recent years with getting children immunized, the reality is that continued immunization of adults for diphtheria, pertussis, and tetanus (DPT) has not kept up. Fear of terroristic use of infectious agents, and the spread of global infections such as avian flu and SARS, have revealed the vulnerability of adults to common illnesses. Have students research the outbreaks of infectious agents for which immunizations are available and correlate them with vulnerable age groups that should receive immunizations. Students can search the Internet for information about national and state efforts to improve immunization rates and compare them with local efforts. (See http://www.cdc.gov for updates on immunization requirements.) This has important global healthcare implications, and thus is a good time to introduce concerns about the easy and swift spread of infectious diseases worldwide. The World Health Organization (http://www.who.org) and the Centers for Disease Control and Prevention (http://www.cdc.gov) are good sources of information on this topic.

Ischemic Heart Disease

Ischemic heart disease is the leading cause of death for men and women. The critical elements of prevention, reduction of recurring events, and optimization of functional capacity should be included in content related to ischemic heart disease. Students should also be asked to explain how these elements apply to their patients. The impact of genetics, diet, exercise, and diversity on this disease are also important content topics.

National Healthcare Quality Report Matrix

The NHQR, as discussed in Part 1, provides important current data describing the status of health care in the United States. The annual National Healthcare Quality Report was designed to do the following (IOM, 2001b, p. 31):

▌ Supply a common understanding of quality and how to measure it that reflects the best current approaches and practices.

▌ Identify aspects of the healthcare system that improve or impede quality.

▌ Generate data associated with major quality initiatives.

▌ Educate the public, the media, and other audiences about the importance of healthcare quality and the current level of quality.

▌ Identify for policy-makers the problem areas in healthcare quality that most need their attention and action, with the understanding that these priorities may change over time and differ by geographic location.

▌ Provide policy-makers, purchasers, healthcare providers, and others with realistic benchmarks for quality of care in the form of national, regional, and population comparisons.

▌ Make it easier to compare the quality of the U.S. healthcare system with that of other nations.

▌ Stimulate the refinement of existing measures and the development of new ones.

▌ Stimulate data collection efforts at the state and local levels (mirroring the national effort) to facilitate targeted quality improvement.

▌ Incorporate improved measures as they become available and practical.

▌ Clarify the many aspects of healthcare quality and how they affect one another and quality as a whole.

▌ Encourage data collection efforts needed to refine quality measures and, ultimately, stimulate the development of a health information infrastructure to support quality measurement and reporting.

The current healthcare quality report uses the matrix described in Figure 5-3, which has been revised since the first matrix was developed for the report by the IOM. This matrix describes the framework for the annual quality report. The matrix attempts to answer the question: what does quality of care look like? The IOM describes quality by using two dimensions. The first dimension includes effectiveness, safety, timeliness, patient-/family-centeredness, access, and efficiency. Introducing these components to students in this framework will help them understand quality. The second dimension focuses on the types of care: preventive, acute, chronic. (See an example of a different care plan that applies IOM aspects of care located in the instructional materials.)

Differences in knowledge base and application will be noted based on the level of the student. Organize learning modules around these dimensions. Ask students to consider these dimensions in pre- and post-conferences, which are golden teaching moments.

Students and nurses alike need to consider how the matrix components relate to their practice and roles:

I Each of these components can be interwoven into content. For example, when discussing the childbearing family, what aspects of nursing care are related to safety, effectiveness, timeliness, patient-/family-centeredness, access, and efficiency?

I When students are in practicum, how do they observe each of these components? Are there differences between acute care and community settings? Why might this be so? Ask students to include these components as they use clinical thinking and clinical reasoning and judgment in care planning or in discussions in post-conferences.

Because patient-centered care is the key core competency, the annual national quality report describes data related to the six dimensions of patient-centered care (Gerteis, Edgman-Levitan, Daley, & Delbanco, 1993, as cited in IOM, 2001a, p. 49): (1) respect for patients' values (cultural, ethnic, and religious preferences) and expressed needs; (2) coordination and integration of care; (3) information, communication, and education; (4) physical comfort; (5) emotional support, relieving fear and anxiety; and (6) involvement of family and friends. These dimensions of patient-centered care should be incorporated into the plan of care, but how can they be used in teaching?

The first National Healthcare Quality Report was published in 2001. Since the first IOM reports acknowledged that health care needed major improvement and that monitoring of care was not ongoing, what has changed, and what is the current status of the nation's care quality? There has been slow improvement. This annual report is a rich source of information for curriculum updates or content for a class, and can be used by students to search data. It is accessible online at www.ahrq.gov/qual/qrdr10.htm.

The quality report matrix is connected to the report *Healthy People in Healthy Communities: A Systematic Approach to Health Improvement*. Figure 5-5 describes the framework for *Healthy People 2020*. This content is typically discussed under community health; faculty should also connect it with the work done by the IOM. (See Teaching–Learning Module 29, National Healthcare Quality Monitoring, for more information about national healthcare monitoring.)

Change Process

QI requires change; to understand QI and the process, students must discuss change. They should be familiar with the change process and be able to apply it in the clinical setting. Discuss change in pre- and post-conferences; ask how change affects individual patients and their families, the patient care unit and its staff, the healthcare organization, and the student. The faculty, however, need to be positive role models by demonstrating the ability to deal with constant flux instead of clinging to the status quo. Content should include the change process, in relation to redesigning care processes based on best practices such as EBP; use of information technology; knowledge management;

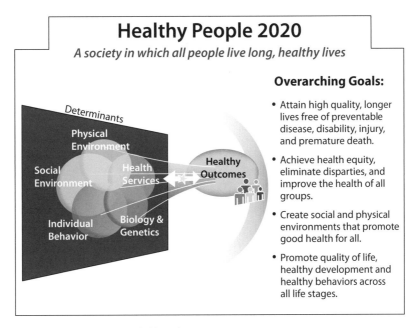

Source: *Healthy People 2020.* Retrieved from http://www.healthypeople.gov

F I G U R E 5 - 5   Healthy People 2020

development of effective teams; coordination of care across patient conditions, services, and settings; performance and outcome measurements; organizational climate; and coping with change. Why are these issues important in health care? How do they affect nursing? What related experiences have students had? (See Teaching–Learning Module 4, Change and Quality Improvement, for more information on this topic.)

Science of Improvement

Berwick (2008) suggests that healthcare professionals need to step back and look at QI research differently from traditional research. Randomized clinical trials (RCTs) are not necessarily the "gold standard" for QI projects. This is not the best way to bring about social change. For "[m]ulticomponent interventions, some of which are interpersonal, all of which are nonlinear, in complex social systems— . . . other, richer, but equally disciplined, ways to learn (such as CMO [context + mechanism = outcome] designs) are needed" (Berwick, 2008, p. 1183). To accelerate improvement of systems of care and practice, we need to (pp. 1183–1184):

- Embrace a wider range of scientific methodologies.
- Reconsider thresholds for action on evidence, and do not favor the status quo ($P < .05$ is not helpful for QI). Some have advised moving cautiously in improvement, but Berwick says, "It is both possible and wise to remain alert and vigilant for problems while testing promising changes very rapidly and with a sense of urgency. A central idea in improvement is to make changes incrementally, learning from experience while doing so: Plan-Do-Study-Act (PDSA)."

- Rethink views about trust and bias. Bias can eliminate local wisdom; those who are making changes in care systems usually know more about the mechanisms and content than a third-party evaluator, and assaults on bias can discourage change agents. The best approach is "to equip the workforce to study the effects of their efforts, actively and objectively, as part of daily work."
- Be careful about mood, affect, and civility in evaluations.

The wrong approach is to ask: "Where is the randomized trial?" The better approach is to ask: "What is everyone learning?"

Berwick, Nolan, and Whittington (2008) emphasize that health care must change to address the Triple Aim: care, health, and cost:

- Improving the experience of care
- Improving the health of population
- Reducing per capita costs of health care

There is still much to be done to ensure care safety, effectiveness, patient-centeredness, timeliness, efficiency, and equity. The three aims are interdependent. The preconditions for meeting the Triple Aim are:

- Specify a population of concern (it does not have to be geographic; it could be based on needs or other criteria).
- Consider policy constraints (reimbursement, for example).
- Use an integrator, an entity that accepts responsibility for all three components of the Triple Aim for a specified population; also, link HCOs.

Patient and Family Roles in Improving Care

We see strong consumer safety initiatives in numerous areas such as the airline industry, and the government is also involved in areas such as product safety. Consumer advocacy is well developed in the United States (Spath, 2008). Strangely, though, health care is one of the weakest areas of consumer safety initiatives. In 1997, the health-care-related Consumer Bill of Rights and Responsibilities stressed consumer access to care that includes information, choice, consumer participation, and grievance and appeals rights when denied services or coverage of services—and yet we still have problems.

The newest issue in consumer health care is not just the importance of consumers (patients, families) participating in healthcare decision-making, but also the role of the patient and families in preventing errors. You do not have to be a healthcare provider to participate in error prevention. The airline industry actively involves travelers in safety prevention; for example, preparing for takeoff and landing and stowing baggage safely to prevent injuries. Why not do the same in health care? Patient-centeredness emphasizes the patient's role, the partnership between the patient and healthcare providers, and empowerment of the patient. Safety improvement should be part of this partnership. Healthcare professionals need to recognize that they are not the only persons involved in healthcare delivery and quality, with the patient totally dependent on healthcare providers. If one agrees that safety is a system property, then the entire healthcare system should be designed to prevent errors. This would include everyone involved—all staff, professional and nonprofessional, and patients and families. Different people may observe different safety issues, enhancing the ability to catch errors before they lead to problems. "Healthcare processes must be made transparent so that everyone (including the patient) knows what is going on and why" (Spath, 2008, p. 25).

What are some examples of situations in which patients should give feedback to prevent errors? Patients and families can easily identify many issues as problems, such as problems with universal precautions, handwashing, medications, cleanliness, slips and falls, clutter, and even medication administration (Spath, 2008). In some hospitals patients and families are encouraged to call rapid response teams if they feel the need for special assistance and are not getting responses from staff. Broader areas that would benefit from patient involvement include reaching an accurate diagnosis; deciding on an appropriate treatment or management strategy; choosing an experienced and safe provider with current appropriate certification and verified training; ensuring that treatment is appropriately administered, monitored, and adhered to; and quickly identifying side effects or adverse events and taking appropriate action (Vincent & Coulter, 2002). The healthcare system should consider the following to improve patient involvement in safety (Spath, 2008):

- Overcome the "culture of individual accountability" that can inhibit collaboration.
- Introduce strategies and techniques for patients to safely navigate a healthcare system.
- Break through barriers caused by low health literacy.
- Overcome legal, cultural, and regulatory issues that affect information sharing and disclosure. Repair adversarial patient–caregiver relationships through patient-centered care and transparency.

(See Teaching–Learning Module 24, Integrating the Patient and Family in Quality Improvement, for more information about this topic.)

Safety: A Critical Component of Quality Improvement

Safety Culture in the Healthcare Organization

Moving to a culture in which everyone is a safety inspector is new for health care. It is easier to blame an individual for an error, as healthcare organizations have done for a long time. However, most errors are due to system, not human, failures. We need to move away from a punitive environment and focus more on learning environments that foster communication about errors and improvement.

In this spirit, HCOs are changing from the Blame Game culture toward a Just Culture approach to errors (Dekker, 2007; Steefel, 2008). This is a nonpunitive, fair, and just system, though there still must be "personal and professional accountability of one's practice actions and accountability for actively engaging in activities that will improve the processes of care" (Steefel, 2008, p. 25). A Just Culture environment is one in which "managers talk to staff about risk factors to safety and contributing factors to errors" (Steefel, 2008, p. 25). All staff are expected to use methods to ensure early recognition of safety risks. The reporting of incidents is seen as a learning opportunity to "trend identifiers that will provide opportunities to address latent safety problems" (Steefel, 2008, p. 25). Human error may require changes in processes, design, procedures, environment, or training. Coaching can reduce at-risk behaviors in staff that may lead them to make errors. Interventions to reduce at-risk behavior include removing incentives for at-risk behaviors, creating incentives for healthy behaviors, and increasing situational awareness.

Some clinical areas are more prone to errors, due to the nature of the care and environment, such as ICUs and ERs. This type of environment requires speed in decisions and actions, which increases the risk of errors (Gaskill, 2008). This calls for greater efforts to prevent errors, but knowing that some will not be prevented is important in establishing a Just Culture. This requires a cultural transformation, rewarding instead of penalizing staff for reporting errors and near misses. Staff need to feel safe to mention near misses and errors and then become part of the solution. Administration needs to recognize that increased reports of errors and near misses is not a bad sign; *not* reporting is much more serious. When students are in high-risk areas, faculty and students both need to be more alert for errors. This should be discussed with students. Ask them for examples of high-risk activities and ways in which errors can be prevented.

What happens when an error occurs and a student and faculty are involved? How comfortable do faculty and students feel about reporting a near miss or an error (disclosure)? Is there a process at the school, similar to the process in the clinical setting, for analyzing errors so students can learn from it, or are errors swept under the rug, with little opportunity for students and faculty to discuss and express their own reactions to making errors? If we do the latter, we are teaching students that this type of response is acceptable in practice after graduation, and it is not. Consider the following with students (and faculty) when errors occur (Banja, 2005, p. 162):

1. What was the nature of my mistake?
2. What are my beliefs about the mistake?
3. What emotions did I experience in the aftermath of the mistake?
4. How did I cope with the mistake?
5. What changes did I make in my practice as a result of the mistake?

When students or faculty are involved in an error and disclosure is necessary, what communication factors should be considered? Newer views of disclosure of errors recommend that the following steps be taken (Banja, 2005, pp. 179–186):

▌ Agree on what happened. All parties should be involved.
▌ The patient's physician should be the principal communicator; the presence of an HCO attorney is not advised.

- Decide where the disclosure should occur. Be as accommodating as possible; privacy without distractions is important.
- Use tape recorders only if the patient wants a recording.
- Anticipate a lawsuit.
- Communicate: Sit and be empathetic; watch body language and defensive posture; talk slowly and avoid overtalking; give the listener time to make comments and ask questions. Answer questions truthfully; listen for cues; and do not interrupt.
- Avoid blaming.
- Apologize.

Certain content should be included in an error disclosure (Banja, 2005, p. 184):

- A description of the nature of the error and the harm it caused
- When and where the error occurred
- Consequences of the harm
- Clinical and institutional actions taken to diminish the seriousness of the harm
- Actions taken to prevent future occurrences of the error
- Responsibility for managing the patient's continuing care
- Identification of systematic elements that contributed to the error
- Responsibility for managing the ongoing communications
- Removal of associated costs of the error from the patient's bill (assuming costs are known)
- Offer of counseling and support

Schools of nursing need an error policy and procedure, and this topic also ought to be discussed with students.

Many HCOs are working to create safety cultures, and students are introduced to this in their practica. Advise students to ask about safety when they seek employment. Provide them with positive examples like the Veterans Administration system. The VA web site (http://www.patientsafety.gov/) describes the VA safety culture, root cause analysis, and more. Ask students to search the Internet for other HCOs with information about safety on their web sites.

Creating and sustaining a culture of safety should include: (1) an understanding of its essential elements, (2) the barriers to creating the culture, (3) strategies to create the safety culture, and (4) evaluation of results or outcomes (IOM, 2004b). Safety orientation is necessary to prepare staff and to maintain the knowledge of safety. Trust is crucial when staff are asked to report errors and near misses: What will be the reaction, and will staff be blamed? Nurses face a major hurdle in accepting this new safety culture because "nurses are trained to believe that clinical perfection is an attainable goal" (Jones, 2002, as cited in IOM, 2004b, p. 298) and that "'good' nurses do not make errors" (Banister, Butt, & Hackel, 1996, as cited in IOM, 2004b, p. 298). Every nursing program should examine its culture periodically and dispel such unrealistic expectations.

Because healthcare organizations periodically review their competency requirements for new staff and update staff over time about safety, schools of nursing should also ensure that safety is included in their student competencies. These should be consistent with the staff competencies established by healthcare organizations. Schools of nursing should use local HCOs' safety requirements and competencies, nursing professional standards, regulations (nurse practice acts), and Joint Commission safety standards and goals and those of other accreditation organizations. These goals change annually, so faculty need to keep up with the changes. (See Teaching–Learning Module 11, Culture of Safety, for more information about this topic.)

Root Cause Analysis

Currently, the root cause analysis is used by most hospitals and many other healthcare organizations to analyze errors. This method supports the view that errors typically have system causes and thus must be understood to improve care. Students need to know about this method, as they will be involved with it when they take nursing positions. They also need to practice using it as students (for example, in simulations). The root cause analysis steps are:

1. What happened (described in detail)?
2. Who was involved?
3. When did it happen?
4. Where did it happen?
5. What is the severity of the actual or potential harm?
6. What is the chance it will happen again?
7. What are the consequences?

An interprofessional team representing key stakeholders should do this analysis. At the end of the process, the team should be able to identify prevention strategies. There are resources on the Internet that can assist faculty in developing content and teaching–learning strategies, such as the web sites of the VA (http://www.patientsafety.gov/rca.html), The Joint Commission (http://www.jointcommission.org), and the Institute for Health Improvement (http://www.ihi.org). (See Teaching–Learning Module 37, Root Cause Analysis, for more information about this topic.)

Stakeholders

Many stakeholders are involved in the healthcare process, and it is important that students understand the identity of the stakeholders and their roles. Ask students about the patient admission process to the hospital and which stakeholders the patient will encounter. How does this affect quality of care, fragmentation of care, care coordination, or the risk of errors?

Current data describe the viewpoints of different stakeholders—and different stakeholders do have different views of quality, as described in the following example. In a 2002 national survey of physicians and consumers about medical errors, 35% of the

831 physicians and 42% of the consumers experienced errors (either in care of self or family members). Neither group viewed errors as an important problem or associated errors with lower-quality care (Blendon et al., 2002). Much literature describes consumer views of quality, but we have less information about how different healthcare professionals view quality (Jennings & McClure, 2004). Nurses are not typically seen as leaders in quality initiatives, but they should be, given nursing's impact on and role in the system (Jennings & McClure, 2004). A national hospital survey on patient safety culture that includes data from almost 400 hospitals, collected from October 2006 to June 2007, indicates: (1) 65% of the patients would definitely recommend their hospital to family and friends; (2) 63% of patients rated their hospitals a score of 9 out of 10; (3) more than 25% of patients said their nurses did not always communicate well with them; (4) many patients said that they were not treated with courtesy and respect by doctors and nurses; (5) patients said they had not received adequate pain medication after surgery; and (6) patients reported that they did not understand discharge directions (Pear, 2008). The ANA polled more than 10,000 nurses on safety and staffing concerns (*Oklahoma's Nursing Times*, 2008, p. 11):

- 73% did not believe that staffing on their unit or shift was sufficient.
- 59.8% said they knew of someone who left direct care nursing because of concerns about safe staffing.
- 51.9% of those polled were considering leaving their current position, and 46% cited inadequate staffing as the reason.
- 51.7% said they thought the quality of nursing care on their unit had declined in the past year.
- 48.2% did not feel confident having someone close to them receiving care in the facility where they worked.

These results indicate serious problems in the nursing profession and the healthcare system that must be addressed. Students in clinical observe nursing care, nurse attitudes and behaviors, and more. Attitudes like those noted in this survey can make students wonder about the profession they are entering. The best response for faculty is to open up discussion so students can express their concerns, discuss the issues, and consider solutions.

Errors and Related Issues

Critical Definitions

The IOM report on patient safety defines *safety* as "freedom from accidental injury" (1999. p. 18) and an *error* as "the failure of a planned action to be completed as intended (for example, error of execution) or the use of a wrong plan to achieve an aim (for example, error of planning)" (Reason, 1990, as cited in IOM, 1999, p. 28). Though the report defines *error*, there is no healthcare consensus on a definition, and there have been disagreements about what actually constitutes an error. Some physicians consider delays in treatment, use of outmoded treatment, failure to use needed diagnostic tests, failure to act on test results, mistakes in administration of treatment, and failure to communicate to be practice variances, suboptimal outcomes, or differences in clinical judgment, not errors. In some situations nurses also agreed that these examples are not errors (Mason, 2004).

There is some controversy about errors and safety. In 2002, the National Coordinating Council for Medication Error Reporting and Prevention (NCC MERP) approved a statement refuting the use of medication error rates. The statement, posted on the council's web site (http://www.nccmerp.org), claims that the "use of medication error rates to compare healthcare organizations is of no value." The council has taken this position for the following reasons:

I Differences in *culture* among healthcare organizations can lead to significant differences in the level of medication error reporting.

I Differences in the *definition* of a medication error among healthcare organizations can lead to significant differences in the reporting and classification of medication errors.

I Differences in the *patient populations* served by various healthcare organizations can lead to significant differences among organizations in the number and severity of medication errors that occur.

I Differences in the *types of reporting and detection systems* for medication errors among healthcare organizations can lead to significant differences in the number of medication errors recorded.

NCC MERP believes that the quality of data is more important than the number of errors; there should be no acceptable incidence rates for medication errors. Given this viewpoint, healthcare organizations should continually improve systems to prevent harm to patients due to medication errors. Monitoring actual and potential medication errors and analysis of the root cause of errors should not stop, and there should be efforts to identify strategies to reduce errors.

Despite the 1999 IOM declaration that the U.S. healthcare system needed improvement and the addition of critical evidence from subsequent reports, errors continue and quality suffers. "From 2004 through 2006, patient safety errors resulted in 238,337 potentially preventable deaths of U.S. Medicare patients and the cost of the Medicare program at $8.8 billion. The overall medical error rate was about 3% for all Medicare patients, which works out to about 1.1 million patient safety incidents during the three years included in the analysis, which included 41 million Medicare patient records. Patients who experienced a patient safety incident had a 20% chance of dying as a result of the incident" (*Washington Post*, 2008). Data from 2010 indicate that 13.5% of hospitalized Medicare patients experienced adverse events that resulted in prolonged hospitalization, required life-sustaining intervention, caused permanent disability, or resulted in death, and an additional 13.5% experienced temporary harm events that required treatment (Levinson, 2012). This report from the HHS Inspector General, which sampled 189 hospitals, identified some key findings that have implications for nursing education (pp. i–ii).

I All sampled hospitals had incident reporting systems to capture events, and the administrators interviewed rely heavily on these systems to identify problems.

- Hospital staff did not report 86% of events to incident reporting systems, partly because of staff misperceptions about what constitutes patient harm.
- Nurses most often reported events, typically identified through the regular course of care; 28 of the 40 reported events led to investigations and 5 led to policy changes.
- Hospital accreditors reported that in evaluating hospital safety practices, they focus on how event information is used rather than how it is collected.

Of the events reported, 11% related to surgery or other procedures; 13% related to medications; 16% to patient care (for example, falls, pressure ulcer, embolism, aspiration, and others); and 16% to infection (pp. 29–30).

Progress has been made in raising awareness about errors, developing reporting systems, and establishing national data collection standards (AHRQ, 2010b). The 2010 National Healthcare Quality Report (NHQR) includes a section devoted to patient safety errors. Students need to understand not only the entire problem area of errors, but also that errors have a major cost impact. Cost due to medical errors was $19.8 billion and total cost per error was $13,000 (2008 estimates; Shreve et al., 2010).

Some error-reduction strategies continue to be important even over a long period of time and are important to consider when designing learning activities related to quality improvement (Leape et al., 1991; Leape, 1994):

- *Reduce reliance on memory*. Make greater use of checklists, computerized decision forms, and protocols.
- *Improve information access*. Make greater use of informatics placed as close to the point of care as possible.
- *Make processes error-proof*. Use processes that force prevention, such as computer safeguards that send up "red flags."
- *Standardize tasks*. Make tasks more consistent.
- *Reduce the number of handoffs*. Reduce handoffs and improve unavoidable handoffs.

Benner, Malloch, and Sheets (2010) discuss individual, practice, and system causes of errors in nursing. Working with the National Council of State Boards of Nursing (NCSBN), they present TERCAP: a Taxonomy of Error, Root Cause Analysis, and Practice Responsibility. The work is based on the standards of safe medication administration, documentation, attentiveness/surveillance, clinical reasoning, prevention, intervention, interpretation of authorized provider orders, and professional responsibility/patient advocacy. The five IOM core competencies are included in this taxonomy. This is an excellent resource for nurse educators; for example, as a guide for the development of student simulation experiences on errors. (See Teaching–Learning Module 12, Disclosure of Errors, and Module 38, Safety and Human Factors, for more information about safety and human factors and errors.)

Near Misses and Students

When near misses occur in the simulation lab or in practicum, ask students to identify the type of near miss error and provide a rationale to support their choice. How did they recognize a near miss? Let students discuss their reactions and feelings. Discuss possible steps to prevent the error. Using a root cause analysis, look at system processes and consider factors such as teaching methods, learning opportunities, faculty experience, or other factors that contributed to the near miss. If an error occurred, this same process can be used to learn more about the error. Give students scenarios to analyze and determine which errors may lead to harm and what type of harm. When students review scenarios, it is easy to jump to the conclusion that there was not enough staff; encourage them to look for many possible causes for the near miss (or error if one occurred), and then discuss possible interventions.

In one study, Dickson and Flynn (2012) examined how staff nurses used clinical reasoning to prevent errors. They noted the following: "Within the overarching theme of clinical reasoning, we identified two safety processes inherent in the data. In the first process of clinical reasoning, maintaining medication safety, we focused on how the nurses kept patients safe from medication errors. Six medication safety practices were identified: educating patients, taking everything into consideration, advocating for patients with pharmacy, coordinating care with physicians, conducting independent medication reconciliation, and verifying with colleagues. The second process of clinical reasoning was managing the clinical environment. Four categories emerged that described how nurses managed the sometimes chaotic environment of a busy hospital medical-surgical unit so as to protect the patients: coping with interruptions and distractions, interpreting physician orders, documenting 'near misses,' and encouraging open communication between disciplines" (p. 7). The investigators used the following definition of clinical reasoning for their study: "Simmons (2010) provided the most relevant definition consistent with our data: 'Clinical reasoning in nursing is a complex cognitive process that uses formal and informal thinking strategies to gather and analyze patient information, evaluate the significance of this information and weigh alternative actions'" (Dickson & Flynn, 2012, p. 1155). We need to examine more thoroughly how clinical reasoning affects a variety of nursing interventions and how it can be used to improve care. The information from this study is highly relevant to nursing education.

Risk for Errors

AHRQ (2003) identified the following as factors that may increase risk for errors:

- Communication problems, verbal and written, among all types of healthcare providers
- Inadequate information flow throughout the continuum of care
- Patient-related issues, such as lack of patient education
- Poor organizational knowledge transfer, such as lack of appropriate orientation, staff education, and so on

- Inadequate staffing patterns, such as inadequate staffing, lack of appropriate supervision in situations that hold high risk for errors, inappropriate staff mix and preparation
- Technical failures, such as of medical equipment; poor maintenance of equipment
- Inadequate policies and procedures

Analyze Errors: A Student Experience

Give students or staff teams the same scenario in which there is an error and ask each team to do a root cause analysis regarding the error. What different solutions can the teams find? Compare the students' proposed solutions. How did each team arrive at its solution? What was the team process? Are there different methods to reach solutions? Students and staff need experience in understanding how errors happen and how best to prevent errors.

In developing an environment of learning rather than blame, and avoiding the Blame Game, staff and students need to learn from near miss and error experiences. Policy and standards must be clear. Communication must be open. Survey the students to find out how they view the learning environment. What do they think will happen if a near miss or an error occurs, and they report it? Do they know the difference between the two? What is their attitude toward errors? What do they see happening related to safety in the healthcare organizations where they go for clinical experience? A school's student nurses association could support a campaign for a safety culture.

Help students analyze errors and identify human factors that may be related to the errors, while reminding them that human factors are not always the cause. Analyze the event, causes, circumstances, conditions, associated procedures, and devices that may be involved. Students need to understand this process well enough to use it in their own clinical practice. Discuss the effects of stressors on error rates, including fatigue, interruptions, noise, job dissatisfaction, burnout, work overload, shift work, family issues, and organizational politics. Include specific examples of legal issues, standards of practice, nurse practice acts, and documentation of errors so that students are aware of the connection between safety and errors and legal and regulatory issues. Discuss the ANA Code of Ethics and standards in relationship to this topic.

As more hospitals have increased QI activities, demands on nurses have also increased (Robert Wood Johnson Foundation, 2008a). A study by the Center for Studying Health System Change (Draper, Felland, Liebhaber, & Melichar, 2008) examined the impact of QI on nurses. Because nurses play a critical role in patient care, it is safe to conclude that they should be an important part of QI. This, however, is a difficult dilemma. Nurses are needed to care for patients and manage care; involving nurses in QI pulls them away from direct care when there is a nursing shortage. QI involves duplicative activities, and data collection is not always the most interesting work. Nurses have inadequate education about QI in their nursing programs, so they are not always prepared to recognize the importance of QI, how they can participate in QI, and how they can assume leadership roles in QI. However, every nurse who provides direct care has QI responsibilities: to ensure that quality care is provided, to prevent or reduced errors, and to monitor care and report critical QI data as needed.

The *Future of Nursing* (2011d) report, discussed earlier, also emphasizes the need for greater nursing leadership in QI—but nurses are not prepared for this, as is clear from earlier IOM reports. Several more recent articles (Shalala & Vladeck, 2011; O'Neil & Chow, 2011) identify areas of practice in which nurses have excelled and could continue to do so. What is of particular interest, and has the most direct connection to the IOM QI effort, is these authors' comments about nurses' roles in integration and coordination of care that lead to care transitions that are safer, more effective, comprehensible, and affordable. This requires leadership—from all nurses, not just ANPs. Staff nurses and nurse managers provide the majority of nursing care, and here is where we need greater QI leadership. Clinical Nurse Specialists also need to assume critical QI oles within the the healthcare delivery system. The RWJ Foundation Executive Nurse Fellows Program identifies the five core leadership competencies of effective leaders: self-knowledge, strategic vision, risk taking and creativity, interpersonal and communication effectiveness, and inspiring and leading change (Morjikian & Bellack, 2005). We need to include more content and learning experiences on leadership. Is it time to look at our placement of leadership and management content in our curricula, which typically comes at the end of our undergraduate programs? We miss many opportunities to reinforce this content and build competency if it is at the end. Where is this content in graduate programs?

Disclosure of Errors/Need for Transparency

"Disclosing a harm-causing medical error can be one of the most anguishing conversations a health professional can have" (Banja, 2005, p. ix). It can be highly stressful psychologically and can even result in staff experiencing physical reactions. The health professional's feelings of control, adequacy, or competence can be threatened. It is difficult to accept that errors are inevitable, but health care is a complex system and errors *will* occur. A nursing study that examined responses to and coping with errors noted that higher proportions of nursing staff experienced more internal than external responses to errors, such as depression, anger, and guilt; however, it is this internal experience that has an impact on improving coping rather than blaming others (Karga, Kiekkas, Diamanto, & Chrisoula, 2011).

The first question is: What should be disclosed? One point of view or assumption is that only the most severe errors should be disclosed; others may be classified as questionable judgment calls, incidents, or misadventures (Banja, 2005). The second question is: Did the error cause harm? This is not always easy to determine; for example, a patient may begin to "crash," but was this caused by an error? Did an error clearly cause the complication, or were other factors involved? This, of course, can be an excuse for nurses to talk themselves out of the error, convincing themselves that it was not a real error.

The third issue is assigning responsibility—not blame, and avoiding the Blame Game. We need to remember that systems facilitate error occurrence. Systems have faults or latent failures that enable errors or fail to stop errors. However, there can be single-point failures when one person fails to do something or does something incorrectly and thus makes an error. The natural tendency is to protect oneself and not reveal an error. As nurse educators, we must try harder to discuss these issues openly with students and in staff education.

If one thinks of the nurse–patient relationship as a contract, this implies that there is a contractual obligation. This is the patient-centered model, and would naturally support disclosure of errors. This contract requires open communication between the parties (nurse and patient). Patients have the right to know about errors that have occurred. Nevertheless, despite this relationship it is easy to use rationalization or blame shifting or even self-deception; a staff member often conceals an error for fear of malpractice charges or fear about impact on performance evaluation (student or staff). Professionalism requires that we take responsibility and that we communicate with patients. Many hospitals and medical centers are trying to figure out the best way to increase disclosure of errors and how staff should communicate errors to patients and families, recognizing that full disclosure is best for practitioners, the organization, and the patient (Shapiro, 2008). Ethical issues and legal concerns are part of this process. Commenting on the ANA Code of Ethics helps students understand the connection between ethics and errors.

Review with students how information is shared with patients or about patients, by whom, and what type of information is shared. Include implications of the Health Insurance Portability and Accountability Act (HIPAA). Why is it important to give patients information? As students participate in procedures, they need to understand informed consent. They should be knowledgeable about organization policies and procedures. The best time to introduce informed consent and the nurse's role is when students learn about procedures. It is important to discuss transparency and sharing information about quality of care.

Medications and Administration: Errors

One of the interventions with a high risk of errors is medication administration, particularly given the increasing number of drugs, unfamiliar drugs, inadequate math proficiency, environmental stresses (interruptions, fatigue, overwork, and miscommunication), illegible orders, lack of patient information, and problems with equipment. Bar codes, unit dose dispensing, smart infusion pumps, reference resources, and drug training can all reduce errors. Administering medications safely is one of the critical competencies that any nursing student learns. Simulation can be very beneficial, and testing competency in simulated experiences allows students to learn without harming patients.

What conditions increase the risk of student nurse errors? A report published in 2008 by Harding and Petrick particularly notes that duality of patient assignments sets up a potential for risk: patients assigned both to students and to staff. This is a necessary situation in the clinical environment, of course, but it is vital to clearly communicate who is administering medications (that is, the student or the staff), what held medications are and when they should be given, and so on. These situations can lead to dose omissions and extra doses. Insulin is among the drugs most frequently involved in student nurse errors. The conditions that lead to most student-nurse errors, with examples of each, are (Institute for Safe Medication Practices, 2007):

I Nonstandard dosage times: A medication is ordered for a time other than two, three, or four times a day.

I Documentation issues: Medications are not properly documented, which can lead to extra doses, dose omissions, and so on.

I Medical administration records (MARs) unavailable: Students should work only with the original MAR, not copies.

I Partial drug administration: Students may not be giving IV medications, but the student needs to confirm this with staff who may be required to administer the medication.

I Held or discontinued medications: Students do not know what the policy is for holding drugs or discontinuing drugs or are not informed of changes.

I Monitoring issues: A patient needs to have vital signs monitored before or after certain medication is administered, with actions taken if vital signs are not in a specified range; or laboratory tests must be reviewed before a medication is administered.

I Nonspecific doses dispensed: Only a multidose source is available, and the student thinks it is a patient-specific dose, so an individual patient dose is not calculated.

I Oral liquids that are only for oral use: The student administers oral liquid medications in a parenteral syringe via intramuscular injection.

A study by Harding and Petrick (2008) examined medication errors made and reported by nursing students. This retrospective review identified three categories of errors:

I *Rights violations*: Does the rights-of-administration approach that we are taught to use and teach students lead to narrow thinking because the rights do not consider the system context? Do we isolate our teaching too much by focusing on patient rights, system parts, and knowledge so that students do not know how to synthesize all of this information? They need greater direction in understanding the process as a whole.

I *System factors*: The full context of the work setting in which medication is administered may contribute to errors. Often errors in this category have something to do with the medical administration record (MAR), but there is much more to it. It includes, for example, the room where medications are prepared: Are there issues with privacy, noise, and interruptions? Are there problems with the pharmacy processes and how the pharmacy interacts with the unit and nurses? Are issues inherent in the entire medication administration process (all steps)? Teaching strategies that are more problem- and simulation-based can improve students' understanding of work-environment issues.

I *Knowledge and understanding*: Gaps in knowledge or understanding can and do lead to errors.

The Joint Commission publishes alerts related to medications and medication administration that are important for faculty to be aware of and use in teaching. The Joint Commission web site (http://www.jointcommission.org/) can be searched for "medication alerts."

Still other factors increase the risk of medication errors (Harding & Petrick, 2008; Wolf, 2001). Students need to recognize that medication administration is a multiphase process (prescribing, transcribing, dispensing, administering, and monitoring), and that each phase has potential for errors. The highest rates of error occur in the ordering phase (49%–56% of the errors), but the second highest is the administration phase (26%–40%) (Ackroyd-Stolarz, Hartnell, & MacKinnon, 2005; Manno, 2006). Wolf (2001) identifies 90 steps in the typical cycle of medication administration. Students report that distractions during administration led to many of their errors. Students need to learn how to cope with distractions. Some of this can be incorporated into simulation experiences. According to studies by Hughes and Ortiz (2005) and Manno (2006), 27% of the errors were due to distraction. Errors of omission are high, at the rate of 34% (Hughes & Ortiz, 2005; Manno, 2006). The common element in many of these errors was the medical administration record, such as inexperience in reading or interpreting the MAR.

Are we focusing too much on the five rights when we teach medication administration? Is this too narrow an approach that ignores the real world (Harding & Petrick, 2008)? Do students understand the system and its parts—from the order, to pharmacy, to unit role, and then to individual patient administration and follow-up? Case scenarios and problem-based teaching strategies may be more effective. We need to do more than just have students administer a medication in a lab setting and then record it on the form or computer MAR that we provide. This separates medication administration from reality. Our simulations must be more realistic, with noise, people demanding information, time pressure, and so on. We should do much more with students to focus them on including the patient. Students need to understand why the patient should be involved and that the patient can help to prevent errors; this also enhances patient-centered care. Some schools of nursing are integrating pharmacology throughout the curriculum, though there are questions about this approach, too. Some faculty believe that there continues to be a need for a stand-alone course on pharmacology (Wolf, 2001). A study by Candela and Bowles (2008) explored recent RN graduates' perceptions of educational preparation. They found that recent graduates felt they lacked sufficient pharmacology content, which is consistent with findings by other researchers (King, 2004). This also has a direct bearing on medication administration. Another study noted success in using a web-based course that integrated pathophysiology and pharmacology and emphasized application and integration rather than memorization (Tse & Lo, 2008).

With more patients taking prescription, over-the-counter, and complementary medications and substances, errors have increased. Students need to learn all the steps of medication administration, use of multiple drugs (both prescribed and over-the-counter), patient and caregiver education and direction, how to question conflicting orders, and assessment of patient medication. Use simulation scenarios that include multiple drug orders for students to identify appropriate orders, drug interactions, dosages, and administration. Discuss typical errors or ask students what they think would be typical errors based on an analysis of the medication procedure. Ask what corrective actions they would take and what might prevent a future error.

Medication Administration Process

Each step in the medication process—prescribing, dispensing, administering, monitoring, and managing—should be included in content and applied to practice. Begin when students first learn about medication administration, and reinforce it throughout the curriculum. Drug name confusion is a common cause of drug errors; provide examples and ask students to distinguish between similarly named drugs. See also Joint Commission recommendations related to medication administration and documentation on its web site (http://www.jointcommission.org/). Inform students about the process for reporting medication errors in the HCO. There is also a system through the U.S. Pharmacopeia (USP) for reporting errors. The Institute for Safe Medication Practices (ISMP, 2007) includes cases and warnings on its web site (http://www.ismp.org). In legal and ethical course content, discuss malpractice and professional liability insurance. Relate this content to the ANA Code of Ethics and standards.

New Approaches to Medication Administration

Dr. Linda Burnes-Bolton initiated a new approach to medication administration at Cedars-Sinai Medical Center of Los Angeles. It blends old and new in a collaborative approach to reduce medication errors, posing four questions (Steefel, 2008):

- What if an RN with advanced knowledge and experience worked in collaboration with pharmacy and medical staff to codesign the medication process?
- What if an RN interviewed all newly admitted patients and set a medication plan?
- What if an RN and a pharmacist co-led the patient or family education process at the unit or clinic level?
- What if nurses applied the "sterile cockpit" approach (no interruptions in the cockpit—in the case of nursing, no interruptions as medications are prepared and administered) to the medication administration process?

Make students aware of these new approaches and ask them use critical thinking in considering different methods to improve the medication process. As RNs, they will not have time to wait for others to come up with solutions.

Medication Reconciliation

The IHI defines *medication reconciliation* as "creating the most accurate list possible of all medications a patient is taking—including drug name, dosage, frequency, and route—and comparing that list against the physician's admission, transfer, and/ or discharge orders with the goal of providing correct medications to the patient at all transition points within the hospital" (IHI, 2008d). To accomplish this, hospitals need policies and procedures that assign primary responsibility for the task, identify time frames for completion of medication reconciliation, use standardized forms that are easily accessible and visible at all times during transfer, and clarify all medication discrepancies with the prescribing physician (Ketchum, Grass, & Padwojski, 2005). How is this relevant for students? They need to know about medication reconciliation; appreciate its importance; and understand the process. This can be discussed during content on medication administration, in simulation, and during clinical experiences; for example, in a home care experience students can review all the medications the patient is taking.

The AHRQ has developed a tool kit, *Medications at Transitions and Clinical Handoffs (MATCH) Toolkit for Medication Reconciliation* (AHRQ, 2011). The toolkit content notes that medication reconciliation is a complex process that affects all patients as they move through healthcare settings (p. 1). It is a comparison of the patient's current medication regimen against the physician's admission, transfer, and/or discharge orders to identify discrepancies. Any discrepancies noted are discussed with the prescriber, and the order is modified, if necessary. Although this toolkit is based on processes developed in acute care settings, the core processes, tools, and resources can be adapted for use in post-acute facilities. The medication reconciliation process can decrease medication errors and patient harm in the following ways:

- Obtaining, verifying, and documenting the patient's current prescription and over-the-counter medications—including vitamins, supplements, eye drops, creams, ointments, and herbals—when the patient is admitted to the hospital or is seen in an outpatient setting.
- Considering the patient's preadmission/home medication list when ordering medicines during a hospital encounter; continuing home medications as appropriate; and comparing the patient's preadmission/home medication list to ordered medicines and treatment plans to identify unintended discrepancies (i.e., those not explained by the patient's clinical condition or formulary status).
- Verifying the patient's home medication list and discussing unintended discrepancies with the physician for resolution.
- Providing an updated medication list and communicating the importance of managing medication information to the patient when he or she is discharged from the hospital or at the end of an outpatient encounter.

This resource (available in PDF format at http://www.ahrq.gov/qual/match/) is an excellent resource on this topic for faculty in developing content and learning strategies, and also for student review. (See Teaching–Learning Module 27, Medication Reconciliation, for more information about this topic.)

Effective Medication Management

The list of priority areas for national action (IOM, 2003f) particularly identified prevention of medication errors and overprescription of antibiotics as critical concerns. Pharmacology courses should explain the purpose of antibiotics, the risk of overprescription, and the results of overprescription. Nurses provide patient and family education in schools, clinics, hospitals, and many other settings where it is easy to incorporate information about appropriate use of antibiotics, especially in pediatrics. What are the consequences for individuals and communities when antibiotics are used inappropriately?

Curriculum and Medication Errors

What do students need to know about medication errors? Key questions that should be included in nursing education and in staff development are:

- What is an error? What are the types of errors? For example: Errors, adverse events, root cause analysis, near misses, and medication administration process and errors
- How frequently do errors occur?
- What factors contribute to errors?
- What are the costs of errors?
- Are public perceptions of safety in health care consistent with the evidence?

Are these questions included in nursing curricula and all clinical experiences in different healthcare settings? Do we consider the following in our curricula? Other sources of medication errors are: human knowledge; chaotic work environment; verbal orders; lack of staff; similar medication packaging, labels, and names; math errors; poor handwriting; lack of a dose verification process; borrowing drugs from a multidose cart; using floor stock medications; not following policies and procedures; human performance; IV solutions that are not premixed; acronyms; typographical mistakes; lack of dose checks for high-risk drugs and pediatric patients' medications; and lack of interprofessional team review of medication errors (Wolf, 2001).

Problem-based teaching of medication error prevention can be effective. Papastrat and Wallace (2003) describe a series of questions and statements that can be used to guide a discussion on a problem-based scenario related to a case on error prevention. These questions include:

- What is known about the problem? From the case scenario; from your previous knowledge; from nursing knowledge?
- What do you need to know? What are the knowledge gaps? What information should spur further research?
- Prioritize the knowledge gaps. What information is the most significant?
- Hypothesize the problem. Identify the knowledge gaps. Describe your recommendations to be included in a quality improvement plan (QIP).

Other Critical Clinical Quality Issues and Methods

There are many critical clinical quality issues today, and different methods have been used to address some of these. The following sections describe some of these issues and related methods to identify the issue/problem and also to analyze and identify solution options.

Failure Modes and Effects Analysis (FMEA)

Failure modes and effects analysis focuses on safety in systems and prevention of accidents (Cohen, Davis, & Sanders, 1994; Wolf, 2001). This focus moves away from the individual to system and interprofessional issues. The approach builds in checkpoints in each step of the process, highlighting "redundancies that serve as safety nets or error traps" (Wolf, 2001, p. 31). Examples include:

- A medication nurse is required to read medication containers three times and may be required to get a second nurse to confirm the order.
- A provider writes a prescription, a unit clerk reads and transcribes the order, and a nurse checks the clerk's transcription.
- An EMR uses a double-check of allergies and sends an alert about a patient's allergy to a drug prescribed.
- A pharmacist dispenses medication, and a nurse checks the pharmacy's dispensing accuracy and medication with the transcribed orders before administering the medication.

"FMEA is a tool that provides a systematic, proactive method for evaluating a process to identify where and how it might fail and to assess the relative impact of different failures in order to identify the parts of the process that are in most need of change" (IHI, 2008c). FMEA software, which can be used to teach students about FMEA analysis, is available at http://www.IHI.org/knowledge/Pages/Tools/ FailureModesandEffectsAnalysisTool.aspx. Give the tool to student teams with case scenarios and ask them apply the tool to the case. (See Teaching–Learning Module 16, Failure Modes with Effects Analysis, for more about FMEA.)

Failure to Rescue (FTR)

Failure to rescue (FTR) is related to quality care and nursing. Hospitals are particularly concerned about this issue today, though it can arise in any patient setting. The "intent of the failure to rescue indicator is to measure the hospital's ability to rescue patients that have developed a serious complication" (Manojlovich & Talsma, 2007, p. 504). The AHRQ and the National Quality Forum (NQF) have described this indicator as a critical performance measure; however, there is no consensus on its definition, and this lack hampers data collection and analysis. What do students know about FTR? How do students understand the relationship between FTR and nursing care?

Two important nursing activities that can prevent failure to rescue are surveillance and taking action when a life-threatening patient complication develops (Clarke & Aiken, 2003). The common causes of failure to rescue are (Jones, DeVita, & Bellomo, 2011, p. 141):

▪ Monitoring technology is used only in the intensive care unit or step-down units.
▪ Hospital-ward monitoring is only intermittent (vital-sign measurements).
▪ Intervals between measurements can easily be 8 hours or longer.
▪ Regular visits by a hospital unit nurse vary in frequency and duration.
▪ Visits by a unit doctor may occur only once a day.
▪ When vital signs are measured, they are sometimes incomplete.
▪ When vital signs are abnormal, there may be no specific criteria for activating a higher-level intervention.
▪ Individual judgment is applied to a crucial decision.
▪ Individual judgment varies in accuracy according to training, experience, professional attitude, working environment, hierarchical position, and previous responses to alerts.
▪ If an alert is issued, the activation process goes through a long chain of command (e.g., nurse to charge nurse, charge nurse to intern, intern to resident, resident to fellow, fellow to attending physician).
▪ Each step in the chain is associated with individual judgment and delays.
▪ In surgical units, doctors are sometimes physically unavailable because they are performing operations.
▪ Modern hospitals provide care for patients with complex disorders and coexisting conditions, and unexpected clinical deterioration may occur while nurses and doctors are busy with other tasks.

Surveillance was identified in *Keeping Patients Safe* (IOM, 2004b) as a critical aspect of care directly related to nursing care. "Surveillance is monitoring patient status . . . . The goal of surveillance is the early identification and prevention of potential problems, which requires behavioral and cognitive skills" (IOM, 2004b, p. 91). The effectiveness of surveillance depends on many variables: competency, staffing levels, skill mix, communication and interprofessional teams and issues, staff stress levels, staff fatigue, documentation, equipment failure, and more. How do we prepare students for surveillance?

The growth in the use of simulation is one method that can work well. Students can experience patient complications in a safe environment and learn to identify factors leading to serious patient complications (Seago, Williamson, & Atwood, 2006). Failure to rescue has been associated with three complications attributable to nursing care: medication errors, falls, and pressure ulcers. As of the fall of 2008, these complications are included in the Medicare and Medicaid Hospital-Acquired Complications (HAC) list. (See Teaching–Learning Module 17, Failure to Rescue, and Module 41, Surveillance, for more information about these two topics.)

Rapid Response Teams (RRTs)

The rapid response team is a team of healthcare clinicians (physicians, nurses, respiratory therapists, and others) who are experts in critical care. The team comes to the bedside to assist staff in making rapid decisions when a patient may be experiencing life-threatening complications. IHI provides excellent content on RRTs at http://www.ihi.org/explore/rapidresponseteams/Pages/default.aspx. IHI notes three system issues that often affect care in critical situations (IHI, 2008f):

▮ Failure in planning (including assessments, treatments, goals) (relates to teamwork)
▮ Failure to communicate (patient to staff, staff to staff, staff to physicians, and so on) (relates to teamwork)
▮ Failure to recognize deteriorating patient condition (relates to patient-centered care; quality improvement)

One study indicates that RRTs may not be all that effective (Chan et al., 2008). This is only one study, but it should not be ignored in evaluating outcomes. Overall hospital death rates did not differ significantly before and after an RRT was implemented. Because these teams are costly and require a change in practice, it is important to investigate outcomes further—and nurses should be involved in this investigation. "Rapid-response systems have been introduced at hospitals in many countries, despite a lack of level 1 evidence that demonstrates their effectiveness. Their introduction has been driven by the belief that they make hospitals safer and prevent serious adverse events after sudden alterations in vital signs in hospital-ward patients. The rationale that early intervention is beneficial in almost all medical emergencies has also provided support for the introduction of rapid-response systems. Moreover, such systems are considered to be consistent with the concept that taking critical care expertise and skills out of the ICU to the patient's bedside (an ICU without walls) as rapidly as possible is physiologically and clinically sound" (Jones, DeVita, & Bellomo, 2011, p. 145).

Students need to explore how are RRTs are used. What impact do RRTs have on staff function? Ask students to search for literature on this topic. How are these teams being used in hospitals? What have been the results? How might RRTs affect quality? (See Teaching–Learning Module 34, Rapid Response Team, for more information about RRTs.)

Handoffs

Patient transfers are considered high-risk error situations. Transfers can involve interruptions in care, miscommunication, and duplication of effort. Interunit transfers have increased. "It is not unusual to see a patient cared for by five different nursing units during one hospital stay—for example, operating room, post-anesthesia care unit (PACU), critical care unit, step-down unit, and general medical-surgical unit—during his or her hospital stay" (IOM, 2004b, p. 251). When might handoffs occur? Some examples are transfer from emergency department to admitting unit; transfer from one unit to another; nurse or physician transferring care to another nurse or physician; transfer to a procedure area; temporary coverage such as for lunch and breaks; anesthesiologist to postanesthesia unit; primary care provider to hospital staff such as intensivist and then reverse at discharge; transfer to home care or to hospice care; transfer to rehab center; transfer to long-term care; and transfer to another hospital. In addition, multiple staff care for the patient in the unit in each 24-hour segment, working varied hours and multiple timeframes for shifts. (See Teaching–Learning Module 19, Handoffs, for more information on this topic.)

A study on patient handoffs (Kitch et al., 2008) indicates that when hand-offs do not provide adequate information, the risk for errors increases. In 2006, Massachusetts General Hospital conducted a survey that included responses from 161 medical or surgical residents. The residents were asked about their experiences with patient handoffs:

- 59% had one or more patients harmed as a result of problematic patient handoffs.
- 12% identified problems that caused significant patient harm, defined as a worsening of clinical status, prolonged harm, disability, or death.
- There is increased risk of poor handoffs when patients are transferred from the emergency department or from another hospital.
- Only 26% of the residents reported that patient handoffs usually or always occurred in quiet settings.
- 37% reported that one or more interruptions occurred frequently or always during the handoff process.

This type of information can be used to plan content and teaching–learning strategies.

Effective handoffs provide "accurate information about a patient's general care plan, treatment, services, current condition, and any recent or anticipated changes" (U.S. Department of Defense, 2005, p. 3). Handoffs should support seamless transitions of care, and this requires a systematic, reliable, and efficient system for transmitting information. Handoffs may be described as follows (p. 3):

- Handoffs are interactive communications providing the opportunity for questioning between the giver and receiver of information about the patient, client, or resident.
- Handoffs include up-to-date information regarding the care, treatment, and services; condition of the patient, client, or resident; and any recent or anticipated changes.
- Interruptions during handoffs are limited to minimize the possibility that information will fail to be conveyed or will be forgotten.
- Handoffs require a process for verification of the received information, including repeat back or read back, as appropriate.
- The receiver of the handoff information has an opportunity to review relevant patient historical data, which may include previous care, treatment, and services.

Though the data in this study focused on the physician perspectives, nurses are involved in handoffs daily and were involved in the examples in this study. Nurses have critical roles in handoffs. Students should consider why transfers increase the risk of errors. Ask them to brainstorm all the possible errors that might occur, and instill in them an awareness of the nurse's role during transfer and the need to consciously prevent errors. What could be changed in the process to reduce risk? (See Teaching–Learning Module 19, Handoffs, for more information on this topic.)

Ambiguity and Workaround Culture

Hospitals are usually organized around functions, and individuals practice in this context. There is ambiguity regarding responsibility: Who does what, when, and how? The healthcare system naturally experiences breakdowns. How do staff (individuals and teams) respond to the signs that a breakdown is occurring? Typically, the response is to try to figure out how to get the work done to stay on schedule, without analyzing at that time what is happening and fixing the problem. This response is a *workaround*. There is a positive aspect of this: many errors are caught before they occur, and one can develop innovative methods to respond to the problem that should be considered to improve care and performance. But the negative result usually is that nothing is learned from the experience, and improvement does not occur. There is just relief that an error was avoided, and then staff move on. The assumption is that workarounds save time, but many of them do not. "All workers—not just those on the front line—need to be coached to learn how to reduce ambiguity systematically and how to continually improve processes through quick, iterative experiments" (Spear, 2005, p. 85). Using this approach, hospitals learn that they can make more effective, long-term change from small changes. The use of simulation to experience workarounds and analysis of the experience can help to determine how to best handle workarounds by asking "not what do we need to do to make the process 'better' but rather what specifics prevent us from performing perfectly" (Spear, 2005, p. 88). The focus should be (p. 82):

- Work is designed as a series of ongoing experiments that immediately reveal problems.
- Problems are addressed immediately through rapid experimentation.
- Solutions are disseminated adaptively through collaborative experimentation.
- People at all levels of the organization are taught to become experimentalists.

(See Teaching–Learning Module 45, Workarounds, for more information about this topic.)

Safety in Every Plan of Care

Faculty should expect that students will include information about safety in the care plans that they develop, and note when they do not. If a standard template is used, include safety in the template to remind students to address it for every patient, as well as to recognize how a patient's safety needs may change. See a sample care plan template in the instructional materials. (See Teaching–Learning Module 38, Safety and Human Factors, for more information about safety in plan of care.)

Checklists: A Method to Reduce Wrong-Site Surgery Errors and Other Errors

The ANA has joined more than 40 organizations to endorse the use of a new Universal Protocol for Preventing Wrong Site, Wrong Procedure and Wrong Person Surgery; more information can be found at http://www.jointcommission.org/standards_information/up.aspx. The protocol includes marking the surgical site, involving the patient in the marking process, and taking a final "time out" in the operating room to recheck with the entire team. This content should be included in clinical content and practicum when surgical patients are assigned to students. In simulation lab, students can demonstrate this protocol through role-play. (See Teaching–Learning Modules 12, Disclosure of Errors and Module 27, Medication Reconciliation, for more information about checklists.)

Patient Falls

Patient falls are a safety concern for all nurses. The ANA National Database of Nursing Quality Indicators (NDNQI) (https://www.nursingquality.org/Default.aspx) reports that falls continue to be a problem on all types of units, and that approximately 30% involved injury (Dunton, Gajewski, Taunton, & Moore, 2004). Content should cover falls, risk assessment including history of falls, medication use and effects, decreased mental status, decreased mobility, physiological effects of aging, external environmental factors, and preventive interventions (Ignatavicius, 2000). Variations in patient populations should be noted in appropriate courses: postsurgery, children, older adults, and so on. This assessment should also be part of the safety element in care plans. This is a good time to introduce the use of restraints and related safety interventions. The NDNQI indicators are available at https://www.nursingquality.org/FAQPage.aspx, and in the following list an asterisk denotes indicators that are also monitored by the NQF:

- Patient falls/Injury falls* (NQF)
- Pressure ulcers:
  - Hospital acquired* (NQF)
  - Unit acquired
- Physical/sexual assault
- Pain assessment/intervention/reassessment cycle
- Peripheral IV infiltration
- Physical restraints* (NQF)
- Healthcare-associated infections:* (NQF)
  - Catheter-associated UTIs
  - Central-line-associated bloodstream infection
  - Ventilator-associated pneumonia

- Staff mix:* (NQF)
  - Registered nurses (RNs)
  - Licensed practical/vocational nurses (LPN/LVNs)
  - Unlicensed assistive personnel (UAPs)
- Nursing care hours provided per patient day* (NQF)
- Nurse turnover:
  - Total
  - Adapted NQF voluntary* (NQF)
  - Magnet controllable
- RN education/certification
- RN Survey:
  - Practice Environment Scales option* (NQF)
  - Job Satisfaction Scales option
  - Job Satisfaction Scales, short form option

(See Teaching–Learning Module 18, Falls and Quality Care, for more information about falls.)

Infectious Diseases

Material on surveillance, prevention, and control of infectious diseases can be introduced when students begin to learn clinical competencies in simulated experiences, included in didactic content, and reinforced in the clinical setting. Let infection control nursing staff teach students. Students need to know and follow the infection control policies and procedures in organizations where they receive clinical experience. Postoperative infections have the most serious consequences of all medical injuries: increased length of stay, treatment costs, and risk of death. Handwashing is critical and must be reinforced with students in the simulation lab and in clinical. The Joint Commission also emphasizes handwashing in its surveys. In simulations, students should be asked what they would assess; in practica, they should identify risks for acquiring and transmitting infectious agents. Students must use handwashing appropriately in all simulated experiences if they are to make this a habit in clinical practice. (See the CDC's Handwashing Guidelines at http://www.cdc.gov/handhygiene/Guidelines.html)

Monitoring patients is a critical element of nursing that can reduce errors, and it should be integrated into all nursing experiences. In clinical, ask students what they should monitor and when. What do monitoring results mean? What interventions should then be taken? There are many studies on this problem, so this is a good issue to emphasize EBP and have students review the studies (if they have had content that enables them to understand the research process) and discuss EBP.

Morbidity and Mortality: Autopsy

Morbidity and mortality (M&M) are common concepts in health care, and students need to understand how the HCO analyzes and uses M&M data. M&M content is often introduced in community health content and epidemiology courses, but the data are also relevant to acute care. The AHRQ, with the University of California at San Francisco, has created WebM&M (http://webmm.ahrq.gov/) as a national forum to discuss and learn from medical errors. This site, which also provides PowerPoint slides for its cases, and changes the cases monthly, can be used to explore the problem of medical errors.

Students will experience patients who die, so they need to understand how autopsies are used to improve care and reduce errors. Open discussion of this topic is essential because it can be a difficult topic for some students. Students also need information about the impact of culture and religion on the topic of autopsies and communication with families. There are also legal issues, as autopsies are required to be performed for some deaths.

High-Risk Areas for Practice and Research Focus

The report on priority areas (IOM, 2003f) listed some critical high-risk areas that should be included in content and discussions with students. The 2011 National Healthcare Quality Report (http://www.ahrq.gov/qual/qrdr11.htm) identifies priority areas of effectiveness of care. Faculty should review this report routinely to ensure that appropriate changes in content and curriculum are made. These are also potential research concerns for nursing (IOM, 2004f, p. 129):

- Widely varied interactions with diagnostic or treatment technology; use of many different types of equipment
- Multiple staff involved in individual patient care, and handoffs of care
- High acuity of patient illness or injury
- Environment prone to distractions or interruptions
- Need for rapid decisions; caregivers being time-pressured
- High-volume or unpredictable patient flow
- Use of diagnostic or therapeutic interventions with a narrow margin of safety
- Communication barriers with patients or coworkers
- Instructional setting for care delivery, with inexperienced caregivers

The 2011 priority areas in effectiveness of care (http://www.ahrq.gov/qual/nhqr10/nhqr10.pdf, p.) include:

- Cancer
- Cardiovascular disease
- Diabetes
- Chronic kidney disease
- HIV disease
- Maternal and child health
- Mental health and substance abuse
- Musculoskeletal disease
- Respiratory diseases
- Lifestyle modification
- Functional status preservation and rehabilitation
- Supportive and palliative care

Other information about the 2011 NHCQ report can be found at http://www.ahrq.gov/qual/nhqr10/nhqr10.pdf

Benchmarking

Benchmarking is an improvement tool whereby a company or organization measures its performance or process against other companies' best practices, determines how those companies achieved their performance levels, and uses the information to improve its own performance (iSixSigma, 2008). Many hospitals and other types of HCOs also use benchmarking. One of the popular benchmarking approaches used by HCOs is SixSigma. "This is a rigorous and a systematic methodology that utilizes information (management by facts) and statistical analysis to measure and improve a company's operational performance, practices, and systems by identifying and preventing 'defects' in manufacturing and service-related processes in order to anticipate and exceed expectations of all stakeholders to accomplish effectiveness" (iSixSigma, 2008). To introduce students to benchmarking, ask staff involved in benchmarking to talk to students about what they do and the impact of benchmarking on QI and the HCO. (See Teaching–Learning Module 2, Benchmarking, for more information on this topic.)

Assessment of Access to Healthcare Services

Access to healthcare services must be monitored and improved. It is an important element of quality care. *Healthy People 2020* views access as a critical need across the country and for all types of health care. When a patient does not have access, the patient's health is at risk and further complications may occur. Access is not a simple concept, though. For example, it can mean any of the following abilities:

- Get to a healthcare appointment (for example, availability of transportation; funds for transportation)
- Get an appointment for care
- Get an appointment in the timeframe needed (for example, appointment times, day of week, wait list)
- Get specialty care when needed
- Get diagnostic tests and reports in a timely manner
- Pay for care or have an outside source for payment such as insurance
- Understand when care is needed
- Understand healthcare information and language (health literacy)
- Access a physical facility (e.g., does the facility have handicap-usable features?)
- Choice of providers
- Childcare problems

Vulnerable populations that often have limited access include low-income, children and adolescents, minorities, homeless, mentally ill, uninsured, disabled, elderly, veterans, immigrants, rural populations, and prisoners. Students need to understand the meaning of access to health care, barriers to access, and the impact of lack of access. Students can review the current national disparities report to learn more about access to care.

Workplace Safety

Workplace safety is a component of healthcare safety. Students need to understand why it is important and how it relates to healthcare safety. Potential positive effects of workplace safety include:

- Reduced cost of care
- Safer care for patients (a patient may be injured in the same incident that injures a nurse)
- Consistent care (reduced risk of sudden nurse absence requiring staff substitution)
- Less stress due to nursing shortage

See also earlier content about staff fatigue.

The ANA position statements related to staff safety include *Assuring Patient Safety: The Employer's Role in Promoting Healthy Nursing Work Hours for Registered Nurses in All Roles and Settings; Assuring Patient Safety: Registered Nurses' Responsibility in All Roles and Settings to Guard against Working When Fatigued,* and others (available at www.nursingworld.org). The ANA is a strong advocate for safety for nurses in all types of healthcare settings. Its position statements on staff safety provide guidelines for work environments. These are excellent resources for students. Discussion of other safety issues for nursing staff follows.

Needlesticks

Healthcare workers (HCWs) suffer between 600,000 and 1 million injuries, and at least 1,000 serious infections, from conventional needles and sharps annually. These exposures can lead to hepatitis B, hepatitis C, and HIV, and mostly affect RNs working at the bedside. More than 80% of needlestick injuries could be prevented by the use of safer needle devices. More disturbing is the fact that less than 15% of U.S. hospitals use them.

Infections

As noted earlier, HCWs are often exposed to communicable diseases via needlesticks. In addition to HIV and hepatitis, these diseases include tuberculosis (the incidence of which is rising in this country), staphylococcus, cytomegalovirus, influenza, and bacteria. Influenza has been linked to suboptimal vaccination levels of HCWs (Polygreen et al., 2008). Bacterial infections have sometimes been linked to glove contamination (Diaz et al., 2008).

Ergonomic Safety

Nurses suffer a significant number of work-related back injuries and other musculoskeletal disorders. Nursing assistants are ranked second in the occupations that experience this type of injury; truck drivers are first, nonconstruction laborers are third, and registered nurses are sixth on the list. Because of these injuries, nurses sometimes must transfer to other units or healthcare settings, and may leave nursing. Typical injuries occur in the neck, shoulder, and back. Nursing requires a lot of patient handling, and the patient's weight, height, body shape, age, dependency, and medical status are important. Weight in the general adult population has increased, and this has raised the risk of injury. The physical setting can also increase risk. Is there enough room to move around when moving the patient? What types of equipment are available to help move patients?

Handle With Care® (De Castro, 2004; ANA, 2003) is a national campaign established by the ANA in September 2003. The goal is a proactive, multifaceted plan to promote safe patient handling and prevent musculoskeletal disorders among nurses in the United States. Through a variety of activities, the campaign seeks to educate, advocate for, and facilitate change from traditional practices of manual patient handling to emerging technology-aided methods. Nursing education is a critical component in exposing nursing students to the most effective patient-handling methods. There also is more emphasis on assistive patient-handling equipment and devices. Students need to learn how to use this equipment safely.

Violence

Violence may not be a typical staff safety concern, nor something that a student would first think of when asked about safety in the healthcare workplace, but it is a concern in HCOs. There is greater risk for violence when working in emergency departments (ED), psychiatric and substance abuse units, and long-term care; however, it can occur anywhere. Patients and families may not be able to control their anger appropriately. The nurse may be where violence occurs even if the violence is not directly related to the nurse or health care—in the home or in the community.

Staff need training so that they can prevent violence when possible. Particularly important subjects include identification of signs of escalation and how to deescalate a situation, and staff also need to know how to protect themselves when violence cannot be prevented. In areas such as psychiatry, this training is more common, though other services (particularly ED) also need this training. Signs of escalation include a sudden change in behavior, clenched jaws or fists, threats, pacing, increased movement, shouting, use of profanity, increased respiration, and staring or pointing. These signs do not mean that the person will inevitably become violent, but rather that the nurse should be more aware of the person's behavior and communication to determine if the person is escalating. Protecting oneself is very important. Students should learn protective actions such as leaving the room; staying near the door or keeping the door open but not standing in the doorway (because the patient may see this as blocking the exit); asking other staff to be present; and calling for security assistance. The Occupational Safety and Health Administration (OSHA) has developed guidelines for preventing workplace violence (OSHA, 2004).

Exposure to Chemicals

An online survey examined workplace exposures and disease conditions among 1,500 nurses. The survey was conducted by the Environmental Working Group (EWG) and Healthcare Without Harm (HCWH), in collaboration with ANA and the Environmental Health Education Center of the University of Maryland's School of Nursing, and was supported by numerous state and specialty nursing organizations. Participating nurses, who were frequently exposed to sterilizing chemicals, housekeeping cleaners, residues from drug preparation, radiation, and other hazardous substances, reported increased rates of asthma, miscarriage, certain cancers, and birth defects. There are workplace safety standards for only six of the hundreds of hazardous substances to which nurses are routinely exposed on the job (EWG, HCWH, ANA, & Environmental Health Education Center, 2007). Specific risks include: anesthetic gases, hand and skin disinfectants, housekeeping chemicals, latex, antiretroviral medications, chemotherapeutic agents, mercury-containing devices, personal care products, radiation, and sterilization and disinfectant agents such as ethylene oxide and glutaraldehyde.

The OSHA and the National Institute for Occupational Safety and Health (NIOSH) should be included in a discussion of the employee health needs. Students can learn more at their web sites (http://www.OSHA.gov and http://www.NIOSH.gov). How do these agencies relate to employers and employees? Some nursing programs use occupational health settings for practica and explore the role of the occupational health nurse. Students can participate in screening efforts and health education programs that might be offered in the work setting. Students can explore the health risks for specific work settings and strategies used to prevent problems in each. Students should understand the worker's compensation system and how it differs from private and other government forms of health insurance. They should also be asked to identify the companies in their area that have dropped health insurance for employees or cut back their contribution to coverage, and evaluate any change in vulnerability of the population to illness and disease. Students should consider the number of uninsured and underinsured in their state and the impact of unemployment on healthcare coverage. They can then compare the percentage of gross national product spent on health care in the United States with that of other countries with better morbidity and mortality rates for childbearing women and children in particular.

Patient Satisfaction with Care

The federal government began a new survey of patient experiences and perceptions of hospital care in the spring of 2008 (U.S. Department of Health and Human Services, 2008). The initial survey data indicate that many patients are dissatisfied with their hospital care and might not recommend the hospital to others. They felt that physicians and nurses did not treat them with courtesy and respect. They did not receive adequate pain medication and did not understand instructions given to them. This type of information should be part of every curriculum, with discussions about patient dissatisfaction and its impact. (See the IOM report on pain management discussed in Part 1.) The survey, produced by the Hospital Quality Alliance (HQA), is now accessible at http://www.hospitalcompare.hhs.gov. There students can access data about hospital process care measures, hospital outcome of care measures, survey of patients' hospital experiences, and Medicare payment and volume.

Another study indicated that patients were generally satisfied with care, but there were still concerns about quality (Jha, Orav, Zheng, & Epstein, 2008). Of the sample, 67% were satisfied; those who were satisfied were generally in hospitals with higher levels of quality. Problem areas were dissatisfaction with pain control and with the discharge process. These two areas are part of nursing care. Discuss with students the impact of patient satisfaction on quality of care and outcomes.

Quality and Cost of Care

Cost

In the fall of 2007, the Centers for Medicare and Medicaid Services (CMS) announced a major change in the inpatient prospective payment system (IPPS) regarding hospital-acquired conditions (HACs; these are preventable hospital-acquired conditions for which treatment is not reimbursable). A white paper, *A Summary of the Impact of Reforms to the Hospital Inpatient Prospective Payment System (IPPS) on Nursing Services*, described the rule change and its effects. "Now, more than ever, hospital leaders need to invest in high-quality nursing care and provide resources to support nurses' ongoing contribution to patient safety and healthcare quality. This rule will have a big effect on how nurses do their jobs" (Centers for Medicare & Medicaid Services, 2007). This change eliminates additional Medicare payments for eight selected HACs, including inpatient pressure ulcers, certain injuries (for example, fractures from falls), catheter-associated urinary tract infections, vascular catheter-associated infections, certain surgical-site infections, objects left in surgery, air embolism, and blood incompatibility. Medicaid has also been added to this initiative.

Nursing is involved in each of these HACs. How hospitals respond will also involve nursing (Robert Wood Johnson Foundation, 2007). The worst response would be to decrease the nursing budget to cover the costs for these complications that will no longer be covered by Medicare or Medicaid. This might lead to reductions in staff or funding for staff education—and neither would be an effective solution. However, this can also be viewed as an opportunity for nursing to demonstrate that it can improve care and control costs. "Nurses know that their care can reduce the incidence of some of these conditions. Reports of nurse-directed interventions that significantly improve the very conditions the payment rule targets have been cited in the literature; risk assessment, surveillance, early diagnosis, treatment, and education have been shown to be effective in lowering rates of pressure ulcers, falls, and infections" (Kurtzman & Buerhaus, 2008, p. 32). As has been noted earlier, chronic disease and care are critical concerns today. "Patients with chronic diseases are even more vulnerable for care errors due to specialization and fragmentation in healthcare delivery" (Suter, 2008, p. 648), and are at higher risk of experiencing one of the nonreimbursable HACs.

Since the CMS announcement, some insurers have also announced that they will not pay for treating these complications. It is not always easy to pinpoint the cause for all of these complications or to determine that all were preventable, so this is likely to lead to some conflicts. Examples on insurers' lists of hospital-acquired complications—which may vary from the CMS list of HACs—include: an object left in the patient after surgery; letting the patient wander or disappear; administering the wrong blood type; artificially inseminating the wrong donor sperm or egg; allowing the patient to fall; operating on the wrong limb; performing the wrong procedure; using contaminated drugs or devices; discharging an infant to the wrong person; a mother's death or serious disability in a low-risk delivery; hospital-acquired bedsores; and patient abduction or sexual assault (Fuhrmans, 2008). This will undoubtedly mean changes in policies and procedures, checklists, documentation, how care is provided, and surveillance. Over time, these lists will change.

Transforming Care at the Bedside (TCAB) is one initiative (IHI, 2008f) that could make a difference in how nursing responds to this new CMS ruling. Other strategies that have already been implemented to reduce these complications so that reimbursement is not affected include (Robert Wood Johnson Foundation, 2008b):

- Recognition that hospitals are not keeping track of who gets urinary catheters and do not do daily checks to determine each patient's need for continuing catheter use
- Changing sterilization technologies
- Using physician assistants (PAs) to monitor staff handwashing compliance
- Monitoring supplies during surgery through bar coding and a "smart" bucket that counts sponges to make sure none are left in the patient

As students go into clinical areas, they need to understand what is happening with reimbursement for care and complications. This is a good opportunity to link expenses, reimbursement, and quality. The complications on both the CMS list and the insurers' list should be emphasized as critical content in curricula. Students need to recognize that medical errors in the United States are expensive. Provide them with real examples of cost.

Other issues related to cost and quality are likewise becoming more important. What is the cost of adverse events and effective levels of staffing? This question was addressed in a study to consider the critical issue of outcomes and costs (Pappas, 2008). Nursing costs are a major part of acute care costs, representing at least 50% of most hospital budgets. Nursing staffing is a critical element in quality care, and staffing is a major portion of the expense. This study "links the occurrence of adverse events to actual patient-level cost per case" (p. 235). Adverse events reflect the level of quality and affect patient outcomes. The Pappas study is an excellent example for students to analyze to better understand the connections among quality, costs, and nursing.

Another study examines the effects of the hospital care environment on patient mortality and nurse outcomes. "Staffing and education have well-documented associations with patient outcomes" (Aiken, Clarke, & Sloane, 2008, p. 223). Patient care environment includes factors such as staff development, quality management, nurse manager ability, leadership, support, and collegial nurse–physician relations. Are "better hospital nurse care environments associated with lower patient mortality and better nurse outcomes independently of nurse staffing and education of the registered nurse workforce in hospitals" (p. 223)? The results indicate that when there are better care environments, nurses have more positive job experiences and fewer concerns about quality, and there are significantly lower risks of death or failure to rescue. Ask students to search for current nursing studies.

Risk Management (RM) and Utilization Management/Review (UR)

Risk management (RM) is a large program in most healthcare organizations. Utilization management/review (UR) is the process of evaluating necessity, appropriateness, and efficiency of healthcare services for specific patients or in patient populations. The goal of risk management is "to maintain a safe and effective healthcare environment and prevent or reduce loss to the healthcare organization" (Pike, Janssen, & Brooks, 2002, p. 3). RM is concerned with decreasing financial loss to the HCO due to legal and malpractice issues. RM programs monitor errors and incidents and collaborate with QI to decrease errors. Data are obtained primarily from medical records to determine necessity, appropriateness, and timeliness of healthcare services.

If there is an error, RM will evaluate the risk for a lawsuit and take appropriate action. HCO attorneys are very involved in RM, and in some HCOs, RNs with a legal background are hired to work in or consult with the RM department. They also often work in UR. RNs have considerable knowledge about healthcare delivery and can be excellent resources for both RM and UR. Students need to know the purposes of RM and UR and how they relate to patient care and nursing roles and responsibilities. This material may be included in management content. If a student makes an error in the clinical setting, the organization's incident report—some schools of nursing also have an incident report form—must be completed. This is a good time to reinforce risk management. Students can also be told why the HCO needs to understand how its services are being used. (See Teaching–Learning Module 35, Risk Management and Utilization Review, for more information on these topics.)

Patients and Families and Quality Improvement

Ask students how patients and families might become more involved in the development of safety standards, and why this is important. Explore initiatives to increase patient and family involvement, like the National Patient Safety Foundation (http://www.npsf.org), AHRQ patient materials (http://www.ahrq.gov), the Institute for Safe Medication Practice (http://www.ismp.org), state patient materials, and the Joint Commission Speak Up campaign (http://www.jointcommission.org). Staff also need to know how to approach patients and families when errors have occurred, so discussing this with students is important to set the standard for professional behavior. They need to consider what an error can mean to a patient or a family, and how the affected individuals might feel: angry, distrustful of staff, or abandoned. What might be the effect the next time the patient seeks care? Why is it important to ask patients more than just dates of past hospitalizations? A bad past experience can affect current treatment. Ask students to put themselves in the place of the patient or family member to gain a better understanding of patient and family responses and how nurses might help them cope. There may be legal ramifications when errors occur, so students need to understand this aspect and to whom they should go for consultation. This should be tied to content on legal issues and the ANA Code of Ethics. (See Teaching–Learning Module 24, Integrating the Patient and Family in Quality Improvement, for more information.)

The Joint Commission and Quality Improvement

Joint Commission Accreditation

Students need to understand the purpose of Joint Commission accreditation and the basic elements of the process. If a local HCO is undergoing accreditation and students are in the organization for practicum, discuss what they can expect during the accreditation survey. Students may be able to attend some of the planning meetings. Invite a staff member who is involved in the accreditation planning to talk about the process and the plan. This is more important today because surveyors are spending more time with staff nurses. Students also need to understand the implications of the professional standards and accreditation. *(See discussion in Part 3.)*

Changes in Joint Commission Standards

Include Joint Commission current annual safety information in course content; for example, under documentation include abbreviations that should not be used based on the current Joint Commission list of prohibited abbreviations. Even after students have completed content about documentation, they need to be informed of changes, to emphasize that even in practice they need to keep up with current safety and documentation requirements. Faculty should stay aware of the changes so that schools of nursing maintain current approaches in their curriculum. This takes monitoring, which might mean that someone is assigned to check regularly for updates, and perhaps post them to a convenient web site for faculty. Updates related to standards, guidelines (AHRQ), safety and QI issues, EBP, FDA drug alerts (http://www.fda.gov), updates on nursing workforce safety (http://www.nursingworld.org), the annual National Healthcare Quality report, and the annual healthcare disparity report also provide faculty with easy access to current and authoritative information.

Joint Commission standards are available online. These provide students with examples of what is evaluated in the accreditation process. The web site (http://www.jointcommission.org/) also includes information that can be used in teaching and for students to explore, such as information about patient safety, sentinel events, root cause analysis, and performance measurement. The site has a number of current public policy reports on topics such as health literacy and patient safety, organ donation, community-wide emergency preparedness, and the nursing shortage. These policy statements change as new issues arise. (See Teaching–Learning Module 26, The Joint Commission, for more information about this topic.)

Schools of Nursing: Setting Safety Standards

Each school of nursing should set minimum safety standards for students. Safety standards established by nursing professional organizations should be incorporated into the curriculum; for example, standards in care of children should be included in pediatric content. Schools of nursing must keep abreast of changes in FDA standards for medical products and safety, so that they can be incorporated into content and practicum. Students and faculty must also follow standards set by the healthcare organizations where students obtain clinical experience. As discussed earlier, the ANA publishes important information about workplace safety. The ANA standards, as well as nursing specialty standards, should be discussed. The Joint Commission Annual Safety Goals, which should be included in nursing curricula, are an important part of practice today. It is also important to discuss the meaning and purpose of standards, policies, and procedures; which develops them; and when they are used. Emphasis should be placed on greater use of evidence to support standards, policies, and procedures (stressing EBP). *(See earlier content on the ANA social policy statement, Code of Ethics, and standards in Part 3.)*

Access to Care Management Programs and Guidelines

Students need to know what care management programs and clinical guidelines are available and where to find them (also patient care protocols, clinical pathways, algorithms, and so on). These are particularly relevant for patients with chronic problems. Standards, policies, and procedures should be evidence based, although at this time there is limited research evidence for many care issues in nursing. Standards, policies, and procedures for nurses and nursing care should not conflict with regulations, such as the state's nurse practice act, and should conform to nursing standards. HCOs need to ensure that staff is competent and meet required regulations, especially regarding licensure and credentialing. Faculty can connect this to QI.

How do these programs and guidelines apply to nursing care? Provide students with examples, which can be found on the Internet, and discuss the implications for nursing. Ask students to identify relevant programs and guidelines for their assigned patients and how they might use those guidelines in providing nursing care. Figure 5-6 describes the continuum from research studies to systematic review to development of clinical guidelines, as described in *Knowing What Works in Healthcare* (IOM, 2008b).

The Nursing Shortage, Staffing, and Quality

It is important for students to understand the relationship between the nursing shortage and its fluctuations, staffing, and quality of care. This issue can be discussed throughout the curriculum and particularly emphasized in leadership and management content. Introduce EBP by exploring evidence related to these three issues and their connections. Do not avoid discussing the nursing shortage because students need a place to talk openly about their concerns. They see the results in clinical, and it can make them

Research Studies

Examples:

- Randomized clinical trials
- Cohort studies
- Case control studies
- Cross-sectional studies
- Case series

Systematic Review
- Identify and assess the quality of individual studies
- Critically appraise the body of evidence
- Develop qualities or quantitative synthesis

Clinical Guidelines and Recommendations

Source: Institute of Medicine. (2008). *Knowing What Works in Healthcare*. Washington, DC: National Academies Press, p. 23. Reprinted with permission.

FIGURE 5-6 Clinical Guidelines and Recommendations

question whether they want to enter this profession. Talking to students about the work environment and how it influences retention is important. What is the impact of management, scheduling difficulties, and departmental relationships, or even the tone and morale in the workplace, on turnover (Christmas, 2008)? Allow students time to understand the work environment, factors such as the ones mentioned, and how they can protect themselves from turnover. With a 27% average voluntary turnover among new graduates, this is a major concern for healthcare organizations and should be for nursing schools (Christmas, 2008). Resolving this problem will require collaboration and partnerships between schools of nursing and HCOs. Nurse externships and residencies, mentioned earlier in the book, are two strategies being used more to increase retention of new graduates.

Nursing Activities and Relationship to Quality

Nurses are very involved in surveillance, which includes assessing or monitoring patients, delivering therapeutic interventions, and coordinating and integrating care from multiple providers (IOM, 2004b). *The Future of Nursing* report (IOM, 2011d) describes the need for more nursing leadership in quality improvement, and an even earlier IOM report (2004b) indicated that nurses are not prepared to do this. Faculty need to ensure that the quality improvement competency is met; nursing students must understand and embrace this role. The nurse's role in HCOs is not static; consequently, nursing education must keep aware of changing roles and modify what is taught. This, of course, must be correlated with current standards of practice. All of this requires that nursing education be able to make changes in curricula and teaching strategies in a timely manner—in sharp contrast to how this process occurs today.

A study published in 2008 explores how efficiency and effectiveness of nursing care are critical to hospital functioning (Hendrich, Chow, Skierczynski, & Zhenqiang). A time-and-motion study was used to identify drivers of inefficiency: nursing practice location, such as the patient room or the nurses' station; unit architecture; distance traveled; variation between shifts; physiological impact; documentation; medication administration; and care coordination. This type of study can be used to illustrate the need for efficiency and to open discussion with students about how inefficiency undermines quality. It can also be used to develop simulations for students so they can experience and discuss how nurses use their time; then they can work on their own time management. (See Teaching–Learning Module 36, Role of the Nurse in Quality Improvement, for more information about this topic.)

National Quality Forum (NQF)

The National Quality Forum (NQF) is a not-for-profit organization whose purpose is to develop and implement a national strategy for healthcare quality measurement and reporting. It is a public–private partnership. Its priorities, which are all directly related to IOM concerns, include (NQF, 2011):

- *Patient safety*: improving the safety and reliability of America's healthcare system. (IOM: Quality improvement)
- *Population health*: improving the health of the population (IOM: Public health)
- *Care coordination*: ensuring that patients receive well-coordinated care within and across all healthcare organizations, settings, and levels of care (IOM: Patient-centered care and interprofessional teams)
- *Patient and family engagement*: engaging patients and families in managing their health and making decisions about their care (IOM: Patient-centered care)
- *Palliative care and end-of-life care*: guaranteeing appropriate and compassionate care for patients with life-limiting illnesses (IOM: Patient-centered care)
- *Overuse*: eliminating overuse while ensuring the delivery of appropriate care (IOM: Quality improvement)
- *Health IT*: Help ensure that care is safer, more affordable, and better coordinated (IOM: Informatics)
- *Disparity reduction:* begins with the provision of culturally appropriate health care, which requires language access, sensitivity to cultural differences, attention to patients' health literacy needs, and consistency across settings, time, and providers (IOM: Patient-centered care)

Quality Improvement: Content and Clinical Experience

Schools of nursing can use the NQF framework to create a learning environment that engenders patient safety. The framework dictates the adoption of safeguards against foreseeable hazards:

- Student safety and quality care competencies incorporated into student evaluation
- Quality of faculty teaching and clinical expertise
- Creating and maintaining a blame-free culture
- Clear communication among faculty and students about courses and learning experiences
- Consistent course content and expectations
- Faculty teamwork and planning
- Up-to-date curriculum (evidence-based practice, IOM reports, AHRQ material, Joint Commission, and so on)
- Evaluation of competency that includes patient safety concerns
- Supportive faculty willing to work with students
- Knowledge of the clinical setting (staffing and qualifications of staff, policies and procedures, culture related to safety, environmental risks that increase errors)
- Integration in care planning
- Integration in the curriculum

The following are specifically mentioned as important elements of nursing content and clinical experience:

- Use a variety of approaches to deliver care, including the provision of care without face-to-face contact.
- Synthesize evidence and communicate it to patients.
- Combine evidence, knowledge about population outcomes, and patient preferences to individualize care.
- Communicate with patients openly to assist them in making decisions and in self-management.
- Use decision support systems and other tools to assist in making decisions to reduce overuse, underuse, waste, and redundancy.
- Identify errors and hazards in care, and understand and implement basic safety design principles.
- Understand the course of illness and the patient's needs and experiences at home (the most critical training need).
- Continually measure quality of care (process and outcomes) and implement best practices.
- Work collaboratively in teams.
- Design processes of care and measure their effectiveness.
- Understand how knowledge continually changes and expands.
- Understand determinants of health, the link between medical care and healthy populations, and professional responsibilities.

Faculty need to ask themselves how this content is currently taught, and how it could be included if it is not. Learning activities should be creative to encourage students to incorporate the ideas and content into their practice. Adding on more lectures is not the answer. In many cases there is no need to add content, but rather a need to redesign learning activities. Quality improvement exercises should be an important part of any papers that students write. Faculty should review current assignments to determine how they reflect QI and how students can better apply it to their practice.

Students first need to understand the ANA National Quality Database, the issues that the ANA and the American Academy of Nursing (AAN) are investigating through NQF, and how The Joint Commission uses the ANA Report Card. These quality indicators have been linked to patient safety outcomes in such areas as medication errors and falls, and they are being integrated into electronic medical records and physician order entry systems. Therefore, it seems reasonable that students and faculty should apply these same measures to nursing education.

Students need to know about The Joint Commission and accreditation, QI, and healthcare quality report cards. They need to know about tools used to monitor quality improvement, such as standards of care, policies and procedures, licensure, risk management and utilization management, benchmarking, clinical pathways and protocols, clinical guidelines, and EBP.

At the University of Connecticut School of Medicine, a program known as Beginning to End (B to E) provides a unique opportunity for medical students to identify examples of less-than-optimal care and to suggest improvement strategies (IHI, 2008a). Each fourth-year student is assigned to observe a patient throughout the patient's hospitalization. The student observes interactions with health professionals and staff that occur in the patient's room and accompanies the patient to other parts of the hospital for procedures or tests. The student records instances of less-than-optimal care as well as those judged as exemplary. Examples of less-than-optimal care include medication errors, unprofessional behavior, long waits for transportation, delayed or incorrect meals, slow nurse response, poor housekeeping, inadequate pain relief, and poor communication. The student then reviews the log with a mentor and discusses possible corrective actions. This same strategy could be used with nursing students. This experience is not just a learning experience; the students' observations about QI become part of the HCO's QI program with the students actively participating and contributing. This type of experience could be used with nursing students and ideally with interprofessional experiences.

Achieving Competence Today (ACT) has been used to help healthcare professions students understand quality improvement and the need for interprofessional collaboration through a Robert Wood Johnson Foundation (RWJF) initiative. ACT includes three components (Ladden, Bednash, Stevens, & Moore, 2006, p. 498):

1. *Getting ready*: a plan with a preceptor for the ACT program
2. *Four course modules*: the structure of health care and how it affects the care you deliver; who pays for care and why it matters; improving the care of individuals, populations, and practices; improving your practice and the health system

3. *Implementing the quality improvement plan (QIP)*: plans vetted by advisory committee; one or more QIPs chosen for implementation; learners work together and with faculty

A good resource for further information is http://www.rwjf.org/pr/product.jsp?id=42368.

A quality improvement plan (QIP) includes a description of a quality problem, a root cause analysis, and an intervention described in a clear business plan. The goal is to have students choose real problems in clinical settings where they might actually make a difference. Interprofessional teams are preferable: students from different healthcare professions working together in collaboration with interprofessional faculty. The student ACT teams may use a variety of tools, such as root cause analysis and the Plan-Do-Study-Act (PDSA) cycle. PDSA is a "continuous quality improvement model consisting of a logical sequence of four repetitive steps for continuous improvement and learning: Plan, Do, Study (Check), and Act. The PDSA cycle (or PDCA) is also known as the Deming Cycle [or] the Deming wheel of continuous improvement spiral" (iSixSigma, 2008).

Core Competency: Use Informatics

Communicate, manage knowledge, mitigate error, and support decision-making using information technology (IOM, 2003b, p. 4).

Use of Computers in Healthcare Organizations

Informatics emphasizes the need to manage patient information, protect the patient against errors, and support healthcare interventions. Information technology (IT) is used not only in providing care, but also in reducing errors. It is an asset in today's healthcare system, but it can also be problematic. Locsin (2005) comments that with the increasing use of medical technology, there is concern about nurses losing the caring aspects of nursing. Help students understand the major contributions of technology to health care, but also discuss the implications for how care is provided and the impact it may have on the nurse–patient relationship. How can the "care" be kept in nursing care in an intensive care unit that is so dependent on medical technology?

"There is a perception that technology will lead to fewer errors than strategies that focus on staff performance; however, technology may in some circumstances lead to more errors. This is particularly true when technology fails to take into account the end users, increases staff time, replicates an already bad process, or is implemented with insufficient training. The best approach is not always clear, and most approaches have advantages and disadvantages" (Finkelman & Kenner, 2007b, p. 55). A report of a study published in 2012 surveyed 16,352 nurses from 316 hospitals in 4 states about the use of EMRs and patient outcomes. The results indicate that the sample believed there was improvement (Kutney-Lee & Deena, 2011). This study is a positive result, and as more healthcare organizations adopt EMRs, there will likely be more studies assessing the outcomes.

We need to learn how to make IT safer and when to rely on people instead. According to the AHRQ, IT can be effective in providing computerized monitoring of adverse drug events, computer-generated reminders for follow-up testing, computerized provider order entry (CPOE), automated dispensing of medication, handheld devices for prescription information, electronic health records (EHR) that can provide portable birth-to-death data, and online support groups for patients (AHRQ, 2003). In addition, the AHRQ recognizes the need to develop IT standards in health care and will lead this effort. Computers are generally used in three ways in health care:

- Computer-based reminder systems
- Access to patient information at the point of care
- Clinical decision support systems

Hospitals and other healthcare settings are moving slowly toward using more informatics. Implementing an electronic medical record (EMR) is costly, but adverse error data are driving some HCOs to move to newer systems faster. Between January 2005 and August 2006, data from six Massachusetts community hospitals showed that 10% of patients had nonfatal preventable adverse drug events. The hospitals adopted a computerized physician order entry system to decrease errors. As a result of decreased errors while using the CPOE system, BlueCross BlueShield of Massachusetts announced in 2008 that it would require its covered hospitals to use CPOE within four years (Robert Wood Johnson Foundation, 2008b). Also in Massachusetts, a study tested whether or not electronic physician alerts could improve medication reconciliation and care coordination for seniors (Robert Wood Johnson Foundation, 2008d).

At the same time that changes are being made in documentation, incentives are also being used to change behavior. In 2008, Medicare began offering physicians incentive payments if they used e-prescriptions: using qualified electronic systems to transmit medication administration for Medicare patients (Robert Wood Johnson Foundation, 2008c). A barrier to seamless coordination is the lack of interoperable computerized records. To improve information sharing and coordination of care, the percentage of physicians using EHRs must increase, and over time this is expected to occur. The expectation is that use of electronic health records will reach 80% by 2016 (Lewis, 2011).

Students need experience working with computers in healthcare settings. Though not all healthcare organizations use the same software, it is critical that students understand the principles of computerized documentation systems. Identifying common errors is helpful. We need to make technology competencies critical skills and terminal objectives of our educational programs. Students need to know how the Health Insurance Portability and Accountability Act (HIPAA) applies to computerized systems. *To Err Is Human* emphasizes the need for shared knowledge and the free flow of information, which should be "interactive, real-time, and prospective" (IOM, 1999, p. 72). This requires effective use of information technology, and students need to begin learning about it in school. (See Teaching–Learning Module 14, Electronic Medical/Health Records in Quality Improvement, for more information about this topic.)

The Digital Divide: Disparities and Informatics

The *digital divide* refers to the problems faced by people with limited access to information technologies (Chang et al., 2004). People with disabilities, rural populations, and those of low socioeconomic status face a barrier between them and the health information and patient-centered care they need. The IOM made it clear that information technology is critical by making informatics one of the five core healthcare profession competencies. *Healthy People 2020* also emphasizes the importance of the Internet in increasing equality. Health literacy is closely tied to informatics as well. Nurses need to understand these issues; recognize the barriers and consider how the barriers might be overcome in communities; and evaluate Internet resources and guide patients in selecting them. Funding is needed to provide more access and to understand how limiting access leads to disparities. Computer literacy is needed across all age groups and for all vulnerable populations. The community should be involved in a plan to improve access. This would be an interesting issue for students in community health to assess; have them propose strategies to reduce inequality, while considering policy, funding, legislative and political issues, education, and more.

Standardized Terminologies

 "Developing and adhering to distinct profession-specific terms may be a manifestation of professionals' desire to preserve identity, status, or control" (IOM, 2003f, p. 123). This problem affects all of the core competencies and the ability to develop educational experiences that meet the competencies across healthcare professions such as nursing, medicine, pharmacy, and allied health. It does not relate only to informatics; however, because informatics is dependent on language, the issue of shared language is even more important here. The IOM recommended that there be an interprofessional group, created by the Department of Health and Human Services (HHS), to develop a common language across health disciplines based "on a core set of competencies that includes patient-centered care, interdisciplinary [interprofessional] teams, evidence-based practice, quality improvement, and informatics" (IOM, 2003f, p. 124). Accomplishing this requires that healthcare professionals be willing to actively work together to achieve this goal.

Once this is done, the next major step is getting different healthcare professionals to accept a universal language. This will require compromises. The use of nursing terminologies such as NIC, NOC, and NANDA must be reconsidered in light of what is the best approach to interprofessional communication methods. Are these effective communication tools or barriers in a time when we need greater interprofessional teamwork and communication? Benner and colleagues (2010) suggest that teaching taxonomies is not applicable in today's healthcare world. Understanding and application of practical knowledge is more critical to providing good patient care, at least as first steps before exploring taxonomies. Meeting this IOM recommendation will not be easy.

Computer-Based Reminder Systems

Students need to understand how computer-based reminder systems work and how they can assist nurses, such as in reminding nurses of risks for patient falls, allergies, and times for medication or specific monitoring. If local HCOs include this support in their information technology, students can appreciate how it can help them provide better care.

Access to Complete Patient Information at the Point of Care

How can access to patient information at the point of care contribute to nursing? Encouraging students to consider this will help them understand how they can use the information, and how this can eliminate errors and near misses and enhance patient-centered care.

Clinical Decision Support Systems

With today's expanding and rapidly changing knowledge, nurses have a difficult time keeping current. Building this knowledge into information technology that helps healthcare professionals make better decisions should be just as important for nurses as for physicians. Students and faculty have installed pharmacology information in their personal digital assistants (PDAs) and smartphones with apps. This is one example of how technology can help in decision-making. Faculty can instruct students in the most effective use of these tools.

Health Insurance Portability and Accountability Act (HIPAA)

The new information infrastructure must meet the requirements of the Health Insurance Portability and Accountability Act. Show students how HIPAA requirements apply to their practice, as students as well as after graduation. Schools of nursing are already very involved in ensuring that HIPAA requirements are met, but these requirements can easily be forgotten, so students need reminders (as do faculty).

IT, Recruitment, and Retention

The California Care Foundation published a report, *Equipped for Efficiency: Improving Nursing Care through Technology*, which examines the critical issue of the impact of health IT on nurses, particularly on recruitment and retention (Turisco & Rhoads, 2008). "New technologies have the potential to create a better work environment for inpatient nurses by improving the efficiency, safety, and quality of care" (p. 2). The project interviewed nurses in a variety of hospitals. Some of the technologies discussed in the report are wireless communication solutions, real-time location systems, delivery robots, wireless patient monitoring, electronic medication administration with bar coding, and electronic clinical documentation with clinical decision support.

The report is a valuable resource for faculty, as it provides information about current technologies with which faculty may not be familiar. The report concludes that health IT can improve the work environment for nurses, improving efficiency, safety, and quality care. The report is available online (http://www.chcf.org/publications/2008/12/equipped-for-efficiency-improving-nursing-care-through-technology).

E-Patients

Patients are more and more involved in use of the Internet and other information technology. Ferguson (2008) refers to these patients as hunters and gatherers of medical information. E-patients can be classified as follows: About 60%–65% of e-patients are well; about 5%–10% are confronting a new medical problem or complications from a current medical problem; and about 30%–35% have stable chronic illness but are not dealing with any medical challenge. Each one of these groups looks for information for different reasons and at different times. Well e-patients are looking for information about staying healthy; e-patients facing a new problem may be looking for information to help them make a decision about their care; and chronic patients may be looking for information for self-management. However, many are also using the Internet to get support or provide it to others with similar health problems. Most patients are satisfied with how the Internet has helped them.

Patients do want additional services available through the Internet, such as physician–patient e-mail, information about the quality of care, the ability to schedule appointments online, information on drugs, information on support, and even free access to fee-only online journals. As was mentioned earlier, access to the Internet is not available to all, and many do not know how to access the Internet, particularly the older generations. Mobile phones can broaden Internet access, but these services do cost money, which puts them out of reach for some patients.

Nurses' Involvement in IT Decisions

Nurses have not been very involved in health IT development and implementation, but this is changing—and it should change. The American Academy of Nursing's Workforce Commission, with support from the Robert Wood Johnson Foundation, surveyed nurses and other healthcare providers at 25 sites nationwide about their work processes and environments (Pulley, 2008). The results show that there is a need for IT tools targeting care coordination, care delivery, communications, discharge processes, documentation, medication administration, patient movement, and supplies and equipment management. Nurses indicated that they wanted all-electronic health records instead of hybrid systems that combine electronic and paper-based reporting; computerized order entry systems to eliminate handwriting legibility issues; touch-screen or voice-activated technology for documentation; and automated networks to collect and download vital patient data. According to the commission's chair, nurses are interested in adding more hands-free tools, particularly wireless technology; greater use of radio-frequency identification technology to track people, supplies, and equipment; robotics to deliver supplies; and smart beds to monitor patient movements, with pressure sensors to reduce the incidence of bedsores. Nurses are important users of IT, so nursing must get involved in application design to improve IT applications (Pulley, 2008).

Nursing Education and Informatics

Informatics must become a curricular thread at all educational levels. Care plans must reflect EMR charting, and teaching should reinforce the process in both its nursing and medical aspects. Students then need opportunities to apply their informatics knowledge in clinical areas. In the classroom, students need to see examples of physician order entry systems, pharmacy orders, and electronic medical records. These technology skills then become part of the critical skills that constitute nursing education expectations and competencies. Technology competencies and a working knowledge of Systematic Nomenclature of Medicine (SNOMED), *International Classification of Diseases, Ninth Revision* (ICD9), and Current Procedural Terminology (CPT) coding are essential; the nurse must understand how a uniform language for all healthcare professions would lead to access to data of nursing actions and how services are reimbursed. At the undergraduate level, this information may be limited to an appreciation of the coding systems, not the practice of coding, whereas advanced practice nursing students need to know about the application of coding.

Nursing education must incorporate the specialty of nursing informatics and its standards of practice. Many schools are doing this during simulation experience, and the practice is likely to expand. Lectures and discussions should include examples and experiences on the web or with screen shots. Students need to know about telenursing and teleconsultations with nurses or physicians; telehome care for monitoring (for example, wound care, skin status using a digital camera, checking BP, checking blood sugar); and teletriage to assess urgency or condition and type of care needed (Lorentz, 2008). Use of all of these methods is growing, and nurses in the future will play more active roles in that use.

Informatics competencies for nurses have been identified but have not yet been effectively incorporated in curricula. A study published in 2005 (McNeil) surveyed 266 BSN and higher programs in the United States out of a possible 677 schools. Approximately half of the undergraduate programs were teaching information literacy skills and requiring students to enter the nursing program with Word and e-mail skills. What was not evident in these programs was content and experience with information system data standards and the nursing role in informatics. About 50% perceived that faculty were novices and advanced beginners. There was no indication of plans to increase the content. Hence, there is still much work to be done to incorporate informatics in nursing programs and ensure that new graduates are ready for informatics in the healthcare setting.

Students must be prepared to use the following in their practice, or at least know about them: EMRs, CPOE, PDAs, clinical decision support systems, computerized monitoring of adverse events, automatic dispensing of medication, bar codes, access to computerized systems at the bedside, computerized reminder systems, wireless voice-activated communication systems to connect staff, wireless laptops, cardiac monitors that communicate directly with badges worn by nurses, telehealth, robots (surgical, courier, multitasking robotic nursing assistant), and much more. Use the IOM report *Health IT and Patient Safety: Building Safer Systems for Better Care* (2011e) to provide additional content about health IT.

Are Nurses in Practice Ready for More IT?

Practicing nurses often lack IT skills and the ability to locate and use online evidence. Hart (2008) conducted a systematic review of literature on the competency of practicing nurses (not new graduates) to use informatics—knowledge and skills—to facilitate EBP and use EMRs effectively. He concluded that although important content has been identified, workplace competencies have not been standardized. Nurses are limited in implementing EBP because they need to build their IT competencies. There is also concern that even new graduates are not as competent in IT as they need to be. "Although nursing attitudes [toward IT] are good, three primary issues cannot be overcome by positive attitudes: Insufficient knowledge, insufficient skills, and insufficient support in terms of training, resources, and time. In addition, it is clear that the capacity for provision of knowledge and skills cannot be left solely to universities because most of the nursing population will not benefit from new advancements in university curriculums" (Hart, 2008, p. 328). Effective EBP requires use of IT. They must be considered together when developing staff competencies.

Another example of the growth of informatics and technology in health care is the new Iowa Medical Center model of an electronic intensive care unit (eICU) to improve patient monitoring (Sagario, 2008). This system allows intensivists at a remote monitoring center to view patients' vital statistics, electrocardiograms, ventilators, and X-ray and lab results. There is also a two-way conference video system so that patients and staff in ICUs at four hospitals can interact. Using the eICU, system experts can be located in one place and then consult with multiple locations and staff. This is particularly useful in providing expert medical consultation and nursing consultation to staff in rural and remote areas; a nurse clinical specialist can view data and consult on patient care with nurses in the various ICUs. The American Association of Critical-Care Nurses has information on this new role on its web site (http://www.aacn.org/wd/certifications/content/ccrn-elanding.pcms?menu=certification), and on certification referred to as CCRN-E Adult Tele-ICU.

Students and Technology

Students expect greater use of IT in their nursing programs as they use it more in their personal lives. iPods, PDAs, Internet tools such as FaceBook and MySpace, and cell phones/smartphones can provide instant information and can be incorporated into very interactive learning experiences. The increased use of social media can be useful in increasing networking and quick sharing of information, but it has its problems, too. Faculty need to talk directly with students about social media and patient confidentiality. Students are very comfortable sharing personal information on the web, but they need to learn what cannot be shared and why. This can also be discussed in the context of ethical and legal issues.

P-Books versus E-books

P-books are paper books, and *e-books* are electronic books. There is growing interest in expanding publication of textbooks in e-book format: either a combination p-book and e-book edition or solely e-book. Walton (2008) compared faculty and student preferences in the use of p-books versus e-books for conducting research, textbook sourcing, and leisure reading. Neither group preferred e-books for leisure reading, though this is rapidly changing today with the increase in methods available for accessing e-books. Nearly a quarter of the students preferred e-books for conducting research and nearly one-fifth for textbooks; the numbers for faculty were 8% and 0%, respectively. Faculty select textbooks, but pressure from students (consumers) and university libraries may have a greater impact over time. Schools are very concerned about the cost of textbooks, so an effective approach must consider costs and accessibility.

There are some technology issues to be resolved, such as what equipment and software are used to read the book: a special book reader (Sony, Amazon's Kindle), a computer (Elsevier), a PDA or other portable digital device, or even a mobile phone. Each has advantages and limitations. There is no doubt that this technology will only continue to expand. It provides portability, interactivity, and options to write notes, highlight, search the content, and more.

Higher education is moving forward in using e-books and digital library collections. However, much work is still needed to set standards for portability and IP protection (Nelson, 2008). The following are key questions that faculty can ask regarding movement to e-book use:

- How are e-books currently used on our campus? What other forms of digital content are being used, particularly by faculty in the classroom? Are students aware of the e-book offerings available to them through the campus library, college store, or other sources?
- What are the cultural and technical barriers to adoption of e-books on our campus? In what ways might we overcome them?
- How can our institution position itself for a future with e-books? What competencies will be required of IT? Libraries? College stores? Faculty? What university pressures will be brought to bear on this issue?

Podcasting

Podcasting can be used to share audio information with students. Faculty can record their lectures prior to class or during class and then make the podcast available to students. Faculty could record cases and follow-up questions with a dialogue about the case, summarize key points weekly, and prepare comments for exam review. Faculty who teach online can use podcasting to personalize contact with students. Students can have the option of listening online or downloading the podcasts to their own iPods for use whenever they want to access the material.

IOM Healthcare Core Competencies Compared to Quality and Safety Education for Nurses Competencies (QSEN)

Quality and Safety Education for Nurses (QSEN) is an initiative funded by the Robert Wood Johnson Foundation to improve nursing care. QSEN alters some of the IOM core competency language. The key message of the IOM core competencies is that all healthcare professions must meet the five core competencies and use the same language to describe them. The language can then be carried into practice, providing a common language for all healthcare professionals to communicate about health care—what do we do and what do we need to improve? Regrettably, when nursing tries to change the language, we separate ourselves from the other healthcare professions at a time when we need to emphasize the interprofessional team.

The most notable difference is that QSEN names six core competencies (separating quality from safety), and deals only with nursing. It identifies the knowledge, skills, and attitudes (KSA) required for each of the competencies (Cronenwett et al., 2007). QSEN has a web site for sharing teaching strategies for each of the QSEN competencies (http://www.qsen.org/). QSEN includes multiple pilots trying new approaches to meet the six QSEN competencies for nursing:

- Patient-centered care
- Teamwork and collaboration (interprofessional teamwork)
- Evidence-based practice
- Quality improvement
- Safety (the IOM includes this in the QI competency)
- Informatics

Summary

Many strategies could be used to respond to the IOM concerns and recommendations. This content should stimulate faculty to be creative in their teaching and encourage greater use of the valuable information and recommendations found in the IOM reports. The digital-only teaching–learning content includes additional materials and strategies related to the IOM reports, all of which provide faculty and instructors with learning module plans on a variety of topics, many of which are mentioned in this chapter and elsewhere in this book. The shorter version of this book, *Learning IOM,* uses much of the same content, but directs it to students.

Part 6

References, Glossary, Acronyms and Abbreviations, and Appendices

References

Ackroyd-Stolarz, S., Hartnell, N., & MacKinnon, N. (2005). Approaches to improving the safety of the medication use system. *Healthcare Quarterly, 8*(Spec. no.), 59–64.

Agency for Healthcare Research and Quality (AHRQ). (2003, December). *AHRQ's patient safety initiative: Building foundations, reducing risk.* Interim Report to the Senate Committee on Appropriations (AHRQ Publication No. 04-RG005). Rockville, MD: AHRQ. Retrieved from http://www.ahrq.gov/qual/pscongrpt

Agency for Healthcare Research and Quality (AHRQ). (2006, February). Patient safety indicators overview. AHRQ Quality Indicators. Retrieved from http://www.qualityindicators.ahrq.gov/psi_overview.htm

Agency for Healthcare Research and Quality (AHRQ). (2010a). *National healthcare disparities report.* Washington, DC: Author. Retrieved from www.ahrq.gov/qual/nhdr10/nhdr10.pdf

Agency for Healthcare Research and Quality (AHRQ). (2010b). *National healthcare quality report.* Rockville, MD: Author.

Agency for Healthcare Research and Quality (AHRQ). (2011). Medications at transitions and clinical handoffs (MATCH) toolkit for medication reconciliation. Retrieved from http://www.ahrq.gov/qual/match/

Aiken, L., Clarke, S., & Sloane, D. (2008). Effects of hospital care environment on patient mortality and nurse outcomes. *Journal of Nursing Administration, 38*(5), 223–229.

American Academy of Nursing (AAN). (2008, November 17). American Academy of Nursing joins movement to transform health care. Retrieved from http://www.aannet.org/i4a/headlines/headlinedetails.cfm?id=167&archive=1

American Academy of Pediatrics. (2007). The National Center of Medical Home Initiatives for Children with Special Needs. Retrieved from http://www.medicalhomeinfo.org/

American Association of Colleges of Nursing (AACN). (2006). *The essentials of doctoral education for advanced nursing practice.* http://www.aacn.nche.edu/DNP/pdf/ Essentials.pdf

American Association of Colleges of Nursing (AACN). (2008a). *Cultural competency in baccalaureate nursing education.* Washington, DC: Author. Retrieved from http://www.aacn.nche.edu/Education/pdf/competency.pdf

American Association of Colleges of Nursing (AACN). (2008b). *The essentials of baccalaureate education for professional nursing practice.* Retrieved from http://www.aacn. nche.edu/Education/pdf/BaccEssentials08.pdf

American Association of Colleges of Nursing (AACN). (2010). *The future of higher education: 2010 annual report.* Washington, DC: Author.

American Association of Colleges of Nursing (AACN). (2011). *The essentials of masters education in nursing.* Washington, DC: Author.

American Association of Colleges of Nursing and Association of American Medical Colleges. (2010). *Lifelong learning in medicine and nursing.* Washington, DC: AACN. Retrieved from www.aacn.nche.edu/education-resources/MacyReport.pdf

American College of Emergency Physicians (ACEP). (2011). The uninsured: Access to medical care. Retrieved from https://www.acep.org/content.aspx?id=45983

American College of Physicians Foundation (ACPF). (2007, October 12). White paper on improving prescription drug container labeling in the United States: A health literacy and medication safety initiative. Retrieved from http://www.acpfoundation.org/files/medlabel/acpfwhitepaper.pdf

American Nurses Association (ANA). (1998). *Shared accountability in today's work environment (Summary of Proceedings, 1998 ANA House of Delegates: June 26–July 1, 1998).* Washington, DC: ANA.

American Nurses Association (ANA). (2003, August). *Handle with care* (fact sheet). http://www.nursingworld.org/MainMenuCategories/OccupationalandEnvironmental/occupationalhealth/handlewithcare/Resources/FactSheet.aspx

American Nurses Association (ANA). (2006a). *Assuring patient safety: The employers' role in promoting healthy nursing work hours for registered nurses in all roles and settings.* Silver Spring, MD: ANA.

American Nurses Association (ANA). (2006b). *Assuring patient safety: Registered nurses' responsibility in all roles and settings to guard against working when fatigued.* Silver Spring, MD: ANA.

American Nurses Association (ANA). (2008). Nurse fatigue. Retrieved from http://www.nursingworld.org/MainMenuCategories/WorkplaceSafety/Work-Environment/NurseFatigue

American Nurses Association (ANA). (2010a). [reissue of 2008 edition]. *Guide to the Code of Ethics for Nurses.* Silver Spring, MD: Nursesbook.org.

American Nurses Association (ANA). (2010b). *Nursing's social policy statement. The essence of the profession.* Silver Spring, MD: Nursesbook.org.

American Nurses Association (ANA). (2010c). *Nursing: Scope and standards of practice.* (2nd. ed.) Silver Spring, MD: Nursesbook.org.

American Organization of Nurse Executives (AONE). (2012). *AONE strategic plan.* Retrieved from www.aone.org/membership/about/docs/2012-2014.AONE.StratPlan.FINAL.doc

Association of American Medical Colleges (AAMC). (2008). *The medical home. A position statement.* Retrieved from https://www.aamc.org/download/60628/data/medicalhome.pdf

Association for Prevention Teaching and Research. (2009). Clinical prevention and population health curriculum framework. Retrieved from www.aptrweb.org/about/pdfs/Revised_CPPH_Framework_2009.pdf

Baker, D. (2007). Health literacy and mortality among elderly persons. *Archives of Internal Medicine, 167*(14), 1503–1509.

Baldwin, D. (2003). Disparities in healthcare: Focusing efforts to eliminate unequal burdens. *Online Journal of Issues in Nursing, 8*(2), 1–16.

Banister, G., Butt, L., & Hackel, R. (1996). How nurses perceive medication errors. *Nursing Management, 27*(1), 31–34.

Banja, J. (2005). *Medical errors and medical narcissism.* Boston, MA: Jones and Bartlett.

Barnsteiner, J., Disch, J., Hall, L., Mayer, D., & Moore, S. (2007). Promoting inter-professional education. *Nursing Outlook, 55*(3), 144–150.

Barr, H., et al. (2005). *Effective interprofessional education: Assumption, argument and evidence.* Oxford, UK: Blackwell Publishing.

Batalden, P. (1998). *Eight domains for the improvement of healthcare.* Boston, MA: Institute for Healthcare Improvement. Retrieved from http://www.ihi.org/IHI/Programs/IHIOpenSchool/EightKnowledgeDomainsForHealthProfessionStudents.htm

Benner, P. (2001). *From novice to expert* (commemorative ed.). Upper Saddle River, NJ: Prentice Hall Health.

Benner, P. (presenter). Colleagues: Sutphen, M., Day, L., Leonard, V., & Rodriguez, L. (2007, June 7). Presentation: *Educating nurses: Teaching and learning for a complex practice of care.* The Carnegie Foundation National Nursing Education Study 6th Annual Conference of State Nursing Workforce Centers. San Francisco, CA.

Benner, P., Malloch, K., & Sheets, V. (Eds.) and the National Council of State Boards of Nursing. (2010). *Nursing pathways for patient safety.* St. Louis, MO: Mosby Elsevier.

Benner, P., Sutphen, M., Leonard, V., & Day, L. (2010). *Educating nurses: A call for radical transformation.* San Francisco, CA: Jossey-Bass.

Berwick, D. (2008). The science of improvement. *Journal of the American Medical Association, 299*(10), 1182–1184.

Berwick, D., Nolan, T., & Whittington, J. (2008). The triple aim: Care, health, and cost. *Health Affairs, 27*(3), 759–769.

Betancourt, J., Green, A., Carrillo, J., & Park, E. (2005). Cultural competence and health care disparities: Key perspectives and trends. *Health Affairs, 24,* 499–505.

Beyea, S., & Kobokovich, L. (2004). Human patient simulation: A teaching strategy. *AORN Journal, 80*(4), 738, 741–742.

Blendon, R., et al. (2002). Views of practicing physicians and the public on medical errors. *New England Journal of Medicine, 347*(24), 1933–1940.

Byrne, M. (2000). *Uncovering racial bias in fundamental nursing textbooks: A critical hermeneutic analysis of the portrayal of African Americans.* Unpublished doctoral dissertation, Georgia State University, Atlanta, GA.

California Endowment. (2003). *Principles and recommended standards for cultural competence education of healthcare professionals.* Woodland, CA: California Endowment.

Campinha-Bacote, J. (2003). *Inventory for assessing the process of cultural competence among healthcare professionals–revised* (IAPCC-R©). Transcultural C.A.R.E. Associates. Retrieved from http://www.transculturalcare.net/

Campinha-Bacote, J. (2008). Transcultural C.A.R.E. Associates. Retrieved from http://www.transculturalcare.net/

Candela, L., & Bowles, C. (2008). Recent RN graduate perceptions of educational preparation. *Nursing Education Perspectives, 29*(5), 266–272.

Carmichael, M. (2008, October 21). ER overload: A new study looks at overcrowding in America's emergency rooms and finds some surprising reasons for those long waits. *Newsweek.* Retrieved from http://www.thedailybeast.com/newsweek/2008/10/21/er-overload.html

Centers for Disease Control and Prevention (CDC). (2011). Chronic disease prevention and health promotion. Retrieved from http://www.cdc.gov/chronicdisease/index.htm

Centers for Medicare and Medicaid Services, U.S. Department of Health and Human Services (CMS). (2007). CMS rule limiting payment for avoidable complications has big implications for nurses. Retrieved from http://www.rwjf.org/pr/product .jsp?id=23434

Chan, S., et al. (2008). Hospital-wide code rates and mortality rates before and after implementation of a rapid response team. *Journal of the American Medical Association, 300*(21), 2506–2509.

Chang, B. L., Bakken, S., Brown, S. S., Houston, T. K., Kreps, G. L., Kukafka, R., et al. (2004). Bridging the digital divide: Reaching vulnerable populations. *Journal of the American Medical Informatics Association, 11*(6), 448–457. doi:10.1197/jamia.M1535

Chassin, M., & Galvin, R. (1998). The urgent need to improve healthcare quality. *Journal of the American Medical Association, 280*(2), 1000–1005.

Christmas, K. (2008). How work environment impacts retention. *Nursing Economics, 26*(5), 316–318.

Classen, D., et al. (2011). "Global trigger tool" shows that adverse events in hospitals may be ten times greater than previously measured. *Health Affairs, 30*(4), 581–589.

Clarke, S., & Aiken, L. (2003). Failure to rescue. *American Journal of Nursing, 103*(1), 42–47.

Cohen, M., Davis, N., & Sanders, J. (1994). Failure modes and effects analysis: A novel approach to avoiding dangerous medication errors and accidents. *Hospital Pharmacy, 29*(4), 319–324, 326–328, 330.

Craig, C., Eby, D., & Whittington, J. (2011). *Care coordination model: Better care at lower cost for people with multiple health and social needs* (IHI Innovation Series white paper). Cambridge, MA: Institute for Healthcare Improvement; available at www.IHI.org

Creech, C. (2008). Are we moving toward an expanded role for part-time faculty? *Nurse Educator, 33*(1), 31–34.

Cronenwett, L., et al. (2007). Quality and safety education for nurses. *Nursing Outlook, 55*(3), 122–131.

Daschle, T., Lambrew, J., and Greenberger, S. (2008). *Critical: What we can do about the health-care crisis.* New York, NY: Thomas Dunne Books.

Davies, D., et al. (2003). The case for knowledge translation: Shortening the journey from evidence to effect. *British Medical Journal, 327*(7405), 33–35.

Davis, K., Schoen, C., & Stremikis, K. (2010). *Mirror, mirror on the wall: How performance of the U.S. health care system compares internationally, 2010 update.* New York, NY: Commonwealth Fund.

De Castro, A. (2004, September 30). Handle With Care©: The American Nurses Association's campaign to address work-related musculoskeletal disorders. *Online Journal of Issues in Nursing, 9*(3). Retrieved from http://www.nursingworld.org/ MainMenuCategories/ANAMarketplace/ANAPeriodicals/OJIN/TableofContents/ Volume92004/No3Sept04/HandleWithCare.aspx

Dekker, S. (2007). *Just culture. Balancing safety and accountability.* Burlington, VT: Ashgate.

DeWalt, C., et al. (2004). Literacy and health outcomes: A systematic review of the literature. *Journal of General Internal Medicine, 19*(12), 1228–1239.

DeWalt, D., & Pignone, M. (2008). Advocacy and patient literacy: What healthcare professionals can do to help patients overcome patient literacy barriers. In J. Earp, E. French, & M. Gilkey (Eds.), *Patient advocacy for healthcare quality* (pp. 215–239). Sudbury, MA: Jones and Bartlett.

Diaz, M., et al. (2008). Contamination of examination gloves in patient rooms and implications for transmission of antimicrobial-resistant micro-organisms. *Infection Control & Hospital Epidemiology, 29*(1), 63–65.

Dickson, G., & Flynn, L. (2012). Nurses' clinical reasoning: Processes and practices of medication safety. *Qualitative Health Research, 22*(1), 3–16.

Donabedian, A. (1980). *Explorations in quality assessment and monitoring: Vol. 1.* Ann Arbor, MI: Health Administration Press.

Donabedian, A. (1988). Quality assessment and assurance: Unity of purpose, diversity of means. *Inquiry, 25,* 173–192.

Donabedian, A. (1996). Evaluating the quality of medical care. *Milbank Quarterly, 44,* 166–203.

Draper, D., Felland, L., Liebhaber, A., & Melichar, L. (2008). The role of nurses in hospital quality improvement. *HSC Research Brief No. 3.* Retrieved from http://www.hschange.com/CONTENT/972/?words=nurses%20QI%202008

Dunton, N., Gajewski, B., Taunton, R., & Moore, J. (2004). Nursing staffing and patient falls in acute care hospital units. *Nursing Outlook, 52*(1), 53–59.

Earp, J., French, E., & Gilkey, M. (Eds.). (2008). *Patient advocacy for healthcare quality.* Boston: Jones and Bartlett.

Enthoven, A. (2008, December 28). Healthcare with a few bucks left over. *New York Times,* p. WK9.

Environmental Working Group (EWG), Healthcare Without Harm (HCWH), American Nurses Association (ANA), & Environmental Health Education Center of the University of Maryland's School of Nursing. (2007). Nurses' health: A survey on health and chemical exposures. Retrieved from http://theluminaryproject.org/downloads/Nurses%20Health%20Survey%20Presentation.pdf

Feagin, J., & Vera, H. (1995). *White racism.* New York, NY: Routledge.

Ferguson, B. (2008). Health literacy and health disparities: The role they play in maternal child health. *Nursing for Women's Health, 12*(4), 286–298.

Fineberg, H. (2012). A successful and sustainable health system—How to get there from here. *New England Journal of Medicine, 366,* 1020–1027.

Finkelman, A., & Kenner, C. (2007a). Commentary: Why should nurse leaders care about the status of nursing education? *Nurse Leader, 5*(6), 23–27.

Finkelman, A., & Kenner, C. (2007b). *Teaching IOM: Implications for nursing education.* Washington, DC: American Nurses Association.

Finkelman, A., & Kenner, C. (2008). Educational and service partnerships: An example of global flattening. *Journal of Professional Nursing, 24*(1), 59–65.

Fox, S. (2006). Online health search 2006. Washington, DC: Pew Internet and American Life Project.

Fox, S. (2007). *E-patients with a disability or chronic disease.* Washington, DC: Pew Internet and American Life Project.

Fuhrmans, V. (2008, January 15). Insurers stop paying for care linked to errors. *Wall Street Journal*, p. D1. Retrieved from http://online.wsj.com/article/SB120035439914089727.html

Gaskill, M. (2008, April 21). Learning from mistakes. Retrieved from http://www.nurse.com

Gerteis, M., Edgman-Levitan, S., Daley, J., & Delbanco, T. (Eds.). (1993). *Through the patient's eyes. Understanding and promoting patient-centered care.* San Francisco, CA: Jossey-Bass.

Gilkey, M., Earp, J., & French, E. (2008). What is patient advocacy? In J. Earp, E. French, & M. Gilkey (Eds.), *Patient advocacy for healthcare quality* (pp. 3–28). Sudbury, MA: Jones and Bartlett Publishers.

Gold, D., et al. (1992). Rotating shift-work, sleep and accidents related to sleepiness in hospital nurses. *American Journal of Public Health, 82*, 1011–1014.

Goldmark, J. (1923). *Nursing and nursing education in the United States.* New York, NY: Macmillan.

Gordon, S. (2005). *Nursing against the odds.* Ithaca, NY: Cornell University Press.

Harding, L., & Petrick, T. (2008). Nursing student medication errors: A retrospective review. *Journal of Nursing Education, 47*(1), 43–47.

Hart, M. (2008). Informatics competency and development within the U.S. nursing population workforce: A systematic review. *CIN: Computers, Informatics, Nursing, 26*(6), 320–329.

Health Resources and Services Administration (HRSA). (2008). Transforming the face of health professions through cultural and linguistic competence education: The role of HRSA Centers of Excellence. Retrieved from http://www.hrsa.gov/culturalcompetence/curriculumguide/ chapter1.htm

Health Resources and Services Administration (HRSA). (2010). *HRSA study finds nursing workforce is growing and more diverse.* Washington, DC: Author.

Hendrich, A., Chow, M., Skierczynski, B., & Zhenqiang, L. (2008, Summer). A hospital time and motion study: How do medical-surgical nurses spend their time? *Permanente Journal, 12*(3). Retrieved from http://xnet.kp.org/permanentejournal/sum08/time-study.html

Hughes, R., & Ortiz, E. (2005). Medication errors: Why they happen, and how they can be prevented. *American Journal of Nursing, 105*(suppl. 3), 14–23.

Hughes, R., & Rogers, A. (2004). Are you tired? Sleep deprivation compromises nurses' health—and jeopardizes patients. *American Journal of Nursing, 104*(3), 15.

Ignatavicius, D. (2000). Do you help staff rise to the fall prevention challenge? *Nursing Management*, (1), 27–30.

Improving Chronic Illness Care. (2003). The chronic care model. Retrieved from http://www.improvingchroniccare.org/index.php?p=The_Chronic_Care_Model&s=2

Improving Chronic Illness Care. (2011). Introduction. Retrieved from http://www.improvingchroniccare.org/

Improvement Science Research Network (ISRN). (2012). University of Texas Health Science Center, School of Nursing, San Antonio, TX. Retrieved from http://www .ISRN.net

Institute for Healthcare Improvement (IHI). (2008a). Beginning to end program. http://www.ihi.org/offerings/IHIOpenSchool/resources/Pages/ImprovementStories/ BeginningtoEndProgram.aspx

Institute for Healthcare Improvement (IHI). (2008b). Establish a rapid response team. http://www.ihi.org/knowledge/Pages/Changes/EstablishaRapidResponseTeam.aspx

Institute for Healthcare Improvement (IHI). (2008c). Failure modes and effects analysis tool. Retrieved from http://app.ihi.org/Workspace/tools/fmea/

Institute for Healthcare Improvement (IHI). (2008d). Medication reconciliation review. Retrieved from http://www.ihi.org/knowledge/Pages/Tools/Medication ReconciliationReview.aspx

Institute for Healthcare Improvement (IHI). (2008e). Self-management support. http:// www.ihi.org/IHI/Topics/PatientCenteredCare/SelfManagementSupport/

Institute for Healthcare Improvement (IHI). (2008f). Transforming care at the bedside. Retrieved from http://www.ihi.org/offerings/Initiatives/PastStrategicInitiatives/ TCAB/Pages/default.aspx

Institute for Healthcare Improvement (IHI). (2011). TCAB. Retrieved from http://www .ihi.org/offerings/Initiatives/PastStrategicInitiatives/TCAB/Pages/default.aspx

Institute for Safe Medication Practices (ISMP). (2007, October 18). Error-prone conditions that lead to student nurse-related errors. Retrieved from http://www.ismp.org/ newsletters/acutecare/articles/20071018.aspInstitute

Institute of Medicine (IOM). (1990). *Medicare: A strategy for quality assurance*. Washington, DC: National Academies Press.

Institute of Medicine (IOM). (1999). *To err is human: Building a safer health system*. Washington, DC: Institute of Medicine and National Academies Press.

Institute of Medicine (IOM). (2001a). *Crossing the quality chasm: A new health system for the 21st century*. Washington, DC: National Academies Press.

Institute of Medicine (IOM). (2001b). *Envisioning the national healthcare quality report*. Washington, DC: National Academies Press.

Institute of Medicine (IOM). (2002). *Guidance for the national healthcare disparities report*. Washington, DC: National Academies Press.

Institute of Medicine (IOM). (2003a). *The future of the public's health in the 21st century*. Washington, DC: National Academies Press.

Institute of Medicine (IOM). (2003b). *Health professions education: A bridge to quality*. Washington, DC: National Academies Press.

Institute of Medicine (IOM). (2003c). *Improving palliative care for cancer: Summary and recommendations*. Washington, DC: National Academies Press.

Institute of Medicine (IOM). (2003d). *Leadership by example: Coordinating government roles in improving healthcare quality*. Washington, DC: National Academies Press.

Institute of Medicine (IOM). (2003e). *Patient safety: Achieving a new standard of care*. Washington, DC: National Academies Press.

Institute of Medicine (IOM). (2003f). *Priority areas for national action: Transforming health care quality.* Washington, DC: National Academies Press.

Institute of Medicine (IOM). (2003g). *Unequal treatment: Confronting racial and ethnic disparities in health care.* Washington, DC: National Academies Press.

Institute of Medicine (IOM). (2003h). *Who will keep the public healthy? Educating public health professionals for the 21st century.* Washington, DC: National Academies Press.

Institute of Medicine (IOM). (2004a). *Health literacy: A prescription to end confusion.* Washington, DC: National Academies Press.

Institute of Medicine (IOM). (2004b). *Keeping patients safe: Transforming the work environment of nurses.* Washington, DC: National Academies Press.

Institute of Medicine (IOM). (2005a). *Preventing childhood obesity: Health in the balance.* Washington, DC: The National Academies Press.

Institute of Medicine (IOM). (2005b). *Quality through collaboration: The future of rural health.* Washington, DC: National Academies Press.

Institute of Medicine (IOM). (2006a). *Emergency medical services at the crossroads.* Washington, DC: National Academies Press.

Institute of Medicine (IOM). (2006b). *From cancer patient to career survivor: Lost in transition.* Washington, DC: National Academies Press.

Institute of Medicine (IOM). (2006c). *Improving the quality of healthcare for mental and substance-use conditions: Quality Chasm Series.* Washington, DC: National Academies Press.

Institute of Medicine (IOM). (2006d). *Preventing medication errors.* Washington, DC: National Academies Press.

Institute of Medicine (IOM). (2007a). *Advancing quality improvement research: Challenges and opportunities* (workshop summary). Washington, DC: National Academies Press.

Institute of Medicine (IOM). (2007b). *America's health care safety net: Intact but endangered.* Washington, DC: National Academies Press.

Institute of Medicine (IOM). (2007c). *Cancer care for the whole patient: Meeting psychosocial needs.* Washington, DC: National Academies Press.

Institute of Medicine (IOM). (2007d). *Emergency care for children: Growing pains.* Washington, DC: National Academies Press.

Institute of Medicine (IOM). (2007e). *Future of emergency care in the United States health system.* Washington, DC: National Academies Press.

Institute of Medicine (IOM). (2007f). *Hospital-based emergency care: At the breaking point.* Washington, DC: National Academies Press.

Institute of Medicine (IOM). (2007g). *Preterm birth: Causes, consequences, and prevention.* Washington, DC: National Academies Press.

Institute of Medicine (IOM). (2007h). *The state of QI and implementation research.* Washington, DC: National Academies Press.

Institute of Medicine (IOM). (2008a). *Engineering a learning healthcare system: A look at the future* (two-day public meeting on April 29–30, 2008). Washington, DC: National Academies Press.

Institute of Medicine (IOM). (2008b). *Knowing what works in health care: A roadmap for the nation.* Washington, DC: National Academies Press.

Institute of Medicine (IOM). (2008c). *Retooling for an aging America: Building the healthcare workforce.* Washington, DC: National Academies Press.

Institute of Medicine (IOM). (2009a). *Health literacy, eHealth, and communication: Putting the consumer first: Workshop summary.* Washington, DC: National Academies Press.

Institute of Medicine (IOM). (2009b). *HHS in the 21st century: Charting a new course for a healthier America.* Rockville, MD: National Academies Press.

Institute of Medicine (IOM). (2010a). *Redesigning continuing education in the health professions.* Washington, DC: National Academies Press.

Institute of Medicine. (IOM). (2010b). *A summary of the February 2010 forum on the future of nursing education.* Washington, DC: National Academies Press.

Institute of Medicine (IOM). (2011a). *Allied health workforce and services: Workshop summary.* Washington, DC: National Academies Press.

Institute of Medicine (IOM). (2011b). *Clinical practice guidelines we can trust.* Washington, DC: National Academies Press.

Institute of Medicine (IOM). (2011c). *Finding what works in health care: Standards for systematic reviews.* Washington, DC: National Academies Press.

Institute of Medicine (IOM). (2011d). *The future of nursing. Leading change, advancing health.* Washington, DC: National Academies Press.

Institute of Medicine (IOM). (2011e). *Health IT and patient safety: Building safer systems for better care* Washington, DC: National Academies Press.

Institute of Medicine (IOM). (2011f). *Learning what works: Infrastructure required for comparative effectiveness research: Workshop summary.* Washington, DC: National Academies Press.

Institute of Medicine (IOM). (2011g). Letter report: Leading health indicators for *Healthy People 2020.* Washington, DC: National Academies Press.

Institute of Medicine (2011h). *Relieving pain in America: A blueprint for transforming prevention, care, education, and research.* Washington, DC: National Academies Press.

Interprofessional Professional Education Collaborative (IPEC). (2011). *Core competencies for interprofessional collaborative practice.* (Collaboration of American Association of Colleges of Nursing, American Association of Colleges of Osteopathic Medicine, American Association of Colleges of Pharmacy, American Dental Education, Association of American Medical Colleges, and Association of Schools of Public Health). Retrieved from www.aacn.nche.edu/education-resources/IPECReport.pdf

iSixSigma. (2008). Deming cycle, PDCA. Retrieved from http://www.isixsigma.com

Issenberg, S., McGaghie, W., Petrusa, E., Gordon, D., & Scalese, R. (2005). Features and uses of high-fidelity medical simulations that lead to effective learning: A BEME systematic review. *Medical Teacher, 27,* 10–28.

Jeffries, P. (Ed.). (2007). *Simulation in nursing education: From conceptualization to evaluation.* New York, NY: National League for Nursing.

Jennings, B., & McClure, M. (2004). Strategies to advance healthcare quality. *Nursing Outlook, 52*(1), 17–22.

Jha, A., DesRoches, C., Kralovec, P., & Joshi, S. (2010). A progress report on electronic health records in U.S. hospitals. *Health Affairs, 29*(10), 1951–1957.

Jha, A., Orav, E., Zheng, J., & Epstein, A. (2008). Patients' perception of hospital care in the United States. *New England Journal of Medicine, 359*(18), 1921–1231.

Johnson, J. (2005). Transforming the face of health professions through cultural & linguistic competence education. Retrieved from http://www.hphnet. org/index.php?option=com_content&view=article&id=50:transform-ing-the-face-of-health-professions-through-cultural-a-linguistic-competence-education&catid=10:library&Itemid=6

Joint Commission. (2005). Root cause analysis matrix. Retrieved from http://www .jointcommission.org/daily_update/joint_commission_daily_update.aspx?k=897

Joint Commission. (2007). "What did the doctor say?" Improving health literacy to protect patient safety. Retrieved from http://www.jointcommission.org/What_Did_the_Doctor_Say

Joint Commission. (2008). *One size does not fit all: Meeting the healthcare needs of diverse populations.* Oakbrook Terrace, IL: Joint Commission. Retrieved from http://www .jointcommission.org/assets/1/6/HLCOneSizeFinal.pdf

Joint Commission. (2011). Healthcare worker fatigue and patient safety. *The Joint Commission Sentinel Event Alert, 48*, 1–3.

Jones, A. (2007). Admitting hospital patients: A qualitative study of an everyday nursing task. *Nursing Inquiry, 14*(3), 212–223.

Jones, B. (2002). Nurses and the code of silence. In M. Rosenthal & K. Sutcliffe (Eds.), *Medical error: What do we know? What do we do?* San Francisco, CA: Jossey-Bass.

Jones, D., DeVita, M., & Bellomo, R. (2011). Rapid-response teams. *New England Journal of Medicine, 365*, 139–146.

Josiah Macy Foundation (JMF), ABIM Foundation, & Robert Wood Johnson Foundation (RWJF). (2011). Team-based Competencies Building a Shared Foundation for Education and Clinical Practice. Retrieved from http://josiahmacyfoundation.org/publications/publication/team-based-competencies-building-a-shared-foundation-for-education-and-clin

Kahn, M. (2008). Etiquette-based medicine. *New England Journal of Medicine, 358*(19), 1988–1989.

Kalisch, B., Begeny, S., & Anderson, C. (2008). The effect of consistent nursing shifts on teamwork and continuity of care. *Journal of Nursing Administration, 38*(3), 132–137.

Karga, M., Kiekkas, P., Diamanto, A., & Chrisoula, L. (2011). Changes in nursing practice: Associations with responses to and coping with errors. *Journal of Clinical Nursing, 20*, 3246–3255.

Ketchum, K., Grass, C., & Padwojski, A. (2005). Medication reconciliation. *American Journal of Nursing, 105*(11), 78–85.

King, R. (2004). Issues and innovations in nursing education: Nurses' perceptions of their pharmacology educational needs. *Journal of Advanced Nursing, 45*(4), 292–400.

Kitch, B., et al. (2008). Handoffs causing patient harm: A survey of medical and surgical house staff. *Joint Commission Journal on Quality and Patient Safety, 34*(10), 563–570.

Koh, H., Nowinski, J., & Piotrowski, J. (2011). A 2020 vision for educating the next generation of public health leaders. *American Journal of Preventive Medicine, 40*(2), 199–202.

Kovner, A., Fine, D., & D'Aquila, R. (Eds.). (2009). *Evidence-based management in health care.* Chicago, IL: Health Administration Press.

Kurtzman, E., & Buerhaus, P. (2008). New Medicare payment rules: Danger or opportunity for nursing. *American Journal of Nursing, 108*(6), 30–35.

Kutney-Lee, A., & Deena, K. (2011). The effect of hospital electronic health record adoption on nurse-assessed quality of care and patient safety. *Journal of Nursing Administration, 41*(11), 466–472.

Ladden, M., Bednash, G., Stevens, D., & Moore, G. (2006). Educating interprofessional learners for quality, safety, and systems improvement. *Journal of Interprofessional Care, 20*(5), 497–505.

Lamb, G., Jennings, B., Mitchell, P., & Lang, N. (2004). Quality agenda: Priorities for action recommendations of the American Academy of Nursing conference on healthcare quality. *Nursing Outlook, 52*(1), 60–65.

Langley, G., Nolan, K., Norman, C., Provost, L., & Nolan, T. (1996). *The improvement guide: A practical approach to enhancing organizational performance.* San Francisco, CA: Jossey-Bass.

Leape, L. (1994). Error in medicine. *Journal of the American Medical Association, 272*(23), 1851–1857.

Leape, L., et al. (1991, February 7). The nature of adverse events in hospitalized patients: Results of the Harvard medical practice study II. *New England Journal of Medicine, 324*(6), 377–384.

Levinson, D. (2012, January). *Hospital incident reporting systems do not capture most patient harm.* Washington, DC: Department of Health and Human Services, Office of the Inspector General.

Lewis, N. (2011, November 28). HER adoption to reach 80% by 2016. *InformationWeek Healthcare.* Retrieved from http://informationweek.com/news/healthcare/EMR/232200275

Li, Y., Glance, L., Yin, J., & Mukamel, D. (2011). Racial disparities in rehospitalization among Medicare patients in skilled nursing facilities. *American Journal of Public Health, 101*(5), 875–882.

Locsin, R. (2005). *Technology competency as caring in nursing.* Indianapolis, IN: Sigma Theta Tau International.

Lohr, K. (Ed.). (1990). *Medicare: A strategy for quality assurance.* Washington, DC: National Academies Press.

Long, K. (2003). The Institute of Medicine report: *Health professions education: A bridge to quality. Policy, Politics, & Nursing Practice, 4*(4), 259–262.

Long, K. (2008, January–February). Managing to keep patients healthier. *Nursing Spectrum (MidWest)*, 26–27.

Lorentz, M. (2008). Telenursing and home healthcare. *Home Healthcare Nurse, 26*(4), 237–243.

Maddox, P., Wakefield, M., & Bull, J. (2001). Patient safety and the need for professional and educational change. *Nursing Outlook, 49*(1), 8–13.

Maeshiro, R., et al. (2011). Using the clinical prevention and population health curriculum framework to encourage curricular change. *American Journal of Preventive Medicine, 40*(2), 232–244.

Manno, M. (2006). Preventing adverse drug events. *Nursing 2006, 36*(3), 56–61.

Manojlovich, M., & Talsma, A. (2007). Identifying nursing processes to reduce failure to rescue. *Journal of Nursing Administration, 37*(11), 504–509.

Marshall, D. (2008). Evidence-based management. *Journal of Nursing Administration, 38*(5), 205–207.

Martin, S., Greenhouse, P., Merryman, T., Shovel, J., Liberi, C., & Konzier, J. (2007). Transforming care at the bedside. *Journal of Nursing Administration, 37*(10), 444–451.

Mason, D. (2004). Who says it's an error? *American Journal of Nursing, 104*(6), 7.

McBride, A. (2005, 4th quarter). Actually achieving our preferred future. *Reflections on Nursing Leadership,* 22–23, 28.

McCloskey, J., & Bulechek, G. (Eds.). (2000). *Nursing interventions classification.* St. Louis, MO: Mosby.

McHugh, M., Kang, R., & Hasnain-Wynia, R. (2009, April 27). Understanding the safety net: Inpatient quality of care varies based on how one defines safety-net hospitals. *Medical Care Research.* Retrieved from http://www.commonwealthfund.org/Publications/In-the-Literature/2009/Aug/Understanding-the-Safety-Net-Inpatient-Quality-of-Care-Varies.aspx

McNeil, B. (2005). Nursing informatics knowledge and competencies: A national survey of nursing education programs in the United States. *International Journal of Medical Informatics, 74*(11–12), 1021–1030.

Meyer, T., & Xu, Y. (2005). Academic and clinical dissonance in nursing education. *Nurse Educator, 30*(2), 76–79.

Michaelsen, L., Knight, A., & Fink, L. (2004). *Team-based learning: A transformative use of small groups in college teaching.* Sterling, VA: Stylus.

Mitchell, P., et al. (2006). Working across boundaries of health professions disciplines in education, research, and service: The University of Washington experience. *Academy of Medicine, 81,* 891–896.

Montalvo, I., & Dunton, N. (2007). *Transforming nursing data into quality care: Profiles of quality improvement in U.S. healthcare facilities.* Silver Spring, MD: American Nurses Association.

Morjikian, R., & Bellack, J. (2005). The RWJ Executive Nurses Fellows Program, part 1. *Journal of Nursing Administration, 35*(10), 431–438.

Morton, P. (1995). Creating a laboratory that simulates the critical care environment. *Critical Care Nurse, 16*(16), 76–81.

Mozes, A. (2008, April). Health insurance premiums skyrocket. *HealthDay News.* Retrieved from http://i.abcnews.com/Health/Healthday/Story?id=4747936&page=3

Mullin, K. (2011). U.S. ranking slips yet again. Professional Patient Advocate Institute. Retrieved from http://patientadvocatetraining.site-ym.com/members/blog_view. asp?id=650743

National Association of Neonatal Nurses (NANN). (2009). *Competencies and orientation toolkit for neonatal nurse practitioners.* Glen View, IL: NANN.

National Center for Education Statistics. (2003). Adult literacy. Retrieved from http:// nces.ed.gov/naal/

National Coordinating Council for Medication Error Reporting and Prevention. (2002, June 11/12). Statement on medication errors. http://www.nccmerp.org

National Council of State Boards of Nursing (NCSBN). (2005, August). *Position paper: Clinical instruction in pre-licensure nursing programs.* Chicago, IL: NCSBN.

National Database of Nursing Quality Indicators (NDNQI). (2010). *NDNQI: Transforming data in quality care.* Kansas City: University of Kansas Medical Center.

National Database of Nursing Quality Indicators (NDNQI). (2011). FAQ. Retrieved from https://www.nursingquality.org/FAQPage.aspx

National Institutes of Health (NIH), NIH Common Fund. (2011). Retrieved from http:// commonfund.nih.gov/interdisciplinary/overview.aspx

National League for Nursing (NLN). (2008, March 3). 2005–06 data. Number of nursing school graduates—including ethnic and racial minorities—on the rise but applications to RN programs dip, reflecting impact of tight admissions. Retrieved from http:// www.nln.org

National League for Nursing (NLN). (2009). *Findings from the latest NLN Annual Survey of Schools of Nursing administered October through December 2009 confirm reported trends.* New York, NY: Author.

National League for Nursing (NLN). (2011, October). *Centers of Excellence handbook.* Retrieved from http://www.nln.org/recognitionprograms/coe/purpose_ goals.htm

National Quality Forum (NQF). (2011). Priorities. Retrieved from http://www .qualityforum.org/Setting_Priorities/Improving_Healthcare_Quality.aspx

Nehring, W. (2008). U.S. boards of nursing and the use of high-fidelity patient simulators in nursing education. *Journal of Professional Nursing, 24*(2), 109–117.

Nehring, W., Ellis, W., & Lashely, F. (2001). Human patient simulators in nursing education: An overview. *Simulation & Gaming, 32,* 194–204.

Nelson, M. (2008, March–April). E-books in higher education: Nearing the end of the era of hype? *EDUCAUSE Review, 43*(2). Retrieved from http://connect.educause. edu/Library/EDUCAUSE+Review/EDUCAUSEReviewMagazineVol/46311

Newhouse, R. (2008). Evidence-based behavioral practice: An exemplar of interprofessional collaboration. *Journal of Nursing Administration, 38*(10), 414–416.

Occupational Safety and Health Administration (OSHA). (2004). Guidelines for preventing workplace violence for health care and social service workers. Retrieved from http://workplaceviolencenews.com/books-2012/books-2011/guidelines-for-preventing-workplace-violence-for-health-care-social-service-workers-kindle-edition

Oklahoma's Nursing Times. (2008, May 30). ANA polls RNs nationwide over safety, staffing concerns. Retrieved from http://www.okcnursingtimes.com/newsletter/newsletter_view.asp?newsid=4557&catid=383&active=0&mode=current

O'Neil, E., & Chow, M. (2011). Leadership action for a new American health system. *Nurse Leader,* (12), 34–37.

Organization for Economic Co-operation and Development (OECD). (2011). *Health data.* Paris, France: OECD, Institute for Research and Information in Health Economics. [Software.]

Orlando Business Journal. (2008, February 29). 250,000 more healthcare workers needed by 2020. Retrieved from http://www.bizjournals.com/orlando/stories/2008/02/25/daily37.html

Paasche-Orlow, M. (2004). The ethics of cultural competence. *Academic Medicine, 79*(4), 347–350.

Paget, L., et al. (2011). *Patient-clinician communication: Basic principles and expectations.* Washington, DC: National Academies Press. Retrieved from http://iom.edu/Activities/Quality/~/media/Files/Activity%20Files/Quality/VSRT/PCCwLogos.pdf

Papastrat, K., & Wallace, S. (2003). Teaching baccalaureate nursing students to prevent medication errors using a problem-based learning approach. *Journal of Nursing Education, 42*(10), 459–464.

Pappas, S. (2008). The cost of nurse-sensitive adverse events. *Journal of Nursing Administration, 38*(5), 230–236.

Patient-Centered Outcomes Research Institute (PCORI). (2012). Retrieved from http://www.pcori.org/

Pear, R. (2008, March 29). Study finds many patients dissatisfied with hospitals. *New York Times* (online). Retrieved from http://www.nytimes.com/2008/03/29/washington/29hospita.html

Pfeffer, J., & Sutton, R. (2006). Evidence-based management. *Harvard Business Review, 84,* 62–74.

Pike, J., Janssen, R., & Brooks, P. (2002). Role and function of a hospital risk manager. *Journal of Legal Nurse Consultants, 13*(2), 3–13.

Pollard, P., Mitra, K., & Mendelson, D. (1996). *Nursing report card for acute care.* Washington, DC: American Nurses Publishing.

Polygreen, P., Chen, Y., Beekmann, S., Srinivasan, A., Neill, M., Gay, T., et al. (2008). Infectious Diseases Society of America's emerging infections network. *Clinical Infectious Diseases, 46*(1), 14–19.

Porter-O'Grady, T. (2005). Leadership for health: Building on the past, creating the future. *Nursing Outlook, 53*(1), 2–3. (Earlier version presented November 2004 at American Academy of Nursing 31st Annual Meeting and Conference, Washington, DC).

The President's Advisory Commission on Consumer Protection and Quality in the Healthcare Industry. (1999). *Quality first: Better healthcare for all Americans.* Washington, DC: U.S. Government Printing Office.

Puchner, L. (1995). Literacy links: Issues in the relationship between early childhood development, health, women, families, and literacy. *International Journal of Educational Development, 15*(3), 307–319.

Pulley, J. (2008, March 13). What nurses want. Retrieved from http://govhealthit.com/articles/2008/03/what-nurses-want_633662646194820028.aspx

Quality and Safety Education for Nurses (QSEN). (2012). About QSEN. Retrieved from www.qsen.org

Reason, J. (1990). *Human error*. Cambridge, UK: Cambridge University Press.

Reinberg, S. (2008, May 13). Quality lags at safety-net hospitals. *The Washington Post*. Retrieved from http://www.washingtonpost.com/wp-dyn/content/article/2008/05/13/AR2008051301951.html

Ridley, R. (2008). The relationship between nurse education level and patient safety. An integrative review. *Journal of Nursing Education, 47*(4), 149–156.

Robert Wood Johnson Foundation (RWJF). (2007, November 8). CMS rule limiting payment for avoidable complications has big implications for nurses. Retrieved from http://www.rwjf.org/qualityequality/product.jsp?id=23434

Robert Wood Johnson Foundation (RWJF). (2007). *A summary of the impact of reforms to the hospital inpatient prospective payment system (IPPS) on nursing services*. Retrieved from http://www.rwjf.org/files/research/ippswhitepaper2007.pdf

Robert Wood Johnson Foundation (RWJF). (2008a, March 20). As more hospitals have increased QI activities this has increased the demands on nurses. Retrieved from http://www.rwjf.org

Robert Wood Johnson Foundation (RWJF). (2008b, February 19). Hospitals taking steps to prevent errors amid reimbursement changes. Retrieved from http://www.rwjf.org

Robert Wood Johnson Foundation (RWJF). (2008c, November 3). Medicare offers physicians e-prescribing bonus. Retrieved from http://www.rwjf.org/qualityequality/digest.jsp ?id=8889&c=EMC-NC142

Robert Wood Johnson Foundation (RWJF). (2008d, February 15). Report highlights medication errors of Massachusetts community hospitals, urges CPOE use. Retrieved from http://www.rwjf.org

Rogers, A., et al. (2004). The working hours of hospital staff nurses and patient safety. *Health Affairs, 23*(4), 202–212.

Sackett, D., Rosenberg, W., & Gray, M. (1996). Evidence based medicine: What it is and what it isn't. *British Medical Journal, 312*, 71–72.

Sagario, D. (2008, February 27). Iowa Medical Center implements eICU to improve patient monitoring. *Des Moines Register*. Retrieved from http://www.desmoinesregister.com/

Salisbury, J. & Byrd, S. (2006). Why diversity matters in healthcare. Retrieved from http://www.csahq.org/pdf/bulletin/issue_12/Diversity.pdf

Salmon, M. (2007). Guest editorial: Care quality and safety: Same old? *Nursing Outlook, 55*(3), 117–119.

Seago, J., Williamson, A., & Atwood, C. (2006). Longitudinal analyses of nurse staffing and patient outcomes: More about failure to rescue. *Journal of Nursing Administration, 36*(1), 13–21.

Seyda, B., Shelton, T., & DiVenere, N. (2008). Family-centered care: Why it is impor-tant, how to provide it, and what parents and children are doing to make it happen. In J. Earp, E. French, & M. Gilkey (Eds.), *Patient advocacy for healthcare quality* (pp. 61–91). Sudbury, MA: Jones and Bartlett.

Shalala, D., & Vladeck, B. (2011). Leading change: How nurses can attract political support for the IOM report on the future of nursing. *Nurse Leader,* (12), 38–39, 45.

Shapiro, E. (2008, March). *Disclosing medical errors: Best practices from the "leading edge."* Unpublished manuscript. Retrieved from http://www.ihi.org/IHI/Topics/PatientSafety/SafetyGeneral/Literature/DisclosingMedicalErrorsBestPracticesLeadingEdge.htm

Shea, K., Shih, A., & Davis, K. (2007). Health care opinion leaders' views on the quality and safety of health care in the United States. New York, NY: Commonwealth Fund.

Shortell, S., Gillies, R., & Anderson, D. (2000). *Remaking healthcare in America* (2nd ed.). San Francisco, CA: Jossey-Bass.

Shreve, J., Van De Bos, J., Gray, T., et al. (2010). *The economic measurement of medical errors.* Schaumberg, IL: Society of Actuaries/Milliman.

Sigma Theta Tau International. (2006). *Implementing evidence-based nursing: Timely articles.* Indianapolis, IN: STTI.

Simmons, B. (2010). Clinical reasoning: Concept analysis. *Journal of Advanced Nursing, 66,* 1151–1158.

Siserhen, L., Blaszak, R., Woods, M., & Smith, C. (2007). Defining family-centered rounds. *Teaching and Learning in Medicine, 19*(3), 319–322.

Smith, J., & Crawford, L. (2003). Report of findings from the practice and professional issues survey: Spring 2002. Chicago, IL: National Council of State Boards of Nursing.

South Carolina Rural Health Research Center. (2009). Rural health. http://rhr.sph.sc.edu/index.phpSpath

Spath, P. (2008). Safety from the patient's point of view. In P. Spath (Ed.), *Engaging patients as safety partners* (pp. 1–34). Chicago, IL: AHA Press.

Spear, S. (2005, September). Fixing healthcare from the inside, today. *Harvard Business Review,* 78–91.

Steefel, L. (2008, March/April). "Just culture" system for nurses takes focus of medical errors from penalties to solutions. Retrieved from http://news.nurse.com/apps/pbcs.dll/article?AID=/20080310/ONC02/303110014

Stevens, K. (2009). *Essential competencies for evidence-based practice in nursing* (2nd ed.). San Antonio, TX: The University of Texas Health Science Center at San Antonio.

Sullivan, L. (2004). *Missing persons: Minorities in the health professions, a report of the Sullivan Commission on diversity in the healthcare workforces.* Retrieved from http://health-equity.pitt.edu/40/

Sullivan, W., & Rosen, M. (2008). *A new agenda for higher education: Shaping the mind for practice.* San Francisco, CA: Jossey-Bass.

Suter, P. (2008). Home care agencies take note: The herald of CMS "Never Events." *Home Healthcare Nurse, 26*(10), 647–648.

Tanner, C. (2003). Building the bridge to quality. *Journal of Nursing Education, 42*(1), 431–432.

Trossman, S. (2011). The practice of ethics. *American Nurse Today, 6*(11), 32–33.

Tse, M., & Lo, L. (2008). A web-based e-learning course: Integration of pathophysiology into pharmacology. *Telemedicine and e-Health, 14*(9), 919–924.

Turisco, F., & Rhoads, J. (2008). *Equipped for efficiency: Improving nursing care through technology.* Oakland, CA: California HealthCare Foundation.

U.S. Department of Defense (DOD). (2005). Patient safety program. In *Healthcare Communications Toolkit to Improve Transitions in Care.* Washington, DC: DOD.

U.S. Department of Health and Human Services (HHS). (2008). Hospital compare survey. Retrieved from http://www.hospitalcompare.hhs.gov

U.S. Department of Health and Human Services (HHS, 2010a). *Healthy People 2020.* Washington, DC: U.S. Government Printing Office.

U.S. Department of Health and Human Services (HHS). (2010b). HHS 2010–1015 strategic plan. Retrieved from http://www.hhs.gov/secretary/about/introduction.html

U.S. Department of Health and Human Services (HHS). (2012). *Healthy people 2020.* Retrieved from http://healthypeople.gov/2020/topicsobjectives2020/overview.aspx?topicid=11

VA Quality Scholars Fellowship (VAQS). (2012). VA national quality scholars. Retrieved from http://vaqs.org/

Vincent, C., & Coulter, A. (2002). Patient safety: What about the patient? *Quality and Safety in Healthcare, 11,* 76–80.

Wachter, R. (2007). *Understanding patient safety.* New York, NY: McGraw-Hill.

Wagner, E. (1998). Chronic disease management: What will it take to improve care for chronic illness? *Effective Clinical Prac*tice, (1), 2–4.

Wakefield, M. (1997). Pioneering new ways to ensure quality healthcare. *Nursing Economics, 15*(4), 225–227.

Walton, E. (2008). E-books in higher education: Near the end of the era of hype. *EDUCAUSE Review,43*(2). Retrieved from net.educause.edu/ir/library/pdf/ERM0822.pdf

Washington Post. (2008, April 8). Medical errors costing U.S. billions. Retrieved from http://www.washingtonpost.com/wp-dyn/content/article/2008/04/08/AR2008040800957.html

Weick, K.E. & Sutcliffe, K.M. (2001). *Managing the unexpected: Assuring high performance in an age of complexity.* San Francisco, CA: Jossey-Bass.

Werner, R., Goldman, L., & Dudley, R. (2008). Comparison of change in quality of care between safety-net and non-safety-net hospitals. *Journal of the American Medical Association, 299*(18), 2180–2187.

Wessling, S. (2008, Summer). Using evidence-based practice to improve minority health outcomes. *Minority Nurse,* 17–22.

Wolf, Z. (2001, May). Understanding medication errors. *Nursing Spectrum Metro Edition,* 31–33.

World Health Organization (WHO). (2010). *Framework for action on interprofessional education and collaborative practice.* Retrieved from http://www.who.int/hrh/resources/framework_action/en/index.html

Young, P. (2007). Caring for the whole patient: The Institute of Medicine proposes a new standard of care. *Community Oncology, 4*(12), 748–751.

Glossary

Accreditation. The establishment of the status, legitimacy, or appropriateness of an institution, program (for example, composite of modules), or module of study.

Acute illness. A rapid and severe onset of illness.

Adverse event. Injuries caused by medical management rather than the underlying condition of the patient.

Blame Game. A punitive environment that blames an individual for errors.

Blog. A web site that provides commentary or news on a particular subject.

Care coordination. An interprofessional approach to the care of a patient.

Caregiver. A person who helps in identifying, preventing, or treating illness or disability.

Chronic illness. A long-term or permanent condition.

Clinical judgment. An application of *clinical reasoning*, using in-depth analysis and evaluation of knowledge and skills, whereby the nurse knows why an intervention is needed, is able to perform the intervention competently, and can justify the clinical decision; allowing the clinician to fit his or her knowledge and experience to an individual patient (individual needs, history, and so on).

Clinical reasoning. An in-depth mental process of analysis and evaluation of knowledge and skills; the process of arriving at problem identification (diagnosis).

Coaching. An expert who draws out what the staff or student knows in a bonded clinical situation.

Collaboration. A team approach among health professionals and family to meet patient needs.

Competency. The ability to perform some task and to meet specified qualifications.

Critical thinking. Actively conceptualizing, applying, analyzing, synthesizing, and evaluating information.

Deep dive. Seeking to improve quality of care by exploring, brainstorming, and prioritizing responses to this critical question: "If you could create the perfect patient and staff experience, what would it look like?"

Delegation. Determining what individual team members should do.

Disclosure of error. Disclosing a harmful medical error, questionable judgment, incident, or misadventure.

Disease management. The coordination and patient-centered use of interventions to decrease length of hospital stay and costs for a disease.

Disparity. Unjustifiable inequality in the treatment of different groups or populations.

Diversity. Racial, cultural, or ethnic variation in the demographics of a place, organization, or profession.

Effective. Designed to provide services with desired outcomes to all who can benefit and refraining from providing services to those not likely to benefit (avoiding underuse and overuse, respectively).

Efficient. Designed to avoid waste of equipment, supplies, ideas, energy, or other resources.

Equitable. Designed to provide care that does not vary in quality because of personal characteristics such as gender, ethnicity, geographic location, and socioeconomic status.

Error. The failure of a planned action to be completed as intended.

Error of omission. An error that occurs because something that should be done is not done.

Evidence-based practice (EBP). The integration of best clinical practice, research evidence, nursing expertise, and the values and preferences of the individuals, families, and communities served.

Evidence-based practice *(IOM core competency).* One of five competencies as defined by the IOM to collect and study data to improve patient-centered care.

Failure to rescue (FTR). The avoidable death of a patient.

Family-centered rounds. Nursing rounds that include the patient's family with the patient's consent.

Handoffs. Accurate information about a patient's general care plan, treatment, services, current condition, and any recent or anticipated changes provided by one healthcare provider to another when the patient changes physical location (such as from one unit to another) or changes healthcare providers.

Health literacy. The degree to which individuals have the capacity to obtain, process, and understand basic information and services needed to make appropriate decisions regarding their health.

Healthcare disparity. Unjustifiable inequality in the health care of different groups or populations.

Healthcare equalities. The absence of disparities in health care.

Healthcare hyperdisparities. Disproportionately low-quality health care provided to a racial and ethnic minority.

High-fidelity simulation equipment. Use of mannequins (human simulators) or equipment common to a particular clinical situation to allow the learner to repeatedly practice appropriate skills in an environment as close to reality as possible.

Iatrogenic error. Adverse effects or complications resulting from medical treatment or advice.

Indicator. A measurement used to assess healthcare structure, process, or outcomes.

Informatics *(IOM core competency).* One of five competencies as defined by the IOM to communicate, manage knowledge, mitigate error, and support decision-making using information technology.

Integrative review. Systematic summaries of appraised studies to provide EBP evidence; a form of EBP literature.

Interdisciplinary/professional teams *(IOM core competency).* One of five competencies as defined by the IOM of healthcare professionals from several fields to cooperate, collaborate, communicate, and integrate care in teams to ensure that care is continuous and reliable.

Interprofessional education (IPE). Joint teaching and learning of students from different professions in order to promote collaborative working in their professional practice.

Just culture. A nonpunitive, fair, and just system that includes personal and professional accountability for one's practice and for actively improving the processes of care, focusing more on system issues and errors rather than individual staff.

Latent failures. Systems faults that allow errors or fail to stop an error.

Medication administration record (MAR). Computer-generated schedule for administering medications to a patient for a defined period, including physician's orders and time of day to administer the agents.

Medication reconciliation. Creating the most accurate list possible of all medications a patient is taking—including drug name, dosage, frequency, and route—and comparing that list against the physician's admission, transfer, and discharge orders with the goal of providing correct medications to the patient at all transition points within the hospital.

Misuse. Improperly applying medications to a patient.

Near miss. An error that was caught before it could occur.

Nurse externship. A program designed to increase the clinical confidence and competence of nursing students, in which they work under the direct supervision of a registered nurse supervisor; usually occurs between the junior and senior years.

Nurse residency. A program designed to transition from nursing student to professional nurse.

Outcome. The effects on health status that are attributable to a planned intervention or series of interventions.

Overuse. Providing more care than needed.

Palliative care. Providing appropriate and compassionate care for patients with life-limiting illnesses.

Patient-centered care *(IOM core competency)*. One of five competencies as defined by the IOM for healthcare professionals: a partnership approach to the planning, delivery, and evaluation of health care to provide better outcomes.

Patient-centered rounds. Regular patient visits in which healthcare professionals are careful to provide medical information to the patient, answer questions, and involve the patient in decisions.

PICO (patient intervention comparison outcome). A model for framing an evidence-based practice question so that an appropriate literature review can be done; derived from **P**atient, **P**opulation, or **P**roblem; area of **I**ntervention or **I**nterest; **C**omparison intervention or **C**ontrol group; desired **O**utcome.

Plan-Do-Study-Act (PDSA). A continuous quality improvement model consisting of a logical sequence of four repeated steps: Plan, Do, Study (Check), and Act.

Process. Methods or functions that are used to achieve an outcome.

Quality. The degree to which health services for individuals and populations increase the likelihood of desired health outcomes and are consistent with current professional knowledge; consists of structure, process, and outcome elements.

Quality improvement (QI). Systematic reduction or elimination of errors and waste and achieving effective care and outcomes for patients.

Quality improvement *(IOM core competency).* One of five competencies as defined by the IOM for healthcare professionals: identify errors and hazards in care; understand and implement basic safety design principles, such as standardization and simplification; continually understand and measure quality of care in terms of structure, process, and outcomes in relation to patient and community needs; and design and test interventions to change processes and systems of care with the objective of improving quality.

Rapid response team (RRT). A team of healthcare clinicians (physicians, nurses, respiratory therapists, and others) and experts in critical care, who come to the bedside to assist staff in making rapid decisions when a patient is in trouble.

Research. Systematic study directed toward fuller scientific knowledge or understanding of the subject.

Risk management (RM). The process of assessing risk and acting in such a manner, or prescribing policies and procedures, as to avoid or minimize risk.

Role model. A nurse who exemplifies the best nursing practice for students or new staff as they transition to a professional nurse.

Root cause analysis. A method designed to examine the causes of an adverse patient event.

Safety. The avoidance of injury or harm when providing care.

Safety-net hospitals. Hospitals that serve a large number of vulnerable patients who have inadequate or no healthcare coverage and poor access to healthcare services.

Self-management. Acceptance by the patient of much of the responsibility for the patient's own care, such as adhering to a prescribed medical regimen or regulating his or her lifestyle.

Sentinel event. An unanticipated event in a healthcare setting that results in death or serious physical or psychological injury to a person, not related to the natural course of the patient's illness.

Simulation. Replication of clinical experiences in a safe environment as part of a student's education

Storytelling. Using stories to present examples to students.

Surveillance. Monitoring of patient status with the goal of early identification and prevention of problems.

Systematic review. A summary of all the published research relevant to a specific question or topic.

Timely. Involving a minimum of waiting or delay for both patients and caregivers.

Transformational leadership. A style of leadership in which the leader engages followers and includes staff in the process.

Underuse. An adverse event caused by failure to provide appropriate care rather than the underlying condition of the patient.

Workaround. A rushed, improvised response to a breakdown in a work process, made without pausing to analyze and correct the underlying problem.

Acronyms and Abbreviations

AACN	American Association of Colleges of Nursing
AACOM	American Association of Colleges of Osteopathic Medicine
AACP	American Association of Colleges of Pharmacy
AAMC	Association of American Medical Colleges
AAN	American Academy of Nursing
AAP	American Academy of Pediatrics
AARP	American Association of Retired Persons
ABNS	American Board of Nursing Specialties
ACPF	American College of Physicians Foundation
ACT	Achieving Competence Today (teaching strategy)
ADE	adverse drug event
ADN	Associate Degree Nurse; Associate Degree Nursing (program)
AHRQ	Agency for Healthcare Research and Quality
ANA	American Nurses Association
ANCC	American Nurses Credentialing Center
ANF	American Nurses Foundation
AONE	American Organization of Nurse Executives
APRN	Advanced Practice Registered Nurse (*as position*); advanced practice registered nurse (*generic*)
APTR	Association for Prevention Teaching and Research
ASPN	Association of Schools of Public Health
BC	board-certified
BHP	Bureau of Health Professions
BMI	body mass index
BSN	Bachelor of Science in Nursing [degree]
C	certified
CAM	complementary and alternative medicine
CDC	Centers for Disease Control and Prevention
CER	comparative effectiveness research
CMO	context + mechanism = outcome (a QI evaluation model)
CMS	Centers for Medicare and Medicaid Services
CNA	Certified Nursing Assistant (*as position*); certified nursing assistant (*generic*)
CNL	Clinical Nurse Leader
CNM	Certified Nurse Midwife
CNP	Certified Nurse Practitioner
CNS	Clinical Nurse Specialist
CPG	clinical practice guideline
CPOE	computerized physician order entry
CPT	Current Procedural Terminology

CRNA	Certified Registered Nurse Anesthetist (*as position*); certified registered nurse anesthetist (*generic*)
DEU	dedicated education unit
DNP	Doctor of Nursing Practice [degree]
DNSc	Doctorate of Nursing Science [degree]
DOD	Department of Defense
DPT	diphtheria, pertussis, and tetanus
DSH	Disproportionate Share Hospital [payment]
EBM	evidence-based management
EBP	evidence-based practice
ED	emergency department
EdD	Doctor of Education [degree]
EHR	electronic health record
EHR/EMR	electronic health record/electronic medical record
ELNEC	End-of-Life Nursing Education Consortium
EMR	electronic medical record
EMS	emergency medical services
EMTALA	Emergency Medical Treatment and Labor Act
EOL	end of life
EWG	Environmental Working Group
FAAN	Fellow of the American Academy of Nursing
FDA	Food and Drug Administration
FEHBP	Federal Employees Health Benefits Program
FMEA	failure modes and effects analysis
FTR	failure to rescue
HAC	hospital-acquired complication/condition
HCO	healthcare organization
HCW	healthcare worker
HCWH	Healthcare Without Harm
HHS	U.S. Department of Health and Human Services
HIPAA	Health Insurance Portability and Accountability Act
HIT	health informatics
HPSA	health professionals shortage area
HQA	Hospital Quality Alliance
HRSA	Health Resources and Services Administration
ICD9	*International Classification of Diseases, Ninth Revision*
ICN	International Council of Nursing
IHI	Institute for Healthcare Improvement
IHS	Indian Health Services
IOM	Institute of Medicine
IPE	interprofessional education
IPEC	Interprofessional Education Collaborative
IPPS	inpatient prospective payment system

IRB	institutional review board(s)
ISMP	Institute for Safe Medication Practices
IT	information technology
JBI	Joanna Briggs Institute
JMF	Josiah Macy Foundation
LPN	licensed practical nurse
LVN	licensed vocational nurse
M&M	morbidity and mortality
MA	Master of Arts [degree]
MAR	medication administration record
MPH	Master of Public Health [degree]
MRSA	methicillin-resistant *Staphylococcus aureas*
MSN	Master of Science in Nursing [degree]
NA	Nurse Anesthetist (*as position*), nurse anesthetis (*generic*)
NAAL	National Assessment of Adult Literacy
NANDA	North American Nursing Diagnosis Association
NCC MERP	National Coordinating Council for Medication Error Reporting and Prevention
NCLEX	National Council Licensure Exam
NCNQ®	National Center for Nursing Quality®
NCNR	National Center for Nursing Research
NCSBN	National Council of State Boards of Nursing
NDNQI	National Database of Nursing Quality Indicators
NHDR	National Healthcare Disparities Report
NHPPD	nursing hours per patient day
NIC	Nursing Interventions Classification
NICU	neonatal intensive care unit
NIH	National Institutes of Health
NINR	National Institute of Nursing Research
NIOSH	National Institute for Occupational Safety and Health
NLN	National League for Nursing
NM	Nurse Midwife (*as position*); nurse midwife (*generic*)
NMDS	nursing minimum data set
NOC	Nursing Outcomes Classification
NONPF	National Organization of Nurse Practitioner Faculties
NP	Nurse Practitioner (*as position*); nurse practitioner (*generic*)
NQF	National Quality Forum
OCNE	Oregon Consortium for Nursing Education
ORHP	Office of Rural Health Policy
OSHA	Occupational and Safety Health Administration
PACU	post-anesthesia care unit
p-book	paper book
PCA	patient-controlled analgesia

PCC	patient-centered care
PCORI	Patient-Centered Outcomes Research Institute
PDA	personal digital assistant
PDSA	plan-do-study-act
PES	practice environment scale
PHR	personal health record
PI	performance improvement
PICO	patient, intervention, comparison, outcome
POES	point-of-entry system
PPP	Preparation for the Professions Program
QI	quality improvement
QIP	quality improvement plan/program
QSEN	Quality and Safety Education for Nurses
RCT	randomized clinical/controlled trial
REALM	Rapid Estimate of Adult Literacy in Medicine
RM	risk management
RN	Registered Nurse (*as position*); registered nurse (*generic*)
RNA	robotic nursing assistant
RRT	rapid response team
RWJF	Robert Wood Johnson Foundation
SAMHSA	Substance Abuse and Mental Health Services Administration
SARS	severe acute respiratory syndrome
SBAR	situation-background-assessment-recommendation
SCHIP	State Children's Health Insurance Program
SIRC	Simulation Innovation Resource Center
SNOMED	Systematic Nomenclature of Medicine
SR	systematic review
TCAB	transforming care at the bedside
TERCAP	Taxonomy of Error, Root Cause Analysis, and Practice Responsibility
UAP	unlicensed assistive personnel
UR	utilization management/review
USP	U.S. Pharmacopeia
VHA	Veterans Health Administration
WHO	World Health Organization

Appendix A
Recommendations from the President's Advisory Commission on Consumer Protection and Quality in the Healthcare Industry

The purpose of the healthcare system must be to continuously reduce the impact and burden of illness, injury, and disability, and to improve the health and functioning of the people of the United States.

Initial Set of National Aims

- Reducing the underlying causes of illness, injury, and disability
- Expanding research on new treatments and evidence on effectiveness
- Ensuring the appropriate use of healthcare services
- Reducing healthcare errors
- Addressing oversupply and undersupply of healthcare resources
- Increasing patients' participation in their care

Measurable objectives need to be specified for each of these aims.

Advancing Quality Measurement and Reporting

A core set of quality measures should be identified for standardized reporting by each sector of the healthcare industry. There should be a stable and predictable mechanism for reporting. Steps should be taken to ensure that comparative information on healthcare quality is valid, reliable, comprehensible, and widely available in the public domain.

Creating Public-Private Partnerships

An advisory council for healthcare quality should be created in the public sector to provide ongoing national leadership in promoting and guiding continuous improvement of healthcare quality. It would track and report on the progress of achieving the national aims for improvement, undertake related quality measurement and reporting, and implement the Consumer Bill of Rights and Responsibilities. A forum for healthcare quality measurement and reporting should be created in the private sector to improve the effectiveness and efficiency of healthcare quality measurement and reporting. Widespread public availability of comparative information on quality care needs to be provided.

Encouraging Action by Group Purchasers

Group purchasers, to the extent feasible, should provide their individual members with a choice of plans. State and federal governments should create further opportunities for small employers to participate in large purchasing pools that, to the extent feasible, make a commitment to individual choice of plans. All public and private group purchasers should use quality as a factor in selecting the plans they will offer to their individual members, employees, or beneficiaries. Group purchasers should implement strategies to stimulate ongoing improvements in healthcare quality.

Strengthening the Hand of Consumers

Widespread and ongoing consumer education should be developed to deliver accurate and reliable information and encourage consumers to consider information on quality when choosing health plans, providers, and treatments. Some consumers will require assistance in making these choices. Further research should be conducted addressing the use of consumer information.

Focusing on Vulnerable Populations

Additional investment should be provided for developing, evaluating, and supporting effective healthcare delivery models designed to meet the specific needs of vulnerable populations.

Promoting Accountability

The Consumer Bill of Rights and Responsibilities should be included in private and public sector contractual and oversight requirements.

Reducing Errors and Increasing Safety in Health Care

Interested parties should work together to develop a healthcare error reporting system to identify errors and prevent their recurrence.

Fostering Evidence-Based Practice and Innovation

Federal funding for healthcare research, including basic, clinical, prevention, and health services research, should be increased and the necessary research infrastructure supported. Collaborative arrangements between researchers and private and public sectors should be developed. Research should target those areas where the greatest improvements in health and functional status of population can occur and where gaps in knowledge exist.

Adapting Organizations for Change

Healthcare organizations should provide strong leadership to confront quality challenges and pursue aims for improvement. They should commit to reducing errors and increasing safety. Organizations need to develop long-term relationships with all stakeholders.

Engaging the Healthcare Workforce

The training of physicians, nurses, and other healthcare workers must change to meet the demands of a changing healthcare industry. Minimum standards for education, training, and supervision of unlicensed paraprofessionals should be established. Steps should be taken to improve the diversity and the cultural competence of the healthcare workforce. Healthcare workers must be encouraged to identify and report clinical errors and instances of improper or dangerous care. Action must be taken to reduce the unacceptably high rate of injury in the healthcare workforce. Efforts must be taken to address the serious morale problems that exist among healthcare workers in many sectors of the industry. Further research should be conducted into how changes in the roles and responsibilities of healthcare workers are affecting quality.

Investing in Information Systems

Purchasers of healthcare services should insist that providers and plans be able to produce quantitative evidence of quality as a means of encouraging investment in information systems.

Source: The President's Advisory Commission on Consumer Protection and Quality in the Healthcare Industry. (1999). *Quality first: Better health care for all Americans.* Washington, DC: U.S. Government Printing Office.

Appendix B

Recommendations from To Err Is Human

Congress should create a Center of Patient Safety with the Agency for Healthcare Policy and Research. This center should:

- Set the national goals for patient safety, track progress in meeting these goals, and issue an annual report to the President and Congress on patient safety; and
- Develop knowledge and understanding of errors in health care by developing a research agenda, funding Centers of Excellence, evaluating methods for identifying and preventing errors, and funding dissemination and communication activities to improve patient safety.

A nationwide mandatory reporting system should be established that provides for the collection of standardized information by state governments about adverse events that result in death or serious harm. Reporting should initially be required of hospitals and eventually be required of other institutional and ambulatory care delivery settings. Congress should:

- Designate the Forum for Healthcare Quality Measurement and Reporting as the entity responsible for promulgating and maintaining a core set of reporting standards to be used by states, including a nomenclature and taxonomy for reporting;
- Require all healthcare organizations to report standardized information on a defined list of adverse events;
- Provide funds and technical expertise for state governments to establish or adapt their current error reporting systems to collect the standardized information, analyze it, and conduct follow-up action as needed with healthcare organizations. Should a state choose not to implement the mandatory reporting system, the Department of Health and Human Services should be designated as the responsible entity; and designate the Center for Patient Safety to:
  - Convene states to share information and expertise, and to evaluate alternative approaches taken for implementing reporting programs, identify best practices for implementation, and assess the impact of state programs; and

- Receive and analyze aggregate reports from states to identify persistent safety issues that require more intensive analysis or a broader-based response (for example, designing prototype systems or requesting a response by agencies, manufacturers, or others).

The development of voluntary reporting efforts should be encouraged. The Center for Patient Safety should:

- Describe and disseminate information on external voluntary reporting programs to encourage greater participation in them and track the development of new reporting systems as they form;
- Convene sponsors and users of external reporting systems to evaluate what works;
- Periodically assess whether additional efforts are needed to address gaps in information, to improve patient safety, and to encourage healthcare organizations to participate in voluntary reporting programs; and
- Fund and evaluate pilot projects for reporting systems, both within individual healthcare organizations and collaborative efforts among healthcare organizations.

Congress should pass legislation to extend peer review protections to data related to patient safety and quality improvement that are collected and analyzed by healthcare organizations for internal use or shared with others solely for purposes of improving safety and quality.

Performance standards and expectations for healthcare organizations should focus greater attention on patient safety.

Regulators and accreditors should require healthcare organizations to implement meaningful patient safety programs with defined executive responsibility.

Public and private purchasers should provide incentives to healthcare organizations to demonstrate continuous improvement in patient safety.

Performance standards and expectations for health professionals should focus greater attention on patient safety.

Health professional licensing bodies should:

- Implement periodic re-examination and re-licensing of doctors, nurses, and other key providers, based on both competence and knowledge of safety practices; and
- Work with certifying and credentialing organizations to develop more effective methods to identify unsafe providers and take action.

Professional societies should make a visible commitment to patient safety by establishing a permanent committee dedicated to safety improvement. The committee should:

- Develop a curriculum on patient safety and encourage its adoption into training and certification requirements;

- Disseminate information on patient safety to members through special sessions at annual conferences; in journal articles, editorials, newsletters, and publications; and on web sites on a regular basis;
- Recognize patient safety considerations in practice guidelines and in standards related to the introduction and diffusion of new technologies, therapies, and drugs;
- Work with the Center for Patient Safety to develop community-based, collaborative initiatives for error reporting and analysis and implementation of patient safety improvements; and
- Collaborate with other professional societies and disciplines in a national summit on the professional's role in patient safety.

The Food and Drug Administration (FDA) should increase attention to the safe use of drugs in both pre- and post-marketing processes through the following actions:

- Develop and enforce standards for the design of drug packaging and labeling that will maximize safety in use;
- Require pharmaceutical companies to test (using FDA-approved methods) proposed drug names to identify and remedy potential sound-alike and look-alike confusion with existing drug names; and
- Work with physicians, pharmacists, consumers, and others to establish appropriate response to problems identified through post-marketing surveillance, especially for concerns perceived to require immediate response to protect the safety of patients.

Healthcare organizations and the professionals affiliated with them should make continually improved patient safety a declared and serious aim by establishing patient safety programs with defined executive responsibility. Patient safety programs should:

- Provide strong, clear, and visible attention to safety;
- Implement nonpunitive systems for reporting and analyzing errors in their organization;
- Incorporate well-understood safety principles, such as standardizing and simplifying equipment, supplies, and processes; and
- Establish interdisciplinary team training programs for providers that incorporate proven methods of team training, such as simulation.

Healthcare organizations should implement proven medication safety practices.

Source: Institute of Medicine (IOM). (1999). *To err is human. Building a safer health system*. Washington, DC: National Academies Press. Reprinted with permission.

Appendix C
Recommendations from Crossing the Quality Chasm

All healthcare constituents, including policy-makers, purchasers, regulators, health professionals, healthcare trustees and management, and consumers, should commit to a national statement of purpose for the healthcare systems as a whole and to a shared agenda of six aims for improvement that can raise the quality of care to unprecedented levels. [*This is related to the six aims or goals identified by the report. This has never been done, and it will not be easy to accomplish. It also requires an interprofessional solution to a multifaceted problem—again an approach never before attempted on a national scale. Nursing education must be part of the interprofessional solution as an active team member working collaboratively with other healthcare educators in fields such as medicine, pharmacy, and allied health.*]

Clinicians and patients, and the healthcare organizations that support care delivery, should adopt a new set of principles to guide the redesign of care processes. [*Identifying critical concerns will be important. Often clinicians, patients, and healthcare organizations do not agree, but consensus will be important for success.*]

The Department of Health and Human Services (DHHS) should identify a set of priority conditions to focus initial efforts, provide resources to stimulate innovation, and initiate the change process. [*A later IOM report,* Priority Areas for National Action *(IOM, 2003f), identifies these conditions.*]

Healthcare organizations should design and implement more effective organizational support processes to make change in the delivery of care possible. [*Change is everpresent, and healthcare organizations and their leaders and staff must learn more effective methods for coping with change.*]

Purchasers, regulators, health professions, educational institutions, key stakeholders, and the DHHS should create an environment that fosters and rewards improvement by:

(1) Creating an infrastructure to support evidence-based practice,
(2) Facilitating the use of information technology (IT),
(3) Aligning payment incentives, and
(4) Preparing the workforce to better serve patients and their families in a world of expanding knowledge and rapid change.

[*There is no doubt that these are key issues. Through its web site, HHS has provided some infrastructure to support evidence-based practice, such as the work done by AHRQ, but more support is needed. As discussed in Part 1, the IOM report* Patient Safety *addresses some of the needs in IT and standards. Financial issues and reimbursement are also areas of deep concern.*]

Source: Institute of Medicine (IOM). (2001). *Crossing the quality chasm*. Washington, DC: National Academies Press. Reprinted with permission.

Appendix D
Recommendations from Leadership by Example

The federal government should assume a strong leadership position in driving the healthcare sector to improve the safety and quality of healthcare services provided to the approximately 100 million beneficiaries of the six major government healthcare programs. Given the leverage of the federal government, this leadership will result in improvements in the safety and quality of health care provided to all Americans.

The federal government should take maximal advantage of its unique position as regulator, healthcare purchaser, healthcare provider, and sponsor of applied health services research to set quality standards for the healthcare sectors. Specifically:

- Regulatory processes should be used to establish clinical data reporting requirements applicable to all six major government healthcare programs.
- All six major government healthcare programs should vigorously pursue purchasing strategies that encourage adoption of best practices through the release of public-domain comparative quality data and the provision of financial and other rewards for providers that achieve high levels of quality.
- Not only should healthcare delivery systems operated by the public programs continue to serve as laboratories for the development of innovative twenty-first century care delivery models, but much greater emphasis should also be placed on the dissemination of the findings and, in the case of information technology, the creation of public-domain products.
- Applied health services research should be expanded and should emphasize the development of knowledge, tools, and strategies that can support quality enhancement in a wide variety of settings.

Congress should direct the Secretaries of the Department of Health and Human Services, Department of Defense, and Department of Veterans Affairs to work together to establish standardized performance measures across the government programs, as well as public reporting requirements for clinicians, institutional providers, and health plans in each program. These requirements should be implemented for all six major government healthcare programs and should be applied fairly and equitably across various financing and delivery options in those programs. The standardized measurement and reporting activities should replace the many performance measurement activities currently under way in the various government programs.

The Quality Interagency Coordination Task Force (QuIC) should promulgate standardized sets of performance measures for five common health conditions in fiscal year (FY) 2003 and another 10 sets in FY 2004.

- Each government healthcare program should pilot test the first set of measures between FY 2003 and FY 2005 in a limited number of sites. These pilot tests should include the collection of patient-level data and the public release of comparative performance reports.
- All six government programs should prepare for full implementation of the 15-set performance measurement and reporting system by FY 2008. Specifically:
  - The government healthcare programs that provide services through the private sector (that is, Medicare, Medicaid, SCHIP, and portions of DOD TRICARE) should inform participating providers that submission of the audited patient-level data necessary for performance measurement will be required for continued participation in FY 2007.
  - The government healthcare programs that provide services directly (that is, VHA, the remainder of DOD, TRICARE, and HIS) should begin work immediately to ensure they have the information technology capabilities to produce the necessary data.

The federal government should take steps immediately to encourage and facilitate the development of the information technology infrastructure that is critical to healthcare quality and safety enhancement, as well as to many of the nation's other priorities, such as bioterrorism surveillance, public health, and research. Specifically:

- Congress should consider potential options to facilitate rapid development of a national health information infrastructure, including tax credits, subsidized loans, and grants.
- Government healthcare programs that deliver services through the private sector (Medicare, Medicaid, SCHIP, and a portion of DOD TRICARE) should adopt both market-based and regulatory options to encourage investment in information technology. Such options might include enhanced or more rapid payments to providers capable of submitting computerized clinical data, a requirement for certain information technology capabilities as a condition of participation, and direct grants.
- VHA, DOD, and HIS should continue implementing clinical and administrative information systems that enable the retrieval of clinical information across their programs and that can communicate directly with each other. Whenever possible, the software and intellectual property developed by these three government programs should rely on web-based language and architecture and be made available in the public domain.

- Starting in FY 2008, each government healthcare program should make comparative quality reports and data available in the public domain. The programs should provide for access to these reports and data in ways that meet the needs of various users, provided that patient privacy is protected.
- The government healthcare programs, working with the Agency for Health Research Quality (AHRQ), should establish a mechanism for pooling performance measurement data across programs in a data repository. Contributions of data from private-sector insurance programs should be encouraged provided such data meet certain standards for validity and reliability. Consumers, healthcare professionals, planners, purchasers, regulators, public health officials, researchers, and others should be afforded access to the repository provided that patient privacy is protected.

The six government healthcare programs should work together to develop a comprehensive health services research agenda that will support the quality enhancement processes of all programs. The QuIC (or some similar interdepartmental structure with representation from each of the government healthcare programs and AHRQ) should be given the authority and resources needed to carry out this responsibility. The agenda for FY 2003–2005 should support the following:

- Establishment of core sets of standardized performance measures.
- Ongoing evaluation of the impact of the use of standardized performance measurement and reporting by the six major government healthcare programs. Development and evaluation of specific strategies that can be used to improve the federal government's capability to leverage the purchaser, regulator, and provider roles to enhance quality.
- Monitoring of national progress in meeting the six national quality aims (safety, effectiveness, patient-centeredness, timeliness, efficiency, and equity).

Source: Institute of Medicine (IOM). (2003). *Leadership by example: Coordinating government roles in improving healthcare quality.* Washington, DC: National Academies Press.

Appendix E
Recommendations from The Future of the Public's Health

Healthcare providers responsible for assuring population health need to focus on the following areas of action and change (IOM, 2003a, p. 4):

- Adopting a population health approach that considers the multiple determinants of health;
- Strengthening the governmental public health infrastructure, which forms the backbone of the public health system;
- Building a new generation of intersectoral partnerships that also draw on the perspectives and resources of diverse communities and actively engage them in health action;
- Developing systems of accountability to assure the quality and availability of public health services;
- Making evidence the foundation of decision-making and the measure of success; and
- Enhancing and facilitating communication in the public health system (for example, among all levels of the governmental public health infrastructure and between public health professionals and community members).

Each of these action areas has relevance to nursing education; baccalaureate level students need some appreciation of how these action areas might be implemented, and graduate students in community health need to be directly involved in activities related to these action areas.

Recommendations for Nursing

Achieving improvement in public health requires an acknowledgement and understanding of trends that affect health. There have been and will continue to be major changes in demographics and population growth, for example, greater diversity, aging population, and disparities. Technology and scientific research are rapidly moving forward, providing opportunities and challenges. Information technology (IT) is discussed in the body of this document, particularly its impact on healthcare delivery, quality, and safety. Use of IT in public health requires consideration of issues such as sharing of information across healthcare organizations, communicable disease data, and more current issues such as the fear of bioterrorism and how this information should be shared in a timely manner.

Globalization has also had an impact on health in the United States. Diversity is one result, but also travel and communication allows U.S. citizens to interact with and share knowledge with others. In addition, there is greater exchange of products, such as pharmaceuticals and food, all of which are positive, but also carry risks such as spread of diseases or contaminated food. Bioterrorism is a critical concern with major implications for public health, and with the movement of greater globalization there is a greater risk. This concern is also changing the way public health is viewed. Prior to September 11, many thought of public health as epidemics, immunizations, and traveler warnings. Since that time the view has been on preparedness, including natural disasters and how we as a nation can respond. It has broadened the definition of public health to include information sharing, knowledge applications, and information networks necessary to speed responses in case of any emergency. This experience has unfortunately pointed out holes in the existing system, including communication problems among agencies and nonexistent databases that "talk" to each other for the purposes of rapid response. Disaster planning and bioterrorism are now included in most nursing curricula. Material has been developed to assist schools of nursing in this effort. For example, the Centers for Disease Control & Prevention (CDC) has funded projects in public health preparedness. They offer curriculum modules free of charge so bioterrorism contact can be used by healthcare organizations and health professionals' education. These can be found through the CDC Office of Workforce Policy and Planning and the Specialty Centers in Public Health Preparedness (S-CPHPs). The Bureau of Health Professions and Department of Health and Human Services Health Resources & Services Administration (BHP and HRSA) have also funded grants to create continuing education programs as well as enhance curricula. Two such grants were awarded in 2004 to the University of Illinois at Chicago. Information on these grants can be found at http://www.hrsa.gov/bioterrorism/cooperative/index.htm

Source: Institute of Medicine (IOM). (2003). *The future of the public's health*. Washington, DC: National Academies Press.

Appendix F

Recommendations from Who Will Keep the Public Healthy?

"A public health professional is a person educated in public health or a related discipline who is employed to improve heath through a population focus" (IOM, 2003b, p. 4). The seven content areas that are important for today's and future public health professions and should be included in nursing curricula are as follows:

- Informatics
- Genomics
- Communication
- Cultural competence
- Community-based participatory research
- Global health, policy, and law
- Public health ethics

These are in addition to the longstanding core components of public health:

- Epidemiology
- Biostatistics
- Environmental health
- Health services administration
- Social and behavioral science

Recommendations for Nursing

- Understanding of public health in the community, health promotion, and disease prevention.
- Undergraduate nursing programs prepare students to understand the ecological model of health, its determinants, and core competencies in population-focused

practice. This level of education and awareness will require that public health agencies to support clinical experiences for nursing students.

▌ "Schools of nursing that offer master's degree programs in public health nursing should be encouraged to partner with schools of public health to ensure that current thinking about public health is integrated into the nursing curricula content, and to facilitate development of interdisciplinary skills and capacities" (IOM, 2003, p. 19). To do so effectively requires educational experiences through interdisciplinary [*interprofessional*] work.

Source: Institute of Medicine (IOM). (2003). *Who will keep the public healthy?* Washington, DC: National Academies Press.

Appendix G
Systematic Review Standards

BOX S-2
Recommended Standards for Initiating
a Systematic Review

Standard 2.1 Establish a team with appropriate expertise and experience to conduct the systematic review

Required elements:

2.1.1 Include expertise in the pertinent clinical content areas

2.1.2 Include expertise in systematic review methods

2.1.3 Include expertise in searching for relevant evidence

2.1.4 Include expertise in quantitative methods

2.1.5 Include other expertise as appropriate

Standard 2.2 Manage bias and conflict of interest (COI) of the team conducting the systematic review

Required elements:

2.2.1 Require each team member to disclose potential COI and professional or intellectual bias

2.2.2 Exclude individuals with a clear financial conflict

2.2.3 Exclude individuals whose professional or intellectual bias would diminish the credibility of the review in the eyes of the intended users

Standard 2.3 Ensure user and stakeholder input as the review is designed and conducted

Required element:

2.3.1 Protect the independence of the review team to make the final decisions about the design, analysis, and reporting of the review

(Continued)

Standard 2.4 Manage bias and COI for individuals providing input into the systematic review

Required elements:

2.4.1 Require individuals to disclose potential COI and professional or intellectual bias

2.4.2 Exclude input from individuals whose COI or bias would diminish the credibility of the review in the eyes of the intended users

Standard 2.5 Fomulate the topic for the systematic review

Required elements:

2.5.1 Confirm the need for a new review

2.5.2 Develop an analytic framework that clearly lays out the chain of logic that links the health intervention to the outcomes of interest and defines the key clinical questions to be addressed by the systematic review

2.5.3 Use a standard format to articulate each clinical question of interest

2.5.4 State the rationale for each clinical question

2.5.5 Refine each question based on user and stakeholder input

Standard 2.6 Develop a systematic review protocol

Required elements:

2.6.1 Describe the context and rationale for the review from both a decision-making and research perspective

2.6.2 Describe the study screening and selection criteria (inclusion/exclusion criteria)

2.6.3 Describe precisely which outcome measures: time points, interventions, and comparison groups will be addressed

2.6.4 Describe the search strategy for identifying relevant evidence

2.6.5 Describe the procedures for study selection

2.6.6 Describe the data extraction strategy

2.6.7 Describe the process for identifying and resolving disagreement between researchers in study selection and data extraction decisions

2.6.8 Describe the approach to critically appraising individual studies

2.6.9 Describe the method for evaluating the body of evidence, including the quantitative and qualitative synthesis strategies

2.6.10 Describe and justify any planned analyses of differential treatment effects according to patient subgroups, how an intervention is delivered, or how an outcome is measured

2.6.11 Describe the proposed timetable for conducting the review

Standard 2.7 Submit the protocol for peer review

Required element:

    2.6.9 Provide a public comment period for the protocol and publicly report on disposition of comments

Standard 2.8 Make the final protocol publicly available, and add any amendments to the protocol in a timely fashion

---

BOX S-3
Recommended Standards for Finding
and Assessing Individual Studies

Standard 3.1 Conduct a comprehensive systematic search for evidence

Required elements:

    3.1.1 Work with a librarian or other information specialist trained in performing systematic reviews to plan the search strategy

    3.1.2 Design the search strategy to address each key research question

    3.1.3 Use an independent librarian or other information specialist to peer review the search strategy

    3.1.4 Search bibliographic databases

    3.1.5 Search citation indexes

    3.1.6 Search literature cited by eligible studies

    3.1.7 Update the search at intervals appropriate to the pace of generation of new information for the research question being addressed

    3.1.8 Search subject-specific databases if other databases are unlikely to provide all relevant evidence

    3.1.9 Search regional bibliographic databases if other databases are unlikely to provide all relevant evidence

Standard 3.2 Take action to address potentially biased reporting of research results

Required elements:

    3.2.1 Search grey literature databases, clinical trial registries, and other sources of unpublished information about studies

    3.2.2 Invite researchers to clarify information about study eligibility, study characteristics, and risk of bias

    3.2.3 Invite all study sponsors and researchers to submit unpublished data, including unreported outcomes, for possible inclusion in the systematic review

(Continued)

3.2.4   Handsearch selected journals and conference abstracts

3.2.5   Conduct a web search

3.2.6   Search for studies reported in languages other than English if appropriate

Standard 3.3 Screen and select studies

Required elements:

3.3.1   Include or exclude studies based on the protocol's prespecified criteria

3.3.2   Use observational studies in addition to randomized clinical trials to evaluate harms of interventions

3.3.3   Use two or more members of the review team, working independently, to screen and select studies

3.3.4   Train screeners using written documentation; test and retest screeners to improve accuracy and consistency

3.3.5   Use one of two strategies to select studies: (1) read all full-text articles identified in the search or (2) screen titles and abstracts of all articles and then read the full texts of articles identified in initial screening

3.3.6   Taking account of the risk of bias, consider using observational studies to address gaps in the evidence from randomized clinical trials on the benefits of interventions

Standard 3.4 Document the search

Required elements:

3.4.1   Provide a line-by-line description of the search strategy, including the date of every search for each database, web browser, etc.

3.4.2   Document the disposition of each report identified including reasons for their exclusion if appropriate

Standard 3.5 Manage data collection

Required elements:

3.5.1   At a minimum, use two or more researchers, working independently, to extract quantitative and other critical data from each study. For other types of data, one individual could extract the data while the second individual independently checks for accuracy and completeness. Establish a fair procedure for resolving discrepancies—do not simply give final decision-making power to the senior reviewer

3.5.2   Link publications from the same study to avoid including data from the same study more than once

3.5.3   Use standard data extraction forms developed for the specific SR

3.5.4   Pilot-test the data extraction forms and process

Standard 3.6 Critically appraise each study
Required elements:
    3.6.1 Systematically assess the risk of bias, using predefined criteria
    3.6.2 Assess the relevance of the study's populations, interventions, and outcome measures
    3.6.3 Assess the fidelity of the implementation of interventions

---

BOX S-4
Recommended Standards for Synthesizing
the Body of Evidence

Standard 4.1 Use a prespecified method to evaluate the body of evidence
Required elements:
    4.1.1 For each outcome, systematically assess the following characteristics of the body of evidence:
- Risk of bias
- Consistency
- Precision
- Directness
- Reporting bias

    4.1.2 For bodies of evidence that include observational research, also systematically assess the following characteristics for each outcome:
- Dose–response association
- Plausible confounding that would change the observed effect
- Strength of association

    4.1.3 For each outcome specified in the protocol, use consistent language to characterize the level of confidence in the estimates of the effect of an intervention

Standard 4.2 Conduct a qualitative synthesis
Required elements:
    4.2.1 Describe the clinical and methodological characteristics of the included studies, including their size, inclusion or exclusion of important subgroups, timeliness, and other relevant factors

---

Source: Institute of Medicine (IOM). 2011. *Finding What Works in Health Care: Standards for Systematic Reviews.* Washington, DC: National Academies Press.

Appendix H

Recommendations from Keeping Patients Safe: Transforming the Work Environment for Nurses

Healthcare organizations (HCOs) should acquire nurse leaders for all levels of management (for example, at the organization-wide and patient care unit levels) who will:

- Participate in executive decisions in the HCO;
- Represent nursing staff to organization management and facilitate their mutual trust;
- Achieve effective communication between nursing and other clinical leadership;
- Facilitate input of direct-care nursing staff into operational decision-making and the design of work processes and work flow; and
- Be provided with organizational resources to support the acquisition, management, and dissemination to nursing staff of the knowledge needed to support their clinical decision-making and actions.

Leaders of HCOs should take action to identify and minimize the potential adverse effects of their decisions on patient safety by:

- Educating board members and senior, midlevel, and line managers about the link between management practices and safety and
- Emphasizing safety to the same extent as productivity and financial goals in internal management planning and reports and in public reports to stakeholders.

HCOs should employ management structures and processes throughout the organization that:

- Provide ongoing vigilance in balancing efficiency and safety,
- Demonstrate trust in workers and promote trust by workers,

- Actively manage the process of change,
- Engage workers in nonhierarchical decision-making and in the design of work processes and work flow, and
- Establish the organization as a "learning organization."

Professional associations, philanthropic organizations, and other professional leaders in the healthcare industry should sponsor collaborative partnerships that incorporate multiple academic and other research-based organizations to support HCOs in the identification and adoption of evidence-based management practices.

The U.S. Department of Health and Human Services (DHHS) should update regulations established in 1990 that specify minimum standards for registered and licensed nurse staffing in nursing homes. Updated minimum standards should:

- Require the presence of at least one RN in the facility at all times;
- Specify staffing levels that increase as the number of patients increase, and that are based on the findings and recommendations of the DHHS report to Congress, Appropriateness of Minimum Nurse Staffing Ratios in Nursing Homes—Phase II Final Report; and
- Address staffing levels for nurse assistants, who provide the majority of patient care.

Hospitals and nursing homes should employ nurse staffing practices that identify needed nurse staffing for each patient care unit per shift. These practices should:

- Incorporate estimates of patient volume that count admissions, discharges, and "less than full-day" patients in addition to a census of patients at a point in time;
- Involve direct-care nursing staff in determining and evaluating the approaches used to determine appropriate unit staffing levels for each shift; and
- Provide for staffing "elasticity" or "slack" in each shift's scheduling to accommodate unpredicted variations in patient volume and acuity and their effect on workload. Methods used to provide slack should give preference to scheduling excess staff and creating cross-trained float pools in the HCO. Use of nurses from external agencies should be avoided.

Hospitals and nursing homes should perform ongoing evaluation of the effectiveness of their nurse staffing practices with respect to patient safety and increase internal oversight of their staffing methods, levels, and effects on patient safety whenever staffing falls below the following levels for a 24-hour day:

- In hospital ICUs: one licensed nurse for every two patients (12 hours of licensed nursing staff per patient day) and
- In nursing homes, for long-term residents: one RN for every 32 patients (0.75 hours per resident day), one licensed nurse for every 18 patients (1.3 hours per resident day), and one nurse assistant for every 8.5 patients (2.8 hours per resident day).

The DHHS should implement a nationwide, publicly accessible system for collecting and managing valid and reliable staffing and turnover data from hospitals and nursing homes. Information on individual hospital and nursing home staffing at the level of individual nursing units and the facility in the aggregate should be disclosed routinely to the public.

Federal and state nursing home report cards should include standardized, case-mix-adjusted information on the average hours per patient day of RN, licensed, and nurse assistant care provided to residents and a comparison with federal and state standards.

During the next three years, public and private sponsors of the new hospital report card to be located on the federal government web sites should undertake an initiative—in collaboration with experts in acute hospital care, nurse staffing, and consumer information—to develop, test, and implement measures of hospital nurse staffing levels for the public.

HCOs should dedicate funds equal to a defined percentage of nursing payroll to support nursing staff in their ongoing acquisition and maintenance of knowledge and skills. These resources should be sufficient for and used to implement policies and practices that:

- Assign experienced nursing staff to precept nurses newly practicing in a clinical area to address gaps in knowledge or skills;
- Annually ensure that each licensed nurse and nurse assistant has an individualized plan and resources for educational development in health care;
- Provide education and training of staff as new technology or changes in the workplace are introduced;
- Provide decision support technology to actively involve direct-care nursing staff in point-of-care learning; and
- Disseminate to individual staff members organizational learning as captured in clinical tools, algorithms, and pathways.

To reduce error-producing fatigue, state regulatory bodies should prohibit nursing staff from providing patient care in any combination of scheduled shifts, mandatory overtime, or voluntary overtime in excess of 12 hours in any given 24-hour period and in excess of 60 hours per seven-day period. To this end:

- HCOs and labor organizations representing nursing staff should establish policies and practices designed to prevent nurses who provide direct patient care from working longer than 12 hours in a 24-hour period and in excess of 60 hours per seven-day period; and
- Schools of nursing, state boards of nursing, and HCOs should educate nurses about the threats to patient safety caused by fatigue.

HCOs should provide nursing leadership with resources that enable them to design the nursing work environment and care processes to reduce errors. These efforts must directly involve direct-care nurses throughout all phases of work design and should concentrate on errors associated with:

■ Surveillance of patient health status;
■ Patient transfers and other patient handoffs;
■ Complex patient care processes; and
■ Non-value-added activities performed by nurses, such as locating and obtaining supplies, looking for personnel, completing redundant or unnecessary documentation, and compensating for poor communication systems.

HCOs should address hand washing and medication administration among their first work design initiatives.

Regulators, leaders in health care, and experts in nursing, law, informatics, and related disciplines should jointly convene to formulate strategies for safely reducing the burden associated with patient and work-related documentation.

HCO boards of directors, managerial leadership, and labor partners should create and sustain cultures of safety by implementing the recommendations presented previously and by:

■ Specifying short- and long-term safety objectives;
■ Continuously reviewing success in meeting these objectives and providing feedback at all levels;
■ Conducting an annual, confidential survey of nursing and other healthcare workers to assess the extent to which a culture of safety exists;
■ Instituting a de-identified, fair, and just reporting system for errors and near misses;
■ Engaging in ongoing employee training in error detection, analysis, and reduction;
■ Implementing procedures for analyzing errors and providing feedback to direct-care workers; and
■ Instituting rewards and incentives for error reduction.

The National Council of State Boards of Nursing, in consultation with patient safety experts and healthcare leaders, should undertake an initiative to design uniform processes across states for better distinguishing human errors from willful negligence and intentional misconduct, along with guidelines for their application by state boards of nursing and other state regulatory bodies with authority over nursing.

Congress should pass legislation to extend peer review protections to data related to patient safety and quality improvement that are collected and analyzed by HCOs for internal use or shared with others solely for purposes of improving safety and quality.

Source: Institute of Medicine (IOM). (2004). *Keeping patients safe. Transforming the work environment of nurses.* Washington, DC: National Academies Press. Reprinted with permission.

Appendix I
Strategies and Recommendations from Health Professions Education: A Bridge to Quality

Strategies

1. Develop a common language and core competencies.

   Vision: Across health professions schools and practice environments, there is a shared definition of key terms and competencies for education healthcare professionals. While the roles of individual health professionals vary with respect to each of the competencies, these shared definitions transcend occupations and enable cross-disciplinary [*cross-professional*] communication. They enable interdisciplinary [*interprofessional*] groups to define and reach consensus around a core set of competencies for health professions education.

2. Integrate core competencies into oversight processes.

   Vision: There is consistency in approach and coordination across the various health professions oversight organizations—including accrediting, licensing, and certification bodies—as the result of a course on an agreed-on set of core competencies. This consistency allows for enhanced communication, integration, and synergy within and across oversight bodies and professions. As a result, educational programs are evaluated based on outcomes, and clinicians' competency is assessed on entry into practice and regularly throughout their career.

3. Motivate and support leaders and monitor progress of the reform effort.

   Vision: An interdisciplinary [*interprofessional*] group of education leaders—from practice environments and academic and continuing education settings, including students—works to create a shared mission for health professions education that relates to but is larger than the five competencies. This reform-minded group monitors progress in integrating the competencies into health professions education, and provides a regular status report to the larger education and quality communities. The group also supports leadership training for education leaders, recognizes and rewards leaders who make a significant contribution to education reform, and continuously assesses changing skill needs for health professionals.

4. Develop evidence-based curricula and teaching approaches.

   Vision: A rich, readily available evidence base exists to make the case for teaching the five competencies to health professions students and clinicians, demonstrating the strong relationship between these competencies and enhanced quality outcomes for patients. This evidence base is integrated across all the health professions through links to profession-specific databases. In addition, those who instruct and mentor health professionals in both academic and continuing education settings have access to a well-developed evidence base regarding the effectiveness of teaching methods and continuously updated best-practices database.

5. Develop faculty as teaching and learning experts.

   Vision: Faculty development programs exist at the national and regional levels for the array of health professional educators, focused on the overarching vision presented in this report. The programs, many of which are interdisciplinary [*interprofessional*], prepare faculty to convey the five competencies, as well as to adopt an evidence-based approach to education.

Recommendations

1. The Department of Health and Human Services (DHHS) and leading foundations should support an interdisciplinary [*interprofessional*] effort focused on developing a common language, with the ultimate aim of achieving consensus across the health professions on a core set of competencies that includes patient-centered care, interdisciplinary [*interprofessional*] teams, evidence-based practice, quality improvement, and informatics.

   Implications for nursing education: These five areas become the curricular framework for guiding didactic and clinical work. They relate to the program's terminal objectives.

2. The DHHS should provide a forum and support for a series of meetings involving the spectrum of oversight organizations across and within the disciplines. Participants in these meetings would be charged with developing strategies for incorporating a core set of competencies into oversight activities, based on definitions shared across the professions. These meetings

would actively solicit the input of health professions associations and the education community.

Implications for nursing education: Discuss internally at schools of nursing the risks and opportunities of actualizing the five core competencies. Identify the stakeholders in making the change—in most states that would be the institution administration—in education and key clinical agencies: chief executive officer (CEO), chief nursing officer (CNO), chief of medicine (COM), deans of the respective health professions colleges, provosts or chancellors, regulatory boards such as the board of nursing or medicine, hospital association, state nursing and medical associations, and board of regents for higher education as well as representatives of community colleges.

3. Building on previous efforts, accreditation bodies should move forward expeditiously to revise their standards so programs are required to demonstrate, through process and outcome measures, that they educate students in both academic and continuing education programs in how to deliver patient care using a core set of competencies. In so doing, these bodies should coordinate their efforts.

Implications for nursing education: Educators must work with clinical agencies and state regulatory agencies to form statewide task forces using the model of the workforce task forces to create a consensus document on accreditation changes needed for the new era of health professions education. Next there must be an action plan developed for implementation.

4. All health professions boards should move toward requiring licensed health professionals to demonstrate periodically their ability to deliver patient care, as defined by the five competencies identified by the committee, through direct measures of technical competence, patient assessment, evaluation of patient outcomes, and other evidence-based assessment methods. These boards should simultaneously evaluate the different assessment methods.

Implications for nursing education: Continued competency in practice may become an expectation for teachers [*faculty*], at least in the clinical courses. While this is true at the advanced practice level, it is not at the undergraduate level.

5. Certification bodies should require their certificate holders to maintain their competence throughout their careers by periodically demonstrating their ability to deliver patient care that reflects the five competencies, among other requirements.

Implications for nursing education: Those who teach clinical at any level must demonstrate continued clinical skills and knowledge. Therefore, this must be part of the performance evaluation criteria for faculty.

6. Foundations, with support from education and practice organizations, should take the lead in developing and funding regional demonstration learning centers, representing partnerships between practice and education. These centers

should leverage existing innovative organizations and be state-of-the-art training centers focused on teaching and assessing the five core competencies.

Implications for nursing education: Create interdisciplinary [*interprofessional*] clinical advisory groups composed of educational institutions (multiple colleges and nursing education systems) and multiple healthcare delivery systems, including state or local health departments, to determine how to develop and implement these learning centers. Key to this implementation is to bring funding agencies into the discussion early to create a cooperative agreement for funding.

7. Through Medicare demonstration projects, the Centers for Medicare and Medicaid Services (CMS) should take the lead in funding experiments to create incentives for health professionals to integrate interdisciplinary [*interprofessional*] approaches in educational or practice settings, with the goal of providing a training ground for students and clinicians that incorporates the five core competencies.

Implications for nursing education: Develop proposals for demonstration projects to examine outcomes of this model. These outcomes would include cost effectiveness, barriers to integration of interdisciplinary interprofessional models, gaps in knowledge regarding the creation and implementation of these centers, and patient outcomes—morbidity and mortality, safety, and satisfaction.

8. The Agency for Healthcare Research and Quality (AHRQ) and private foundations should support the ongoing research projects addressing the five core competencies and their association with individual and population health, as well as research into the link between the competencies and evidence-based education. Such projects should involve researchers across two or more disciplines.

Implications for nursing education: Recognize that health policy is an essential tool for nurses at any level. Use this skill by attending open forums held by AHRQ to voice the new funding needs. Respond to interdisciplinary [*interprofessional*] Requests for Proposals (RFPs) from AHRQ leveraging partnerships with other colleges or healthcare institutions.

9. The AHRQ should work with a representative group of healthcare leaders to develop measures reflecting the core set of competencies, set national goals for improvement, and issue a report to the public evaluating progress toward these goals. The AHRQ should issue the first report, focused on clinical educational institutions, in 2005 and produce annual reports thereafter.

Implications for nursing education: Involve nursing at the grassroots level to follow the national discussion, determine stakeholders in the state or region, and collectively make a strong voice to AHRQ through the open forums and meetings with key representatives of the agency to shape the agenda for the future.

10. Beginning in 2004, a biennial interdisciplinary [*interprofessional*] summit should be held involving healthcare leaders in education, oversight processes, practice, and other areas. This summit should focus on both reviewing progress against explicit targets and setting goals for the next phase with regard to the five competencies and other areas necessary to prepare professionals for the twenty-first-century health system.

Implication for nursing education: Use key representatives to lobby the nursing and healthcare organizations as well as educational and regulatory bodies to develop state or regional summits to gain an understanding of the needs at these levels. Then take these recommendations to the national level through state medical, nursing, pharmacy, and allied health, and hospital associations so that national summits can be held. The caveat is that this cannot be a 10-year process.

Source: Institute of Medicine (IOM). (2003). *Health professions education. A bridge to quality*. Washington, DC: National Academies Press. Reprinted with permission.

Appendix J

Ace Star Model of the Cycle of Knowledge Transformation

ACE Star Model of Knowledge Transformation©

Academic Center for Evidence-Based Practice
The University of Texas Health Science Center at San Antonio

Background

The health care we provide does not reflect current knowledge due to a number of hurdles. In order to achieve science-based care, two principal hurdles must be addressed: the complexity of knowledge, including volume, and the form of available knowledge.

HURDLES AND SOLUTIONS

Hurdle: Complexity of Literature

One obstacle in moving research rapidly into patient care is the growing complexity of science and technology. "No unaided human being can read, recall, and act effectively on the volume of clinically relevant scientific literature" (IOM, 2001, 25).

EBP Solution

Evidence summaries, including systematic reviews and other forms, reduce the *complexity and volume* of evidence by integrating all research on a given topic into a single, meaningful whole.

Hurdle: Form of Knowledge

Not only is the volume of literature a hurdle, but the *form* of the knowledge is a hurdle as well. Literature contains a variety of knowledge forms, many of which are NOT suitable for direct practice application.

EBP Solution

From the point of discovery, knowledge can be transformed through a series of stages to increase meaning to the clinician and utility in clinical decision-making. The stages of converting knowledge are explained by the ACE Star Model of Knowledge Transformation.

The Star Model of Knowledge Transformation© is a model for understanding the cycles, nature, and characteristics of *knowledge* that are utilized in various aspects of evidence-based practice (EBP). The Star Model organizes both old and new concepts of improving care into a whole and provides a framework with which to organize EBP processes and approaches. Known as the **ACE Star Model**, it is a simple, parsimonious depiction of the relationships between various stages of knowledge transformation, as newly discovered knowledge is moved into practice. It is inclusive of familiar processes and also emphasizes the unique aspects of EBP. The ACE Star Model places nursing's previous scientific work within the context of EBP, serves as an organizer for examining and applying EBP, and mainstreams nursing into the formal network of EBP.

ACE Star Model of Knowledge Transformation

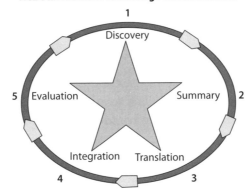

The Star Model depicts various *forms* of knowledge in a relative sequence, as research evidence is moved through several cycles, combined with other knowledge and integrated into practice. The ACE Star Model provides a framework for systematically putting evidence-based practice processes into operation.

Configured as a simple 5-point star, the model illustrates five major stages of knowledge transformation: (1) knowledge discovery, (2) evidence summary, (3) translation into practice recommendations, (4) integration into practice, and (5) evaluation. Evidence-based processes and methods vary from one point on the Star Model to the next.

Definition of Knowledge Transformation—the conversion of research findings from primary research results, through a series of stages and forms, to impact on health outcomes by way of EB care.

Underlying Premises of Knowledge Transformation

1. Knowledge transformation is necessary before research results are useable in clinical decision-making.
2. Knowledge derives from a variety of sources. In health care, sources of knowledge include research evidence, experience, authority, trial and error, and theoretical principles.

3. The most stable and generalizable knowledge is discovered through systematic processes that control bias, namely, the research process.
4. Evidence can be classified into a hierarchy of strength of evidence. Relative strength of evidence is largely dependent on the rigor of the scientific design that produced the evidence. The value of rigor is that it strengthens cause-and-effect relationships.
5. Knowledge exists in a variety of forms. As research evidence is converted through systematic steps, knowledge from other sources (expertise, patient preference) is added, creating yet another form of knowledge.
6. The form ("package") in which knowledge exists can be referenced to its use; in the case of EBP, the ultimate use is application in health care.
7. The form of knowledge determines its usability in clinical decision-making. For example, research results from a primary investigation are less useful to decision making than an evidence-based clinical practice guideline.
8. Knowledge is transformed through the following processes:
   - summarization into a single statement about the state of the science
   - translation of the state of the science into clinical recommendations, with addition of clinical expertise, application of theoretical principles, and client preferences
   - integration of recommendations through organizational and individual actions
   - evaluation of impact of actions on targeted outcomes

Explanation of Each Stage

Star point 1. Discovery

This is a knowledge generating stage. In this stage, new knowledge is discovered through the traditional research methodologies and scientific inquiry. Research results are generated through the conduct of a single study. This may be called a *primary research study* and research designs range from descriptive to correlational to causal; and from randomized control trials to qualitative. This stage builds the corpus of research about clinical actions.

Star point 2. Evidence Summary

Evidence summary is the first unique step in EBP—the task is to synthesize the corpus of research knowledge into a single, meaningful statement of the state of the science. The most advanced EBP methods to date are those used to develop evidence summaries (i.e., evidence synthesis, systematic reviews, e.g., the systematic review methods outlined in the Cochrane Handbook) from randomized control trials. Some evidence summaries employ more rigorous methods than others, yielding more credible and reproducible results.

This stage is also considered a knowledge generating stage, which occurs simultaneously with the summarization. Evidence summaries produce new knowledge by combining findings from all studies to identify bias and limit chance effects in the conclusions. The systematic methodology also increases reliability and reproducibility of results. The following terms are used to refer to various forms of evidence summaries: *evidence synthesis* (Agency for Healthcare Research and Quality), *systematic review* (Cochrane Collaboration), *meta analysis* (a statistical procedure), *integrative review, review of literature,* and *state of the science review* (less rigorous and therefore less reliable summary process). This field of science is referred to as the "science of research synthesis."

The rigorous evidence summary step distinguishes EBP from the old paradigm of research utilization. Largely due to the work of the Cochrane Collaboration, rigorous methods for systematic reviews have been greatly advanced, using meta analytic techniques and developing other statistical summary strategies, such as Number Needed to Treat (NNT).

Advantages of an Evidence Summary

An evidence summary has the following advantages:

▪ Reduces large quantities of information into a manageable form
▪ Establishes generalizability across participants, settings, treatment variations, and study designs
▪ Assesses consistency and explains inconsistencies of findings across studies
▪ Increases power in suggesting the cause-and-effect relationship
▪ Reduces bias from random and systematic error, improving true reflection of reality
▪ Integrates existing information for decisions about clinical care, economic decisions, future research design, and policy formation
▪ Increases efficiency in time between research and clinical implementation
▪ Provides a basis for continuous updates with new evidence (Mulrow, 1994)

Star point 3. Translation

The transformation of evidence summaries into actual practice requires two stages: *translation* of evidence into practice recommendations and *integration* into practice.

The aim of translation is to provide a useful and relevant package of summarized evidence to clinicians and clients in a form that suits the time, cost, and care standard. Recommendations are generically termed *clinical practice guidelines (CPGs)* and may be represented or embedded in care standards, clinical pathways, protocols, and algorithms.

CPGs are tools to support informed clinical decisions for clinician, organization, and client. Well-developed CPGs state benefits, harms, and costs of various decision options. The strongest CPGs are developed systematically using a process that is explicit and reproducible. Summarized research evidence is interpreted and combined with other sources of knowledge (such as clinical expertise and theoretical guides) and then contextualized to the specific client population and setting. Evidence-based CPGs explicitly articulate the link between the clinical recommendation and the strength of supporting evidence and/or strength of recommendation.

Star point 4. Integration

Integration is perhaps the most familiar stage in health care because of society's long-standing expectation that health care be based on most current knowledge, thus, requiring implementation of innovations. This step involves changing both individual and organizational practices through formal and informal channels. Major aspects addressed in this stage are factors that affect individual and organizational rate of adoption of innovation and factors that affect integration of the change into sustainable systems.

Star point 5. Evaluation

The final stage in knowledge transformation is evaluation. In EBP, a broad array of endpoints and outcomes are evaluated. These include evaluation of the impact of EBP on patient health outcomes, provider and patient satisfaction, efficacy, efficiency, economic analysis, and health status impact.

As new knowledge is transformed through the five stages, the final outcome is evidence-based quality improvement of health care.

Source: Stevens, K. R. (2004). *ACE Star Model of EBP: Knowledge Transformation.* Academic Center for Evidence-Based Practice. The University of Texas Health Science Center at San Antonio. www.acestar.uthscsa.edu

Index

integration, knowledge transformation, 262, 264, 265

integrative review, 264
    defined, 220

interdisciplinary teams and teamwork
    Achieving Competence Today (ACT), 129
    continuing education, 130
    as IOM core competency, 119–130, 220
    learning, xxi
    need for, 22
    teams, 119–120

International Classification of Diseases, 197

Internet. *See also* informatics
    familiarity with, 196
    podcasting, 199
    presentations, 40

interpreters for facilitating healthcare communication, 111

Interprofessional Education Collaborative (IPEC), 17

interprofessional education (IPE), 85, 128–130
    action framework, 80
    core competencies, 80–81
    defined, 220
    issues, 17
    literature on, 81
    need for, 78–81

Interprofessional Professional Education Collaborative, 80

interprofessional teamwork, 53, 55, 56, 192. *See also* interdisciplinary teams and teamwork

interventions, health literacy and, 111–112

IOM. *See* Institute of Medicine (IOM) reports

IPE. *See* interprofessional education (IPE)

IPEC. *See* Interprofessional Education Collaborative (IPEC)

ischemic heart disease, 150

ISMP. *See* Institute for Safe Medication Practices (ISMP)

IT, recruitment, and retention, 195–196

J

JBI. *See* Joanna Briggs Institute (JBI)

JMF. *See* Josiah Macy Foundation (JMF)

Joanna Briggs Institute (JBI), 133

joint appointments, 69

Joint Commission
    ANA Report Card, 191
    communications and, 123
    diversity and, 103–104
    handwashing and, 177
    health literacy improvements, 109–110
    medications and, 167, 168
    pain assessment, 146
    quality improvement and standards change, 186
    root cause analysis, 141–142
    safety standards, 158, 186–187

Joint Commission Annual Safety Goals, 187

Joint Commission Speak Up campaign, 185

Josiah Macy Foundation (JMF), 17

Just Culture approach, 155–156
    defined, 221

K

Keeping Patients Safe: Transforming the Work Environment for Nurses, 21–23, 39, 123
    acquisition and maintenance, 22, 251, 253
    recommendations, 125, 251–254
    on surveillance, 172

Knowing What Works in Healthcare: A Roadmap for the Nation, 15–16, 18, 136, 187

knowledge and understanding, errors and, 166. *See also* errors

knowledge generating stage, 263, 264

knowledge transformation
    ACE Star Model, 261–265
    complexity of literature and, 261
    defined, 262
    evidence-based practice and, 261, 262
    form of knowledge and, 261
    hurdles and solutions, 261
    processes, 263
    stages of, 262, 263–265
    underlying premises of, 262–263

L

language and languages, 119
    common language for healthcare professionals, 62, 129, 200, 255, 256
    health literacy and, 111, 179
    interpreters for patients, 111
    interprofessional learning and, 128–129
    patient self-management and, 100